Amyloidosis

CONTEMPORARY HEMATOLOGY

Judith E. Karp, SERIES EDITOR

For other titles published in this series, go to
www.springer.com/series/7681

Amyloidosis

Diagnosis and Treatment

Edited by

Morie A. Gertz

Mayo Clinic
Rochester, MN
USA

S. Vincent Rajkumar

Mayo Clinic
Rochester, MN
USA

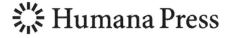

Editors
Morie A. Gertz
Mayo Clinic
200 First Street SW
Rochester, MN 55905
USA
gertz.morie@mayo.edu

S. Vincent Rajkumar
Mayo Clinic
200 First Street SW
Rochester, MN 55905
USA
rajkumar.vincent@mayo.edu

ISBN 978-1-60761-630-6   e-ISBN 978-1-60761-631-3
DOI 10.1007/978-1-60761-631-3
Springer New York Dordrecht Heidelberg London

Library of Congress Control Number: 2010927445

Printed on acid-free paper

Humana Press is part of Springer Science+Business Media (www.springer.com)

Preface

Amyloidosis is a term that represents a wide spectrum of protein folding disorders. The disease may be localized or systemic. The systemic amyloidoses can be either immunoglobulin light chain derived, related to the deposition of amyloid A protein in chronic inflammatory conditions, or an inherited disorder usually related to mutant transthyretin. Normal proteins are known to misfold into amyloid, the clinically most important being native transthyretin in the form of senile systemic amyloidosis. This text attempts to comprehensively provide a framework to clinicians seeing these patients and scientists studying the disorder, with an in-depth treatment of selected world's literature, as well as newest developments in the disorder. Because amyloidosis is so rare, many practicing clinicians are uncomfortable in the diagnosis, management, classification, prognostication, and therapy of the amyloidoses. This book calls on the clinical and scientific expertise of the world's noted experts in the protein folding disorders.

To understand the protein folding disorders, knowledge of fibril structure and fibrillogenesis is essential. Drs. Martin, Randles, and Ramirez-Alvarado cover the essentials in the identification of amyloid fibrils, recognition of the kinetics of fibril formation, the issues associated with thermodynamic instability, and the mechanism by which the beta-pleated sheet forms. Whether it is the fully formed fibril or soluble oligomers which are responsible for the complications of the disease is also dealt with.

Drs. Palladini, Merlini, and Perlini cover what is known about the in vivo imaging of amyloid fibrils. Unlike most hematologic disorders where sensitive imaging techniques exist to stage the extent of the disease, the identification and imaging of amyloid fibrils in vivo have been a challenge for four decades. The chapter covers radionuclide imaging with SAP, ultrasound, magnetic resonance imaging, and computerized tomography and its role in identifying amyloid deposits.

Drs. Grateau and Stankovic review the diagnosis and classification of amyloidosis, reviewing correct nomenclature and clues to an appropriate clinical diagnosis. A review of available clinical techniques to establish the diagnosis, the pitfalls of histochemical staining, and the classification of the amyloidosis is dealt with.

Drs. Lavatelli, Palladini, and Merlini review the pathogenesis of systemic amyloidosis, dealing with the cellular control mechanisms that regulate misfolding and the role of the non-fibrillar components of amyloid, including serum amyloid P, glycosaminoglycans, and the impact of molecular crowding.

Drs. Lacy and Leung review supportive care for patients with amyloidosis, dealing with the role of cardiotropic agents, anti-arrhythmics, implantable defibrillators, and cardiac transplant. Renal involvement is dealt with in depth, using medical strategies to reduce proteinuria, the role of renal transplant for amyloidosis, and the management of common complications such as pleural effusions that are recurrent.

Dr. Dispenzieri discusses response assessment and prognosis in evaluating patients with immunoglobulin light chain amyloidosis, both in terms of the hematologic response and the role of the immunoglobulin free light chain, and defining organ response. The use of a clinically relevant staging system is presented.

Since cardiac failure is the most common cause of death in systemic amyloidosis, special treatment is given to amyloid heart disease by Drs. Falk and Dubrey with specifics on the treatment of cardiac amyloidosis. Transthyretin-inherited cardiac amyloidosis and transthyretin senile systemic amyloidosis are treated independently and in depth.

Drs. Bajwa and Kelly deal with the complex issues associated with amyloid neuropathy, clinical manifestations, differential diagnosis, and the role of the sural nerve biopsy.

Dr. Gertz discusses the conventional treatment of immunoglobulin light chain amyloidosis from the first use of melphalan and prednisone through the use of the newest novel agents and their role in suppressing the light chain production by the clonal plasma cells responsible for the morbidity of the disease.

Drs. Cohen and Comenzo deal with the increasingly important role of high-dose therapy with stem cell replacement in the management of amyloidosis, including the key issues of patient selection, risk-adapted therapy, and the role of post-transplant maintenance therapy.

Dr. Zeldenrust deals with transthyretin amyloidosis, covering the diagnosis, the prognosis, and the available therapies with in-depth treatise on the use of liver transplantation to manage this devastating disorder.

Dr. Benson draws on his in-depth experience with the rarest forms of amyloid, including apolipoprotein, lysozyme, and fibrinogen amyloidosis. Without awareness of these rare forms of amyloidosis, the diagnosis is frequently overlooked and the patient is not correctly managed.

It is our hope that by comprehensively covering all forms of amyloidosis, from pathogenesis to therapy, this book can serve as a long-lasting reference volume for practicing physicians and scientists directly involved in the care of patients with amyloidosis, ultimately benefitting the patient population by shortening the diagnostic evaluation and allowing appropriate timing of necessary therapies.

Rochester, Minnesota, USA

Morie A. Gertz, MD
S. Vincent Rajkumar, MD

Contents

Contributors

Harman P.S. Bajwa, MD
Department of Neurology, George Washington University, Washington, DC, USA

Merrill D. Benson, MD
Departments of Pathology and Laboratory Medicine, Medicine, and Medical and Molecular Genetics, Indiana University School of Medicine, Indianapolis, IN, USA

Francis Buadi, MB, ChB
Division of Hematology, Department of Medicine, Mayo Clinic, Rochester, MN, USA

Adam D. Cohen, MD
Department of Medical Oncology, Fox Chase Cancer Center, Philadelphia, PA, USA

Raymond L. Comenzo, MD
Blood Bank and Neely Cell Processing and Collection Center, Tufts Medical Center, Boston, MA, USA

Laura M. Dember, MD
Renal Section, Evans Biomedical Research Center, Boston University School of Medicine, Boston, MA, USA

Angela Dispenzieri, MD
Department of Medicine and Laboratory Medicine and Pathology, Mayo Clinic College of Medicine, Rochester, MN, USA

Simon W. Dubrey, MD, FRCP
Department of Cardiology, Hillingdon Hospital, Middlesex, UK

Rodney H. Falk, MD, FACC
Department of Medicine, Harvard Medical School, Cardiac Amyloidosis Program, Brigham and Women's Hospital, Harvard Vanguard Medical Associates, Boston, MA, USA

Morie A. Gertz, MD
Division of Hematology, Department of Medicine, Mayo Clinic, Rochester, MN, USA

Gilles Grateau, MD
Department of Internal Medicine, National Reference Center of Rare Diseases for Inflammatory Amyloidosis and Familial Mediterranean Fever, Hôpital Tenon, Assistance publique, Hôpitaux de Paris, Paris, France

John J. Kelly, MD
Departments of Neurology and Neurosurgery, School of Medicine and Health Care
Sciences, The George Washington University, Washington, DC, USA

Helen J. Lachmann, MD, FRCP
Division of Medicine, UK National Amyloidosis Centre, University College London
Medical School, London, UK

Martha Q. Lacy, MD
Division of Hematology, Department of Medicine, Mayo Clinic, Rochester, MN,
USA

Francesca Lavatelli, MD
Biotechnology Research Laboratories, Biomedical Informatics Laboratory,
Fondazione Istituto di Ricovero e Cura a Carattere Scientifico Policlinico San
Matteo, Amyloid Research and Treatment Center, University of Pavia, Pavia, Italy

Nelson Leung, MD
Department of Nephrology and Hypertension, Mayo Clinic College of Medicine,
Rochester, MN, USA

Douglas J. Martin, BS
Department of Biochemistry and Molecular Biology, Mayo Clinic College of
Medicine, Rochester, MN, USA

Giampaolo Merlini, MD
Biotechnology Research Laboratories, Departments of Biochemistry and Internal
Medicine, Amyloidosis Research and Treatment Center, Fondazione IRCCS
Policlinico San Matteo, University of Pavia, Pavia, Italy

Giovanni Palladini, MD, PhD
Biotechnology Research Laboratories, Department of Biochemistry, Amyloidosis
Research and Treatment Center, Fondazione IRCCS Policlinico San Matteo,
University of Pavia, Pavia, Italy

Stefano Perlini, MD
Biotechnology Research Laboratories, Department of Biochemistry, Amyloidosis
Research and Treatment Center, Fondazione IRCCS Policlinico San Matteo,
University of Pavia, Pavia, Italy; Department of Internal Medicine, Fondazione
IRCCS Policlinico San Matteo, University of Pavia, Pavia, Italy

Marina Ramirez-Alvarado, PhD
Department of Biochemistry and Molecular Biology, Mayo Clinic College of
Medicine, Rochester, MN, USA

Edward G. Randles, PhD
Department of Biochemistry and Molecular Biology, Mayo Clinic College of
Medicine, Rochester, MN, USA; Laboratory for Neurophysics and Intelligence
Modeling, Department of Biochemistry, Boston University School of Medicine,
Boston, MA, USA

Katia Stankovic, MD
Department of Internal Medicine, National Reference Center of Rare Diseases for
Inflammatory Amyloidosis and Familial Mediterranean Fever, Hôpital Tenon,
Assistance publique, Hôpitaux de Paris, Paris, France

Steven R. Zeldenrust, MD, PhD
Division of Hematology, Department of Medicine, Mayo Clinic, Rochester, MN,
USA

Chapter 1

Fibril Structure and Fibrillogenesis

Douglas J. Martin, Edward G. Randles, and Marina Ramirez-Alvarado

Abstract Amyloid fibrils are protein aggregates with a characteristic cross-β structure found in association with many human diseases. This chapter begins with a review of some basics of protein biochemistry and the theory of amyloid formation. The rest of the chapter focuses on the biophysical understanding of amyloid formation, touching on the kinetics and thermodynamics of fibril formation, different tools that can be used to probe fibril formation, and current theories on the mechanism of fibril formation. Finally, we discuss current structural approaches for the study of amyloid fibrils and several structural models that have been proposed as a result of these studies.

Keywords Amyloid structure, Fibril formation mechanism, Kinetics of fibril formation, Thermodynamics of fibril formation, Spectroscopy, In vitro amyloid formation, Structural models

Introduction

Amyloidosis

The amyloidoses are a diverse group of disorders whose effects are felt in every part of the body and every corner of the globe. The hallmark of these diseases is the aggregation and deposition of misfolded protein as insoluble amyloid fibrils. In each case, the deposits are derived from a different precursor protein: transthyretin (TTR) in familial amyloidosis, amyloid β (Aβ) in Alzheimer disease, prion protein (PrP) in Creutzfeldt–Jakob disease, the immunoglobulin light chain in light chain amyloidosis (AL), and β2-microglobulin (β2m) in dialysis-related amyloidosis (DRA), for example. In spite of their diverse origins, all of these amyloid deposits have a basic common structure and share many deposited cofactors such as serum amyloid P component, apolipoprotein-E, and heparan sulfate proteoglycans [1]. This isomorphism in such a heterogeneous group of proteins and diseases is unprecedented and suggests a common pathogenesis. Consequently, physicians and researchers around the world have devoted a great deal of time and energy to understanding this family of disease proteins.

Like all other proteins, these disease proteins are composed of a linear chain of amino acids joined together by amide bonds. Each of the 20 amino acids has a different side chain, ranging in complexity from the single hydrogen atom of glycine to the indole group of tryptophan. These different amino acids in a unique sequence determine the three-dimensional structure of the protein and the type of chemistry

From: *Amyloidosis*, Contemporary Hematology,
Edited by: M.A. Gertz and S.V. Rajkumar, DOI 10.1007/978-1-60761-631-3_1,
© Springer Science+Business Media, LLC 2010

it can perform [2]. It is well known that virtually all of the chemical reactions and structures that make up a living organism are derived from the interaction of these 20 functional groups [3]. The three-dimensional structures of proteins are restrained to certain patterns, or secondary structures, by the geometry of chemical bonds and the steric hindrance of atoms, with the two most common patterns being the α-helix and the β-sheet [3]. The study of amyloid is primarily the study of the β-sheet. Indeed, the common structure of all amyloid fibrils is called the cross-β motif [4], in which a series of β-strands are arrayed perpendicularly to the long axis of the fibril (Fig. 1-1). And though there are amyloidogenic proteins that are either natively unfolded or contain α-helical structures in addition to the many β-sheet amyloid precursors, in these instances either the entire protein or a portion of it undergoes a conformational switch and transforms into a β-sheet en route to amyloid formation [5, 6].

It is also important to recall that a protein is not a static structure frozen in a vacuum. In a living organism or even in solution in a test tube, a protein bends, twists, and vibrates, colliding with hundreds or thousands of molecules every second. What we call the structure of the protein is only the most likely state where the energetic interactions between the amino acid groups are at their most stable. Proteins move and collide on a timescale we can barely fathom [3]. It is this violent molecular dance that gives rise to the conformations that can act as amyloid nuclei. The currently accepted dogma of amyloid formation is that sequence and solution conditions cause a partial unfolding of the precursor protein from its native state in such a way as to encourage the formation of a fibril nucleus. Once the nucleus has formed, it can interact with native precursor proteins and add them to the growing fibril (Fig. 1-1) [7]. This dogma provides the framework for our discussion of fibril structure and fibrillogenesis.

Before we go further, we must define precisely what distinguishes an amyloid fibril from other protein aggregates. The traditional, histopathological definition of amyloid is an extracellular, proteinaceous deposit characterized by apple green birefringence when stained with Congo red and viewed under polarized light [8]. A more

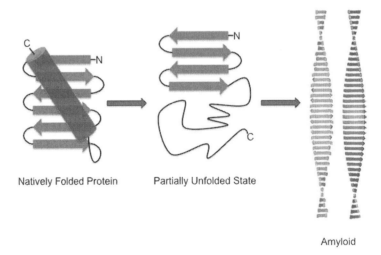

Natively Folded Protein   Partially Unfolded State

Amyloid

Fig. 1-1. A hypothetical α/β protein transition from its native state to amyloid. The native structure first undergoes a partial unfolding of its C-terminus before forming the characteristic cross-β structure. The cross-β structure shows two possible arrangements for the β-strands; antiparallel β-strands are shown in green and parallel β-strands are shown in purple. Cross-β structure adapted from [27].

recent biophysical definition is broader, including any polypeptide that polymerizes to form a cross-β structure, whether in vivo or in vitro [9]. Some polypeptides, although demonstrably cross-β in structure, fail one of the tissue-based tests of amyloid such as the Congo red birefringence test. This new definition is especially important in light of the discovery that many nonpathogenic proteins can form amyloid-like fibrils and will be the definition used in this discussion.

Here we intend to highlight recent findings in amyloid fibril structure and fibrillo-genesis. We will review some of the techniques used in amyloid research, the kinetic and thermodynamic considerations of fibril formation, and existing models of fib-ril structure. Finally we will consider how these findings are contributing to current therapeutic solutions.

Amyloid Basics

Because of their shared physical and chemical properties, the information derived from the study of one amyloidogenic protein is frequently if not always illuminating for the study of other amyloidogenic proteins. This is important to bear in mind as we talk about the basic research that has been done on amyloid structure because many studies and models we will reference have not yet been done for more than one or two amyloid disorders. Understanding fibril formation in simpler, experimentally tractable systems is a necessary first step to the understanding of the more general problem. This section will emphasize the macro view of amyloid fibrils, beginning with the various methods used to identify amyloid fibrils and then discussing the kinetics and thermodynamics of fibril formation.

Identifying Amyloid Fibrils

The study of fibril formation typically uses either the fluorescent thioflavin T (ThT) molecule or light scattering to track the progress of the reaction. ThT specifically binds amyloid fibril species in aqueous samples, resulting in a large increase in the fluorescence emission around 480 nm [10], while light scattering uses the ability of amyloid fibrils (and any solid particles in solution) to scatter light of an appropriate wavelength in order to detect fibril formation. Both techniques have their advantages and disadvantages. ThT is not absolutely specific for fibrils, so the presence of fib-rils must be verified independently [10]. In addition, ThT loses signal over time due to photobleaching of the dye and inner-filter effects resulting from the presence of fibrils in solution [11]. Light scattering can give you additional information about the size of the particles being formed but it has the significant disadvantage that it does not distinguish between amyloid fibrils and amorphous aggregates or even non-proteinaceous solids suspended in solution [11]. The end result is that fibril formation tracked by either light scattering or ThT must also be confirmed by an alternative tech-nique. Electron microscopy, specifically transmission electron microscopy (TEM), is most frequently used to confirm the presence of fibrils in these sorts of studies. TEM involves a high-voltage electron beam emitted by an electron gun, usually fitted with a tungsten filament cathode as the electron source. Stains used in TEM consist of compounds of heavy metals such as tungsten, osmium, lead, or uranium that selec-tively deposit electron-dense atoms in or on the sample. These electron-dense metal atoms and ions enhance contrast by scattering electrons out of the beam. In the case of amyloid samples, uranyl acetate is commonly used as a contrast agent. Amyloid fibrils display a characteristic morphology when properly stained and visualized by TEM, and basic properties like the length and diameter of the fibrils can be mea-sured (Fig. 1-2a) [12]. TEM studies first revealed the hierarchy of amyloid assembly

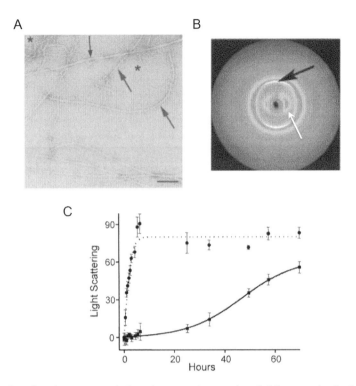

Fig. 1-2. Panel a shows transmission electron micrographs of Aβ$_{1-40}$ stained with uranyl formate. The *asterisks* indicate protofibrils, while the *red* and *black arrows* indicate fibrils with different degrees of twist. **Panel b** shows a representative synchrotron X-ray diffraction pattern of amyloid fibrils from a patient with familial amyloidosis (TTR). The *black arrow* points to the 4.7 Å intrastrand spacing, while the *white arrow* indicates the approximately 10 Å intersheet distance. **Panel c** is an example of the classic nucleated polymerization kinetics seen in most fibril formation reactions. The *solid line* shows the course of polyglutamine aggregation without seeds, while the *dotted line* shows a seeded reaction. Note in particular the extended lag phase seen without seeding. **Panel a** adapted from [12], **panel b** from [4], and **panel c** from [15].

[13]. Typically, oligomers are the first visible structures formed from a solution of soluble protein; the oligomers then rearrange into small 'wormlike' structures termed protofibrils. Protofibrils then mature into protofilaments, the first structures that show the characteristics of amyloid fibrils. These protofilaments then form the higher order structures that we term fibrils by twisting around one another [14]. Fibrils formed in vitro do not always show the same higher order structure of tissue-derived amyloid fibrils, but the spectroscopic and physical properties are indistinguishable.

In most instances, a combination of positive ThT fluorescence and TEM imaging can confirm that a protein aggregate is amyloid. However, if additional proof is needed or desired, there are several other methods available. The dye Congo red, best known for its use in the histological detection of amyloid fibrils, is also able to bind fibrils in vitro [11]. This binding can be observed as a red shift (i.e., a shift of the peak absorbance to a longer wavelength) in the absorbance spectrum upon binding to amyloid. This effect is more subtle than the increase in signal found with either ThT or light scattering, so Congo red remains most used in the histopathological diagnosis of amyloid disorders. X-ray diffraction (XRD) of amyloid fibrils may be used to uniquely identify a protein aggregate as amyloid. XRD measures the reflections created by the interaction of an aligned fibril sample with a beam of X-radiation. These reflections are normally very weak, but the atoms that are aligned in specific planes within the sample can create an interference pattern where particular reflections are enhanced or diminished based on their position relative to the detector. In the diffraction of aligned fibrils there are two characteristic signals produced at 4.7 and 10 Å (0.47 and 1.0 nm), corresponding to the intrastrand and stacking distances in β-sheets (Fig. 1-2b) [4]. These reflections were the first evidence that amyloid fibrils assumed a cross-β structure and first established that fibrils derived from different proteins were structurally isomorphic, sharing the cross-β structure.

Fibril Formation Kinetics

As was mentioned earlier, ThT fluorescence and light scattering are the most common techniques used to track ongoing fibril formation reactions, as in the case of fibril kinetics. Regardless of the technique, the kinetics of amyloid fibril formation are generally those of a classical nucleated polymerization reaction, which consists of a lag phase of variable length followed by a rapid elongation phase and a plateau (Fig. 1-2c) [15]. In this type of reaction, the rate-limiting step is the formation of a nucleus, or seed, during the lag phase, from which the reaction can proceed. The nucleus has a high conformational energy and thus is highly unstable, making its appearance under normal conditions frustratingly rare. Critically for the timely in vitro study of fibril formation, this lag phase can be abolished by the addition of preformed seeds to a solution of precursor protein. This allows study of the elongation phase of the reaction by itself and greatly speeds up the process of fibril formation. In terms of human disease, this phenomenon helps us to understand the transmissibility of certain aggregates such as prions through the ingestion of preformed fibrils: fibrils ingested orally can act as seeds for the formation of larger aggregates using the soluble native protein [16]. It has been shown that the ability of a protein to seed amyloid formation in another protein (the seeding efficiency) is proportional to the sequence identity of the two proteins, allowing for transmission between individuals and across species [17]. Studies in yeast have also implicated conformational variations in the fibrils as being key factors in the efficiency of seeding [18].

Another characteristic of nucleated polymerization is the direct dependence of the reaction rate on the concentration of the precursor (soluble protein in the case of amyloid fibrils) [15]. Simply put, if you increase the initial protein concentration, you will increase the rate of fibril formation. This relationship is an easy way to determine if a process follows a nucleated polymerization pathway. With AL protein SMA, for example, it has been shown that there is an inverse concentration dependence for fibril formation rather than a direct dependence [19]. There are several possible explanations for this behavior, the most likely being the parallel formation of amorphous aggregates of the AL proteins [20]. This amorphous aggregation could take the form of generic off-pathway aggregation or it could signify a more specific protective mechanism against fibril formation arising from the light chain's ability to homodimerize [19]. Further studies are necessary to distinguish between the two possibilities. Fibril formation kinetics can also be used to determine the size of the nucleus. In a nucleated polymerization reaction, the size of the nucleus can be calculated from a plot of the fibril formation half-life versus the natural log of the concentration. This analysis has not been done yet for AL but has been done for the related Ig domains of titin and shows a dimeric nucleus [21]. In a different amyloidogenic protein, α-synuclein, studies have calculated a monomeric nucleus, indicating that the nucleus is an alternate conformer of the native protein and not a multimer [15]. Taken together, these results reinforce the idea that conformational changes in the protein are key for fibril formation and emphasize the significant degree of polymorphism in the pathway to amyloid fibrils.

Thermodynamics

Perhaps the most unique property of amyloid fibrils in the spectrum of human disease is their remarkable stability. Fibrils of amyloidogenic proteins, including the prion protein, have been shown to survive high temperatures and pressures as well as extremes of pH and denaturant without perturbing their structure [22]. It is the stability of the fibril structure that prevents the body from effectively clearing the deposits as it would any other protein deposit. In recent years a method has been developed to quantitatively assess the thermodynamic stability of amyloid fibrils. This method makes use of the fact that a reaction in thermodynamic equilibrium cannot progress to absolute completion. Thus, even in the case of the highly favorable formation of amyloid, there must be some amount of monomer that is not incorporated into the amyloid fibrils. By measuring the concentration of monomer, termed the critical concentration, we can determine the equilibrium constant and the free energy (ΔG) for a fibril formation reaction. From a clinical perspective, it is important to note from this observation that all aggregates are theoretically reversible. This gives hope that small molecule or peptide-based inhibitors of fibril formation could not only halt the spread of the fibrils but also lead to the dissolution of previously formed deposits.

Thermodynamics also plays an important role in the earlier stages of fibril formation. It has been shown on multiple occasions that less stable proteins have a higher tendency to form amyloid, whether we are discussing amyloidogenic or non-disease proteins [23–26]. Since a partial unfolding of the precursor protein is needed for aggregation to occur, less stable proteins have a thermodynamic predisposition for fibril formation independent of cofactors or other sequence considerations. This is especially pertinent in AL, where the precursor proteins are almost universally mutated due to somatic hypermutation.

All of these studies have combined to give us a good picture of the general features of amyloid structure and fibril formation. However, they have not enabled us to understand how the diseases are initiated and how they progress at a molecular level. There are fundamental questions regarding the structure of fibrils, the identity of the toxic species, and the molecular steps by which a monomeric or multimeric protein can transition to an insoluble fibril. We will next look at the progress that has been made in assessing these questions using newer techniques for the analysis of fibril structure.

Amyloid Structure

Low-resolution data on fibril structure from X-ray diffraction and electron microscopy identified the cross-β structure and roughly established the dimensions of amyloid fibrils, but higher resolution data have not been forthcoming. Technical factors have prevented the application of the most common structural biology techniques (X-ray crystallography and nuclear magnetic resonance (NMR) spectroscopy), but several new techniques have arisen in the past decade that are allowing the creation of increasingly more detailed structural models of amyloid fibrils.

Solid-State NMR

The most prominent structural technique used in recent years has been solid-state nuclear magnetic resonance spectroscopy (ssNMR). Conventional NMR utilizes the magnetic spin of an atomic nucleus to establish the distances and angles between residues of a protein. These measurements then serve as constraints on molecular dynamics simulations of the protein. By probing multiple nuclei (^{1}H, ^{15}N, ^{13}C) in two-dimensional (two different nuclei) and three-dimensional (three different nuclei) experiments, one can acquire enough data to completely solve the protein's three-dimensional structure to atomic resolution. The size and insolubility of amyloid aggregates have necessitated the use of ssNMR instead of conventional solution-phase NMR spectroscopy. While ssNMR is not yet able to give as high a resolution as conventional NMR can, the technique provides much greater detail than prior methods, and technical advances in the field continue to push the resolution higher [27]. Because ssNMR cannot show atomic detail of the protein structure, several competing models of amyloid fibril structure have arisen to explain the constraints measured so far. We will discuss the three most prominent models: the β-sheet model, the β-helix model, and the α-sheet model. It is important to note that these models are highly dependent on the conditions under which the fibrils were grown in vitro and are not necessarily mutually exclusive. In fact, it is only once researchers were able to study fibril structure at a higher resolution that they began to appreciate how much small variation, or polymorphism, is present in fibril samples, even in those grown under similar conditions.

The β-Sheet Model

The β-sheet model has been most thoroughly investigated using fibrils derived from the Aβ$_{1-40}$ or Aβ$_{1-42}$ peptides, which are found in Alzheimer disease. Using well-characterized in vitro fibril formation conditions it has been possible to reproducibly gather high-resolution NMR data and generate full structural models for Aβ$_{1-40}$ fibrils. From ^{13}C NMR chemical shift data it is observed that residues 10–22 and 30–40 form β-strands, while amino acids outside of this region show either a disordered structure or non-β-strand conformations. Detailed examination shows that the Aβ$_{1-40}$ protofilament appears to be stabilized primarily by hydrophobic interactions at the interface between β-sheets and at the interface between the two layers (Fig. 1-3) [28]. Polar and charged side chains are distributed on the outer surface of the protofila-

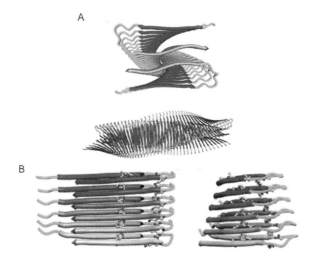

Fig. 1-3. A model of amyloid fibril structure from solid-state NMR data. **Panel a** shows two views of Aβ$_{1-40}$, modeled in an antiparallel arrangement. The structure is based on constraints derived from ^{13}C–^{13}C magic angle spinning ssNMR. *Red* and *blue* ribbons indicate β-strand residues 10–22 and 30–40, while *green* segments indicate turns or disordered regions. **Panel b** demonstrates the concept of staggering in amyloid fibrils. The β-strand shown in *blue* is shifted one residue out of phase with the hydrogen bonds in the *red* strand, leaving a one-residue overhang at the N-terminus of the *red* strand. Figure adapted from [28].

ment, with the exception of a pair of oppositely charged side chains that form a salt bridge, D23 and K28. This salt bridge formation is consistent with NMR experiments showing a distance of ~3.7 Å between the β-strands, approximately the same value obtained from X-ray diffraction data. Transmission electron microscopy images also support this model of fibril structure with a 5 nm protofilament diameter, requiring two layers of Aβ$_{1-40}$ molecules [28, 29].

There are three additional criteria for the β-sheet model addressed by ssNMR data. In this model, the β-strands can be arranged either parallel or antiparallel to one another, their hydrogen bonds can be either in or out of register, and there may be differing degrees of staggering between β-sheets along the axis of the fibril (Fig. 1-3). The β-sheet model shown in Fig. 1-3 for Aβ$_{1-40}$ shows an in-register, parallel β-sheet structure. This differs from previous models, which included antiparallel β-sheets, β-hairpins [30, 31], or only the C-terminal β-strand in the cross-β motif of the fibril [32]. It has been speculated that changes in these higher order properties of the fibril could account for the newly discovered structural polymorphism of amyloid fibrils. Though the bulk of the research has been performed on Aβ, this model could be applicable to many other amyloid-forming proteins. This β-sheet model has considerable flexibility and dynamic range to encompass a variety of cross-β conformations.

The β-Helical Model

The β-helix is a structural motif found in a variety of proteins with many diverse functions [33]. The peptide chain in a β-helix contains multiple β-strands of about four to six residues in length that are separated by one to two residue bend or loop segments (Fig. 1-4a) [34]. The peptide chain winds itself into many turns of a right-handed or left-handed spiral, roughly triangular in cross-section, and is stabilized through backbone-mediated hydrogen bonding. β-helices can be 5–10 nm in length and ~2–3 nm in width, resembling filamentous subunits in certain amyloid fibrils. The directions of β-strands and inter-strand hydrogen bonds in β-helices would be consistent with cross-β fiber diffraction. The β-helix model has been proposed for

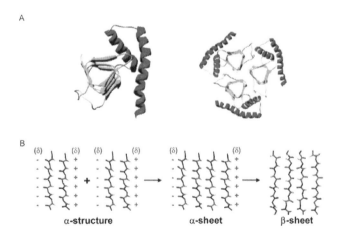

Fig. 1-4. Two alternatives to the β-sheet model of amyloid fibril structure. **Panel a** shows a β-helical structure derived from the human prion protein, including both the monomeric subunit and the proposed trimeric arrangement. β-strands are shown in *green* and α-helices in *blue*. **Panel b** shows the α-sheet structure and mechanism of fibril formation as proposed by Armen et al. + and −δ indicate the charge distribution of the structure. **Panel a** adapted from [34], **panel b** from [40].

the human prion protein (PrP) [35], several glutamine- and asparagine-rich model peptides [36], and the yeast transcription factor Sup35 (another prion protein) [37].

The β-helix has not yet been explicitly shown in high-resolution structures. It seems that in several cases, using ssNMR data, some structures are actually better described as layered β-sheet structures with staggering. Recently, a structure of Aβ$_{1-40}$ fibrils was published that showed a structure grossly similar to a β-helix, with threefold symmetry about the fibril axis [38]. These fibrils were grown under different conditions and displaying a twisted morphology by EM. All of these structures and proposed structures approximate a β-helix in the sense that they have a roughly threefold axis, but they do not meet the precise criteria for the β-helix as described in natively folded proteins. Still, the β-helix model has not been explicitly ruled out as a possibility for amyloid formation.

The α-Sheet Model

Daggett and coworkers have carried out molecular dynamics simulations of the unfolding of monomeric PrP, lysozyme, TTR, and β2-microglobulin (all of which are known to form amyloid fibrils) at high temperatures and have observed transient formation of α-sheet structures [39, 40]. Based on these simulations, Daggett and coworkers propose that α-sheets may be important intermediates in the conversion of globular proteins to amyloid fibrils. They also raise the possibility that amyloid fibrils themselves may contain α-sheets.

An α-sheet resembles a β-sheet in that the peptide segments comprising an α-sheet have an extended, linear conformation and are linked by backbone hydrogen bonds, forming a planar assembly (Fig. 1-4b). As in a β-sheet, successive side chains in each segment are located on alternating sides of the α-sheet. An α-sheet differs from a β-sheet in that all backbone carbonyl groups point in the same direction, rather than alternating directions in each peptide segment. This structure might be consistent with the cross-β X-ray fibril diffraction patterns observed for amyloid fibrils, as well as with TEM and STEM data, but it is unclear whether an α-sheet would be consistent with the experimental infrared and circular dichroism spectra of amyloid fibrils. While α-sheets may well occur in partially unfolded proteins or non-fibrillar aggregates that represent precursors to fibril formation, existing experimental data do not support the presence of α-sheets in amyloid fibrils.

Steric Zippers

There are many methods beyond solid-state NMR that have been used to probe the structure of amyloid fibrils. A common theme in structural studies today is the idea of short amyloidogenic sequences within a larger protein. The theory is that a small region of the protein sequence drives amyloid formation and the rest of the protein is insignificant (from the perspective of amyloid) [41]. Based on this theory, several computer programs have been designed to search protein sequences for these amyloidogenic elements in the hope of identifying novel fibril-forming peptides [42–45]. In addition, several groups have begun to study the structure and fibrillogenesis of these sequences by themselves. David Eisenberg's group has been a leader in this field, studying the structure and fibril-forming properties of many of these sequences. Beginning in 2005, the group found that a number of these sequences form microcrystals whose structures were determined using X-ray crystallography (Fig. 1-5) [46, 47]. These sequences share a common basic fold, which they termed the steric zipper, where the sequences form a tightly interacting stack of β-sheets that exclude water from its core. If the structures of these peptides can be shown to be equivalent to the amyloid fold of larger peptides and proteins, then these images would be the

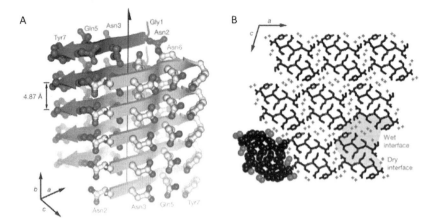

Fig. 1-5. Steric zippers as shown in [46]. In **panel a**, we see a model of the crystal structure of the GNNQQNY peptide solved to 1.8 Å resolution. **Panel b** shows the wet and dry interfaces of the steric zipper structure, with the β-strands shown in *black* and water molecules in *red*.

first atomic resolution images of amyloid structure. However, at this time that has not been shown and it is not clear whether these peptides are necessary and sufficient to drive fibril formation in the larger precursor proteins.

Atomic Force Microscopy

Atomic force microscopy (AFM) is a very high-resolution type of scanning probe microscopy, with resolution in the order of fractions of a nanometer. Although it is termed microscopy, the image is not directly derived from light but rather by 'feeling' the surface of a sample with a mechanical probe. AFM has proven useful for addressing questions of fibril polymorphism. Looking at fibrils of the AL protein SMA, it was observed that there are two distinct fibril types formed under normal growth conditions, mirroring the polymorphism of other amyloidogenic proteins and possibly indicating multiple pathways of fibril formation for this protein [48]. In an ingenious study, two forms of the yeast prion protein Sup35 were engineered, one containing a hemagglutinin (HA) tag and the other containing a mutant tag that would not recognize an HA-specific antibody. Addition of the HA antibody to these fibrils resulted in an easily observable increase in the width of fibrils derived from the HA-tagged protein. Using this system, it was possible to track the growth of single fibrils and observe that the different yeast prion strains propagate faithfully, possibly due to undetectable conformational variants [49].

Hydrogen/Deuterium Exchange

Hydrogen/deuterium (H/D) exchange studies are an excellent source of dynamic information on fibrils and their soluble precursors and thus make an excellent complement to the types of structural studies discussed previously. The frequency with which the backbone amide protons (N–H) of a protein exchange with the protons of water is a function of pH and the solvent accessibility of the protein backbone. This exchange can be limited if other residues shield the amide proton (as in the hydrophobic core of a protein) or if the amide proton is involved in a hydrogen bond. By taking a protein or fibril sample and transferring it into a solution of D_2O at the proper pH, one can measure how frequently the protons exchange in different parts of the protein backbone. H/D exchange can be coupled with either mass spectrometry or NMR; in mass spectrometry, you look at the rate of mass increase in different fragments of the protein, while in NMR you can track the replacement of hydrogen by deuterium residue by residue [50]. This information can provide detailed, global snapshots of an amyloidogenic protein's changing conformation in a particular time frame.

H/D exchange studies have been done with many amyloidogenic proteins. In particular, studies of Aβ fibril structure by this method have been shown to support the β-sheet model of amyloid fibril formation. These experiments show slow exchange times and therefore high levels of protection for residues primarily localized at position 15–23 and 27–35, making it likely that these residues are locked in a very stable arrangement (such as the core of an amyloid fibril) [51, 52].

In summary, all of these structural techniques have combined to give us a reasonable idea of what a fully formed amyloid fibril looks like. A core of β-strands is arranged in either an antiparallel or a parallel manner, depending on the protein. These strands interact with the strand above and below via hydrogen bonding and with the facing sheet through either hydrophobic interactions or a polar zipper. Beyond the residues that make up the fibril core, the remainder of the protein may still retain a native-like structure and function, but this is largely uncertain. The fibrils are characterized by a very low error rate, having very few misplaced residues despite their long length and apparent polymorphism. Once a fibril has formed, it propagates its structure faithfully regardless of the growth conditions.

Analysis of Soluble Proteins

At least as important as structural analysis of fibrils themselves is the analysis of how soluble, folded proteins convert into insoluble aggregates. In many ways, these studies face the opposite problem from the analysis of fully formed fibrils; there are many techniques that can be utilized to collect information, but the intermediate structures populated during fibril formation are so transient that observation is nigh impossible. Nevertheless, there have been many recent studies analyzing the solution properties of amyloidogenic proteins in order to determine what factors predispose them to fibril formation. Much work has focused on the structure and dynamics of native (non-amyloidogenic) β-sheet proteins. It has been observed that these proteins prevent aggregation through negative design elements such as 'capping' of exposed hydrogen bonding sites and the placement of charged amino acids at key positions [53, 54]. Analysis of these elements has led some groups to design β-breaker peptides for the inhibition of fibril formation [55]. In AL, analysis of the crystal structure of a κI O18/O8 germline amyloidogenic light chain designated AL-09 has shown a drastic alteration in the dimer interface. Restoration of one of the mutations in AL-09 is sufficient to stabilize the protein and restore the dimer interface to that of the germline, suggesting a role for the light chain homodimer in fibrillogenesis [25, 56]. Work in β2-microglobulin has shown that copper (II) binding at the surface of that protein leads to the formation of a hexameric assembly through which fibril formation is thought to occur [57]. There have been additional studies, too numerous to mention here, utilizing every technique from molecular dynamics simulations to mass spectrometry, but the central idea is that if we can somehow identify the key intermediates we will better understand how fibrils form and how to prevent this process in vivo.

Clinical Ramifications

A great deal of progress has been made in understanding the in vitro behavior of amyloidogenic proteins and amyloid fibrils, but important questions abound. High-resolution studies have enabled the creation of several plausible models of amyloid structure; which (if any) represents the true fibril structure? Much has been made of the discovery that 'non-amyloidogenic' proteins can form fibrils [58], does this mean that the amyloid fold is accessible to all proteins under the proper conditions? We have seen both the isomorphism and the polymorphism of amyloid fibrils; are there common pathways that every protein must take to form amyloid structure? Which of the lessons learned in the in vitro study of amyloid fibrils will translate in vivo, or better yet, can we leverage this knowledge into mechanistic understanding and/or new therapies? This last question is particularly important, as the reasons for amyloid-associated toxicity are unclear. There is an emerging school of thought that pre-fibrillar oligomers, rather than mature amyloid fibrils, cause cell death [59, 60]. If confirmed, this would drastically change our view of fibril formation, but there is still a clear need for a greater understanding of how amyloid fibrils form and interact within biological systems. The great hope is that understanding fibrillogenesis and the factors that influence it will lead to the development of effective therapeutics, as has been the case in familial amyloidosis [61].

References

1. Alexandrescu AT. Amyloid accomplices and enforcers. Protein Sci. 2005;14:1–12.
2. Anfinsen CB. Principles that govern the folding of protein chains. Science 1973;181: 223–30.
3. Creighton TE. Proteins. New York: W.H. Freeman and Company; 1993.
4. Sunde M, et al. Common core structure of amyloid fibrils by synchrotron X-ray diffraction. J Mol Biol. 1997;273:729–39.
5. Gross M. Proteins that convert from alpha helix to beta sheet: implications for folding and disease. Curr Protein Pept Sci. 2000;1:339–47.
6. Kumar S, Udgaonkar JB. Conformational conversion may precede or follow aggregate elongation on alternative pathways of amyloid protofibril formation. J Mol Biol. 2009;385:1266–76.
7. Chiti F, Dobson CM. Protein misfolding, functional amyloid, and human disease. Annu Rev Biochem. 2006;75:333–66.
8. Sipe JD. Amyloidosis. Crit Rev Clin Lab Sci. 1994;31:325–54.
9. Nilsson MR. Techniques to study amyloid fibril formation in vitro. Methods. 2004;34:151–60.
10. Eisert R, Felau L, Brown LR. Methods for enhancing the accuracy and reproducibility of Congo red and thioflavin T assays. Anal Biochem. 2006;353:144–6.
11. Hawe A, Sutter M, Jiskoot W. Extrinsic fluorescent dyes as tools for protein characterization. Pharm Res. 2008;25:1487–99.
12. Goldsbury C, Frey P, Olivieri V, Aebi U, Muller SA. Multiple assembly pathways underlie amyloid-beta fibril polymorphisms. J Mol Biol. 2005;352:282–98.
13. Shirahama T, Cohen AS. High-resolution electron microscopic analysis of the amyloid fibril. J Cell Biol. 1967;33:679–708.
14. Kodali R, Wetzel R. Polymorphism in the intermediates and products of amyloid assembly. Curr Opin Struct Biol. 2007;17:48–57.
15. Wetzel R. Kinetics and thermodynamics of amyloid fibril assembly. Acc Chem Res. 2006;39:671–9.
16. Scott MR, Supattapone S, Nguyen HO, DeArmond SJ, Prusiner SB. Transgenic models of prion disease. Arch Virol Suppl. 2000;16:113–24.
17. Krebs MR, Morozova-Roche LA, Daniel K, Robinson CV, Dobson CM. Observation of sequence specificity in the seeding of protein amyloid fibrils. Protein Sci. 2004;13: 1933–8.
18. Tanaka M, Chien P, Naber N, Cooke R, Weissman JS. Conformational variations in an infectious protein determine prion strain differences. Nature 2004;428:323–8.

19. Qin Z, Hu D, Zhu M, Fink AL. Structural characterization of the partially folded intermediates of an immunoglobulin light chain leading to amyloid fibrillation and amorphous aggregation. Biochemistry 2007;46:3521–31.

20. Powers ET, Powers DL. Mechanisms of protein fibril formation: nucleated polymerization with competing off-pathway aggregation. Biophys J. 2008;94:379–91.

21. Wright CF, Teichmann SA, Clarke J, Dobson CM. The importance of sequence diversity in the aggregation and evolution of proteins. Nature 2005;438:878–81.

22. Prusiner SB. Prions. Proc Natl Acad Sci USA. 1998;95:13363–83.

23. Kim Y, et al. Thermodynamic modulation of light chain amyloid fibril formation. J Biol Chem. 2000;275:1570–4.

24. Wall JS, et al. Structural basis of light chain amyloidogenicity: comparison of the thermodynamic properties, fibrillogenic potential and tertiary structural features of four Vlambda6 proteins. J Mol Recognit. 2004;17:323–31.

25. Baden EM, et al. Altered dimer interface decreases stability in an amyloidogenic protein. J Biol Chem. 2008;283:15853–60.

26. Ramirez-Alvarado M, Merkel JS, Regan L. A systematic exploration of the influence of the protein stability on amyloid fibril formation in vitro. Proc Natl Acad Sci USA. 2000;97:8979–84.

27. Tycko R. Molecular structure of amyloid fibrils: insights from solid-state NMR. Q Rev Biophys. 2006;39:1–55.

28. Petkova AT, Yau WM, Tycko R. Experimental constraints on quaternary structure in Alzheimer's beta-amyloid fibrils. Biochemistry 2006;45:498–512.

29. Petkova AT, et al. A structural model for Alzheimer's beta-amyloid fibrils based on experimental constraints from solid state NMR. Proc Natl Acad Sci USA 2002;99:16742–7.

30. George AR, Howlett DR. Computationally derived structural models of the beta-amyloid found in Alzheimer's disease plaques and the interaction with possible aggregation inhibitors. Biopolymers 1999;50:733–41.

31. Tjernberg LO, et al. A molecular model of Alzheimer amyloid beta-peptide fibril formation. J Biol Chem. 1999;274:12619–25.

32. Chaney MO, Webster SD, Kuo YM, Roher AE. Molecular modeling of the Abeta1-42 peptide from Alzheimer's disease. Protein Eng. 1998;11:761–67.

33. Jenkins J, Pickersgill R. The architecture of parallel beta-helices and related folds. Prog Biophys Mol Biol. 2001;77:111–75.

34. DeMarco ML, Silveira J, Caughey B, Daggett V. Structural properties of prion protofibrils and fibrils: an experimental assessment of atomic models. Biochemistry 2006;45:15573–82.

35. Govaerts C, Wille H, Prusiner SB, Cohen FE. Evidence for assembly of prions with left-handed beta-helices into trimers. Proc Natl Acad Sci USA. 2004;101:8342–7.

36. Perutz MF, Finch JT, Berriman J, Lesk A. Amyloid fibers are water-filled nanotubes. Proc Natl Acad Sci USA. 2002;99:5591–5.

37. Krishnan R, Lindquist SL. Structural insights into a yeast prion illuminate nucleation and strain diversity. Nature 2005;435:765–72.

38. Paravastu AK, Leapman RD, Yau WM, Tycko R. Molecular structural basis for polymorphism in Alzheimer's beta-amyloid fibrils. Proc Natl Acad Sci USA. 2008;105:18349–54.

39. Armen RS, Alonso DO, Daggett V. Anatomy of an amyloidogenic intermediate: conversion of beta-sheet to alpha-sheet structure in transthyretin at acidic pH. Structure 2004;12:1847–63.

40. Armen RS, DeMarco ML, Alonso DO, Daggett V. Pauling and Corey's alpha-pleated sheet structure may define the prefibrillar amyloidogenic intermediate in amyloid disease. Proc Natl Acad Sci USA. 2004;101:11622–7.

41. Balbirnie M, Grothe R, Eisenberg DS. An amyloid-forming peptide from the yeast prion Sup35 reveals a dehydrated beta-sheet structure for amyloid. Proc Natl Acad Sci USA. 2001;98:2375–80.

42. Thompson MJ, et al. The 3D profile method for identifying fibril-forming segments of proteins. Proc Natl Acad Sci USA. 2006;103:4074–8.

14   D.J. Martin et al.

43. Trovato A, Seno F, Tosatto SC. The PASTA server for protein aggregation prediction. Protein Eng Des Sel. 2007;20:521–3.
44. Galzitskaya OV, Garbuzynskiy SO, Lobanov MY. Prediction of amyloidogenic and disordered regions in protein chains. PLoS Comput Biol. 2006;2:e177.
45. Tartaglia GG, et al. Prediction of aggregation-prone regions in structured proteins. J Mol Biol. 2008;380:425–36.
46. Nelson R, et al. Structure of the cross-beta spine of amyloid-like fibrils. Nature 2005;435:773–8.
47. Sawaya MR, et al. Atomic structures of amyloid cross-beta spines reveal varied steric zippers. Nature 2007;447:453–7.
48. Ionescu-Zanetti C, et al. Monitoring the assembly of Ig light-chain amyloid fibrils by atomic force microscopy. Proc Natl Acad Sci USA. 1999;96:13175–9.
49. DePace AH, Weissman JS. Origins and kinetic consequences of diversity in Sup35 yeast prion fibers. Nat Struct Biol. 2002;9:389–96.
50. Kheterpal I, Wetzel R. Hydrogen/deuterium exchange mass spectrometry—a window into amyloid structure. Acc Chem Res. 2006;39:584–93.
51. Kheterpal I, Williams A, Murphy C, Bledsoe B, Wetzel R. Structural features of the Abeta amyloid fibril elucidated by limited proteolysis. Biochemistry 2001;40:11757–67.
52. Whittemore NA, et al. Hydrogen–deuterium (H/D) exchange mapping of Abeta 1-40 amyloid fibril secondary structure using nuclear magnetic resonance spectroscopy. Biochemistry 2005;44:4434–41.
53. Soldi G, Bemporad F, Chiti F. The degree of structural protection at the edge beta-strands determines the pathway of amyloid formation in globular proteins. J Am Chem Soc. 2008;130:4295–302.
54. Richardson JS, Richardson DC. Natural beta-sheet proteins use negative design to avoid edge-to-edge aggregation. Proc Natl Acad Sci USA. 2002;99:2754–9.
55. Soto C, et al. Reversion of prion protein conformational changes by synthetic beta-sheet breaker peptides. Lancet 2000;355:192–7.
56. Baden EM, Randles EG, Aboagye AK, Thompson JR, Ramirez-Alvarado M. Structural insights into the role of mutations in amyloidogenesis. J Biol Chem. 2008;283:30950–6.
57. Calabrese MF, Eakin CM, Wang JM, Miranker AD. A regulatable switch mediates self-association in an immunoglobulin fold. Nat Struct Mol Biol. 2008;15:965–71.
58. Guijarro JI, Sunde M, Jones JA, Campbell ID, Dobson CM. Amyloid fibril formation by an SH3 domain. Proc Natl Acad Sci USA. 1998;95:4224–8.
59. Kayed R, et al. Common structure of soluble amyloid oligomers implies common mechanism of pathogenesis. Science 2003;300:486–9.
60. Bucciantini M, et al. Inherent toxicity of aggregates implies a common mechanism for protein misfolding diseases. Nature 2002;416:507–11.
61. Sekijima Y, Dendle MA, Kelly JW. Orally administered diflunisal stabilizes transthyretin against dissociation required for amyloidogenesis. Amyloid 2006;13:236–49.

Chapter 2

Imaging of Systemic Amyloidosis

Giovanni Palladini, Stefano Perlini, and Giampaolo Merlini

Abstract In systemic amyloidosis, several imaging techniques can be used to detect the presence, extent, and localization of amyloid deposits, to monitor their progression and regression, and to assess organ involvement and dysfunction. The presence of heart involvement is the main prognostic determinant and most efforts have been directed to the evaluation of cardiac amyloidosis. Heart involvement is classically diagnosed based on increased ventricular wall thickness and myocardial echogenicity (often referred to as "granular sparkling") at echocardiography. However, more refined echocardiographic techniques, such as myocardial integrated backscatter, tissue Doppler, and strain imaging can provide evidence of early heart involvement and add functional and prognostic information. Magnetic resonance imaging (MRI) and cardiac scintigraphy with radiolabeled phosphate derivatives showed good sensitivity and specificity in the detection of heart involvement. In particular, scintigraphy with radiolabeled aprotinin can detect early amyloid deposits in the heart. Scintigraphy has the advantage of specific tissue characterization. The prototype of a specific amyloid tracer is iodinated serum amyloid P component (I-SAP). Scintigraphy with I-SAP is a useful complement for the diagnosis and provides an estimation of amyloid load, and serial studies can reveal disease progression and regression. However, I-SAP scintigraphy cannot image the heart. Anatomo-functional imaging, via ultrasound, computed tomography, and MRI scanning, is useful in the diagnosis and follow-up of localized amyloidosis. Accurate imaging of amyloid deposits can now be combined with the biochemical assessment of organ, particularly cardiac, damage and with reliable measurement of the circulating precursors. This will improve the care of patients with amyloidosis and shed light on the pathogenesis of organ damage.

Keywords Amyloidosis, Imaging, Diagnosis, Scintigraphy, I-SAP, Aprotinin, Ultrasound scan, Echocardiography, Magnetic resonance imaging, Computed tomography

Introduction

The ability to image a pathologic process provides with an objective means to assess the presence and extent of a disease, as well as to monitor response to treatment or determine whether relapse has occurred. Several imaging modalities have been developed for systemic amyloidosis with the purpose to detect organ involvement, to determine its extent, to monitor progression and regression of amyloid deposits, and to characterize known lesions, differentiating them from other pathologies. More recently, refined imaging techniques have been used to provide functional information

From: *Amyloidosis*, Contemporary Hematology,
Edited by: M.A. Gertz and S.V. Rajkumar, DOI 10.1007/978-1-60761-631-3_2,
© Springer Science+Business Media, LLC 2010

on the organs involved by amyloidosis. In systemic amyloidoses, one of the most important prognostic determinants is the presence of heart involvement that can be detected and studied by echocardiographic techniques and magnetic resonance imaging. Scintigraphy with amyloid-specific tracers is a useful complement in diagnosing amyloidosis and an accurate means to assess amyloid load at diagnosis and during the course of the disease. Anatomic imaging, such as computed tomography and magnetic resonance imaging, is useful in the diagnosis and follow-up of localized extracardiac amyloidosis.

In this chapter, we review the specific tools that have been developed to image amyloid deposits and the applications of common imaging techniques to amyloidosis.

Nuclear Imaging

Scintigraphy is a biochemical imaging modality and has the potential advantage of specific tissue characterization over anatomical imaging, such as computed tomography, ultrasound scan, and magnetic resonance imaging. The clinical impact of nuclear imaging in amyloidosis is mainly contingent upon the specificity of radiotracers for amyloid deposits. In the last two decades, the scintigraphic scan of amyloid deposits in vivo has been attempted with several tracers, some specifically designed for imaging amyloidosis and others originally developed for different purposes, like bone tracers, that proved useful also in studying amyloid deposits, particularly in the heart. Several tracers have been proposed to identify myocardial amyloid involvement that were recently reviewed [1]. Amyloid deposits can be identified by the use of ^{99m}Tc (technetium)-aprotinin, ^{99m}Tc-(pyro)phosphate, ^{67}Ga (gallium), and ^{111}In (indium)-antimyosin antibody, whereas cardiac innervation can be evaluated by ^{123}I-MIBG (metaiodobenzylguanidine) scintigraphy. Myocardial perfusion can be evaluated with ^{99m}Tc-sestamibi and ^{201}Tl (thallium), and ventricular function has been characterized by the use of conventional radionuclide ventriculography.

In recent years, the combination of amyloid-specific tracers with tomographic techniques, such as single photon emission computed tomography (SPECT) and positron emission tomography (PET), was used to provide accurate high-resolution localization of amyloid deposits.

Serum Amyloid P Component Scintigraphy

The prototype of a specific amyloid tracer is radiolabeled serum amyloid P component (SAP). All amyloid deposits contain SAP, a glycoprotein that reversibly binds amyloid fibrils independently from the protein of origin [2]. The circulating SAP is in constant dynamic equilibrium with the SAP bound to amyloid deposits, the latter representing as much as 200 times in quantity the blood pool in patients with systemic amyloidosis [3]. Serum amyloid P component can be conjugated with the short half-life ^{123}I that is used for scintigraphic imaging [4] or with the longer half-life ^{125}I for metabolic studies [3]. In patients with amyloidosis, ^{123}I-SAP localizes rapidly to the amyloid deposits, in proportion to their quantity, and persists there, whereas in healthy subjects and in patients with diseases other than amyloidosis, it is almost exclusively confined to the blood and is rapidly catabolized in the liver, and the associated radioactivity is released back in the circulation and excreted in the urine within 14 days [3]. In patients with amyloidosis, I-SAP is initially cleared from the blood more rapidly reflecting extravascular localization to the deposits [3]. This specific dilution phenomenon, due to the constant equilibrium between SAP bound to amyloid deposits and the blood pool, renders it possible to use I-SAP to evaluate amyloid deposits quantitatively and repeatedly in vivo. In particular, the combination of whole-body γ counting with measurement of radioactivity in 24-h urine collection allows to derive the size of the extravascular compartment [5].

Scintigraphy with ^{123}I-SAP was developed by Pepys and Hawkins and its use in patients was first reported in 1988 [6]. Since then, several thousands of scans have been performed by the London group. Scintigraphy with ^{123}I-SAP can demonstrate amyloid deposits in the kidneys, liver, bones, spleen, and adrenal glands. The organ distribution of amyloid deposits detected by ^{123}I-SAP scan can sometimes suggest a particular type of amyloidosis. For example, bone uptake is pathognomonic of immunoglobulin light-chain (AL) amyloidosis [4]. However, SAP scintigraphy cannot detect amyloid deposits in the heart, due to blood pool content, movement, intense uptake of I-SAP into the adjacent spleen, and lack of a fenestrated endothelium in the myocardium, hindering the access of the large 127 kDa tracer within the timescale determined by the short half-life of ^{123}I [7]. Myocardial uptake has been demonstrated using the longer half-life ^{131}I that, however, is unsuitable for routine clinical studies [8].

It has been reported that SAP scintigraphy can demonstrate articular β_2-microglobulin amyloid deposits [9, 10], but interpretation is difficult, because synovial effusion found in pathological joints represents an extension of the blood pool I-SAP background. Localized amyloid deposits are not imaged by I-SAP scans [11], and the chief value of SAP scintigraphy in localized amyloidosis is to rule out systemic disease [12].

Although the diagnosis of amyloidosis needs to be based on a tissue biopsy [13], given the very high specificity of ^{123}I-SAP for amyloid deposits, SAP scintigraphy has been proposed as a diagnostic tool. In a study on 189 consecutive patients with systemic amyloidosis, the diagnostic sensitivity of ^{123}I-SAP in AL amyloidosis and amyloidosis reactive to chronic inflammation (AA) was 90% [11]. Conversely, in patients with hereditary transthyretin (ATTR) amyloidosis, sensitivity was much lower (48%), particularly in subjects carrying non-Met30 TTR mutations (sensitivity 13%) [11]. Indeed, in patients with ATTR amyloidosis, typically involving the heart and peripheral nervous system, that cannot be imaged by SAP scintigraphy, amyloid deposits can be identified only if they are also present in other organs, such as the spleen and kidneys. On the other hand, SAP scintigraphy demonstrates that the distribution of amyloid within individual organs can be inhomogeneous, accounting for false negative biopsy results [14]. Moreover, SAP scintigraphy provides information on the distribution and amount of amyloid that cannot be derived from tissue biopsies. The diagnostic sensitivity of SAP scintigraphy can be improved by combination with the determination of the extravascular compartment, which is greatly increased in patients with systemic amyloidosis. Increased extravascular retention of ^{123}I-SAP alone had a 65, 61, and 22% diagnostic sensitivity in AA, AL, and ATTR amyloidosis, respectively [5].

Serum amyloid P component scans can identify extensive amyloid deposits in organs in which they have not been suspected clinically [11, 14]. For example, in the study by Hazenberg et al., 86% of patients with AA amyloidosis and 76% of patients with AL had amyloid deposits in the spleen that were clinically relevant only in 8 and 18% of subjects, respectively [11]. Adrenal uptake was seen in 20% of patients with AA amyloidosis, but adrenal failure was present just in 3% [11]. Although certain organs can continue to function in a normal way despite the presence of substantial amyloid deposits, they may nevertheless fail under stress, and the possibility of recognizing asymptomatic amyloid deposits may improve the assessment of eligibility to toxic therapies, thus preventing otherwise unexpected treatment-related toxicity. Conversely, in some cases, clinically relevant organ involvement may not be accompanied by significant tracer uptake. In the same study, 90% of AA and 83% of AL patients had clinical signs of renal involvement, but kidney I-SAP uptake was detected only in 67 and 31% of cases, respectively [11]. Moreover, SAP scintigraphy revealed a poor correlation between the quantity of amyloid present in a particular organ and the severity of organ dysfunction [14]. These observations support the hypothesis that, in AL and AA amyloidoses, the amount of amyloid deposited is not the only determinant of organ dysfunction.

Scintigraphy with ^{123}I-SAP also provides prognostic information. Measurements of whole-body amyloid load by SAP scintigraphy correlate with the risk of death and progression to end-stage renal disease in AA amyloidosis [15]. Additional prognostic information may come from the determination of I-SAP tissue retention [7]. Hazenberg et al. demonstrated that in AL amyloidosis extravascular retention of ^{123}I-SAP has a prognostic impact that is independent from the presence of cardiac involvement [5]. Moreover, serial SAP scans demonstrate regression of amyloid deposits in a significant proportion of patients in whom it has been possible to reduce or eliminate the supply of the amyloidogenic precursor. This includes reduction of serum amyloid A protein (SAA) by control of the underlying inflammatory disease in AA amyloidosis [15]; effective chemotherapy with reduction of the involved circulating free light chains (FLC) in AL amyloidosis [16]; liver transplantation in ATTR amyloidosis [17], in hereditary fibrinogen amyloidosis (AFib) [18], and in familial apolipoprotein AI amyloidosis (AApoAI) [19]; and renal transplantation in β_2-microglobulin dialysis-associated amyloidosis (Aβ_2m) [20].

Despite the useful diagnostic and prognostic information it can provide, the clinical use of SAP scintigraphy is hampered by several important limitations, such as the inability to image cardiac amyloid deposits and the unavailability of I-SAP in most centers. Availability of I-SAP is limited because it is not a commercial product, SAP is isolated from human sera, and ^{123}I-SAP is produced at a high cost. Attempts of labeling SAP with the cheaper ^{99m}Tc have been made, but conjugation of SAP with ^{99m}Tc is technically difficult. Moreover, ^{99m}Tc-SAP is a less specific ligand of amyloid fibrils than I-SAP, part of the ^{99m}Tc separates from SAP in the circulation, and ^{99m}Tc-labeled degradation products are cleared incompletely, increasing the background signal in the kidneys and liver [14].

[99m]Tc-Aprotinin Scintigraphy for Cardiac Imaging

The observation of the presence of antiproteases in amyloid deposits led our group to hypothesize that a radiolabeled antiprotease could be a specific tracer for amyloid deposits. We chose ^{99m}Tc-conjugated aprotinin, a low molecular weight protease inhibitor that was used as a cortical renal tracer. It has been reported that aprotinin binds specifically to amyloid fibrils, probably through pairing of the β structures of the antiprotease with exposed structures of the same type on the amyloid deposits [21]. Aprotinin is known to accumulate in the kidneys masking the whole abdominal area, thus, we evaluated the capability of ^{99m}Tc-aprotinin to detect extra-abdominal, particularly cardiac, amyloid deposits (Fig. 2-1) [22]. In 1995, in a first series of 25 patients with systemic amyloidosis, we observed cardiac uptake in 10 of 14 (71%) subjects fulfilling echocardiographic criteria of heart involvement and in 1 patient who subsequently developed overt cardiac amyloidosis. Cardiac biopsies were available in four cases (three positive and one negative) and were all concordant with ^{99m}Tc-aprotinin uptake [22]. In the same study, localization to the neck

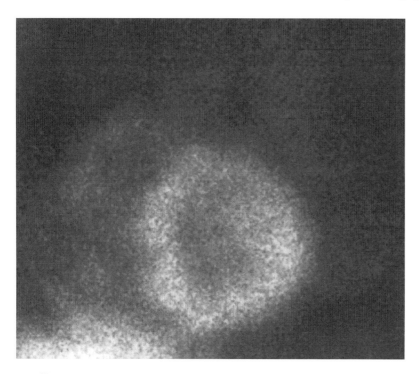

Fig. 2-1. ^{99m}Tc-aprotinin scintigraphy of the heart in a patient with AL amyloidosis and cardiac involvement.

region (thyroid, salivary glands, and tongue) was also detected in eight patients with AL amyloidosis [22]. In 2001, in a subsequent study on 78 patients with systemic AL amyloidosis followed for a median of 31 months, the sensitivity and specificity of ^{99m}Tc-aprotinin scintigraphy to detect cardiac involvement were 95 and 97%, respectively, and the scans were able to detect cardiac involvement before it became apparent at echocardiography [23, 24]. Further clinical studies at our center were hampered by a ban on bovine derivates that precluded further use of aprotinin in patients. In 2002 Schaadt and coworkers found ^{99m}Tc-aprotinin uptake in several localizations (heart, tongue, submandibular glands, intestines, lymph nodes, liver, spleen, pleura, lungs, joints) in 22 of 23 patients with known or suspected amyloidosis [25]. Biopsy or autopsy evaluations were available for 20 of the 90 detected localizations and confirmed the presence of amyloid deposits [25]. Asymptomatic uptake accounted for approximately 50% of detected lesions and, notably, in five patients, preceded clinical symptoms [25]. In a more recent retrospective study, involving 18 patients with biopsy-proven amyloidosis and 17 controls, Han et al. showed myocardial uptake of ^{99m}Tc-aprotinin in all the five patients who had amyloid cardiac involvement as assessed by clinical, echocardiographic, and magnetic resonance criteria [26]. Four of these five patients eventually died due to cardiac amyloidosis [26]. In none of the other 30 patients, who had no signs of cardiac involvement, thoracic uptake of ^{99m}Tc-aprotinin was detected [26]. The available data indicate that ^{99m}Tc-aprotinin is a very promising radiotracer for cardiac amyloidosis, with high sensitivity and specificity and able to detect early cardiac involvement before it becomes detectable by echocardiography.

Scintigraphy with ^{99m}Tc-Labeled Phosphate Derivatives

Radiolabeled phosphate derivates were developed as bone tracers and they are believed to localize to amyloid deposits because of their relevant calcium content. In 1977 Kula et al. visualized calcifications in amyloid deposits with ^{99m}Tc-diphosphonate [27]. Since then, several phosphate derivatives have been tested in cardiac amyloidosis, including ^{99m}Tc-pyrophosphate (^{99m}Tc-PYP) [27–32], ^{99m}Tc-(hydroxy)methylene diphosphonate (^{99m}Tc-MDP or ^{99m}Tc-HMDP) [33], and ^{99m}Tc-3,3-diphosphono-1,2-propanodicarboxylic acid (^{99m}Tc-DPD) [34, 35]. The latter was also shown to help in differentiating AL- and ATTR-type cardiac amyloidosis, suggesting a role of ^{99m}Tc-DPD scintigraphy in the evaluation of cardiac amyloidosis etiology [34].

Overall, although ^{99m}Tc-labeled phosphate myocardial scanning seems to be a sensitive test for the diagnosis of cardiac amyloidosis in patients with congestive heart failure, it does not appear to be of value for the early detection of cardiac involvement in patients with known amyloidosis. Differently from aprotinin scintigraphy, positive phosphate scanning seems to correlate with high amounts of amyloid fibrils in the heart, but this occurs at an advanced stage of the disease, when clinical symptoms of cardiomyopathy are already apparent. Thus, the clinical relevance of ^{99m}Tc-labeled phosphate myocardial scintigraphy remains uncertain, and according to Eriksson et al., a high threshold amount of amyloid is probably required to produce an abnormal scintigram, although lesions with less amyloid can evidently be identified by echocardiography [36], a finding that was confirmed by Lee et al. [37]. In the same line, Hartmann et al. showed that ^{99m}Tc-PYP scintigraphy is not useful in screening patients for cardiac involvement in amyloidosis, but that first-pass studies yield valuable information about diastolic function impairment [38].

Beyond being used to image cardiac amyloidosis, radiolabeled phosphate derivates have also been reported to localize in extracardiac amyloid deposits, such as amyloid deposits in the bronchi [39], soft tissues [40], testicles [41], liver [42], and lungs [43]. In patients with amyloidosis localized to the airways, SPECT and PET techniques with radiolabeled phosphate derivates can provide accurate anatomical localization [44, 45].

Assessment of Cardiac Innervation with ^{123}I-Metaiodobenzylguanidine

Metaiodobenzylguanidine (MIBG), a structural analogue of the "false" neurotransmitter guanethidine, shares noradrenaline uptake and storage mechanisms in the sympathetic nerve endings, allowing to visualize cardiac innervation when labeled with ^{123}I. The use of ^{123}I-MIBG in patients with amyloidosis was reported for the first time by Nakata et al. in 1995 [46], who found decreased myocardial activity of ^{123}I-MIBG in all cardiac regions in a patient with severe peripheral neuropathy due to a TTR-related familial amyloidotic polyneuropathy. Subsequently, a high incidence of myocardial denervation by ^{123}I-MIBG imaging, even in the presence of normal LV wall thickness and systolic function, was shown in ATTR patients [47, 48]. Similar findings were reported in patients with AL amyloidosis, who show signs ranging from presynaptic sympathetic dysfunction to overt myocardial denervation according to the degree of congestive heart failure and cardiac autonomic dysfunction [49].

^{99m}Tc Pentavalent Dimercaptosuccinic Acid Scintigraphy

^{99m}Tc pentavalent dimercaptosuccinic acid (^{99m}Tc-(V)-DMSA) is a tumor tracer used in medullary thyroid cancer and soft tissues tumors, which is taken up by cancer cells probably due to the structural similarity with the phosphate ion. Initially, the possibility of imaging plasmacitomas associated with localized AL amyloid deposits with this tracer has been reported and could be explained by uptake by plasma cells [50]. However, in a patient with systemic AL amyloidosis, ^{99m}Tc-(V)-DMSA uptake was observed in the heart, kidney, liver, spleen, and thyroid and correlated with autopsy findings [51]. Moreover, cases of myocardial uptake of ^{99m}Tc-(V)-DMSA in patients with systemic amyloidosis and heart involvement have been described [52]. However, the possibility to image myocardium with ^{99m}Tc-(V)-DMSA is hampered by a strong signal from the blood pool.

Radiolabeled β_2-Microglobulin

Since conventional techniques, such as joint ultrasonography, X-ray, CT, or MRI, lack specificity in evaluating lesions caused by dialysis-related amyloidosis (Aβ_2m), imaging of β_2-microglobulin deposits has been attempted using β_2-microglobulin labeled with ^{131}I as a radiotracer [53–55]. Tracer accumulations correspond to the typical distribution pattern of Aβ_2m deposits [53, 54]. ^{111}In (indium)–β_2-microglobulin reduces the radiation exposure and improves the optical resolution of this scan [53, 54, 56]. Recombinant β_2-microglobulin has been produced for use as a radiotracer [53, 54, 56]. A limitation of β_2-microglobulin scintigraphy is that it cannot be performed in case of residual renal function, because the tracer is rapidly cleared in the urine.

β_2-Microglobulin amyloid deposits can be also imaged by ^{201}Tl (thallium) and ^{67}Ga (gallium) scintigraphy [57].

Radioimaging with Fibril-Reactive Monoclonal Antibodies

Researchers at the University of Tennessee observed that certain murine anti-human light chain antibodies recognize a conformational epitope common to fibrils formed from light chain as well as other amyloidogenic precursors such as SAA, TTR, and ApoAI [58]. Hence, the same group developed a radiolabeled fibril-reactive monoclonal antibody (mAb), conjugated with ^{125}I or ^{124}I, that was tested in mice. In an amyloidoma mouse model the radioiodinated mAb localized predominantly in the tumor and could be accurately imaged by SPECT and PET [59]. Combination of high-resolution SPECT with the radioiodinated mAb and I-SAP with computed tomography allows accurate anatomical localization of amyloid deposits in AL and AA mouse models [59].

Other Scintigraphic Tracers

^{67}Ga (gallium) has been proposed to image cardiac involvement in systemic amyloidosis, but it proved less sensitive than ^{99m}Tc-PYP in this setting [60, 61]. ^{111}In (indium)-labeled antimyosin antibodies that bind specifically to areas of myocardial necrosis were used to image cardiac amyloid deposits [62, 63].

Ultrasound Imaging

The echocardiographic features of advanced cardiac amyloidosis are distinctive, with non-dilated ventricles showing marked thickening of the left and right ventricular walls, as well as of the interventricular and interatrial septa. Amyloid infiltration gives a characteristic aspect to the myocardial texture, which has been described as "granular sparkling" [64–68], due to the granular appearance of the myocardium.

In the attempt of quantifying the subjective evaluation of increased myocardial echoreflectivity, tissue characterization can be achieved by cycle-dependent variation of myocardial integrated backscatter, a measure that has been shown to have a prognostic potential [69].

Also valve leaflets are often thickened showing increased echogenicity. Concentric left ventricular geometry is almost invariably present [70] due to increased wall thickness with normal or reduced ventricular diameters, with normal or near-normal global left ventricular function as assessed by ejection fraction. In the many patients with reduced end-diastolic diameters and volumes, this leads to reduced stroke volume that is often associated with increased heart rate to maintain cardiac output. Wall thickening is disproportionate to the degree of current or prior arterial hypertension or valve disease, due to myocardial infiltration rather than to cardiomyocyte hypertrophy (Fig. 2-2). As a consequence, the ECG limb lead voltages tend to decrease as the ventricle wall thickens, resulting in a decreased ratio of voltage to echo-derived left ventricular mass, a finding that strongly suggests an infiltrative cardiomyopathy [68]. Indeed, a low-voltage pattern (defined as all limb lead voltage <5 mm) is found in a high proportion of patients.

In a minority of patients (that has been estimated around 5%), the echocardiographic aspect may mimic hypertrophic cardiomyopathy [71–75], with normal or even mildly hyperdynamic left ventricular function and normal voltages on the 12-lead ECG. However, at variance with "true" hypertrophic cardiomyopathy, mitral valve systolic anterior motion is very uncommon and ECG limb lead voltages are not in the ventricular hypertrophy range.

Diastolic function is abnormal in both myocardial relaxation and ventricular compliance, with Doppler transmitral velocity profile ranging from an impaired distensibility to a clear-cut restrictive pattern, and Doppler serial studies demonstrate a progression of diastolic dysfunction as myocardial infiltration progresses [66]. In advanced disease, left ventricular filling restrictive physiology can be identified by

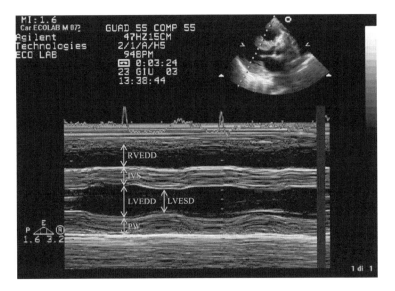

Fig. 2-2. Two-dimensional directed M-mode imaging of the right and left ventricular cavities in a patient with cardiac AL amyloidosis. RVEDD: right ventricular end-diastolic diameter; IVS: end-diastolic interventricular septum thickness; LVEDD: left ventricular end-diastolic diameter; PW: end-diastolic posterior wall thickness; LVESD: left ventricular end-systolic diameter.

combined Doppler studies evaluating transmitral and pulmonary venous flow velocities. Such a profound alteration in filling dynamics is caused by the association of left ventricular diastolic dysfunction and impaired atrial contraction, both due to myocardial amyloid infiltration [64, 76–83]. As a consequence, the Doppler transmitral flow velocity profile shows increased peak early (E) to peak atrial (A) velocity ratio, reduced E-wave deceleration time, and low-velocity A wave.

Beyond allowing further insights into cardiac diastolic dysfunction in cardiac amyloidosis, pulsed tissue Doppler imaging can demonstrate the presence of longitudinal systolic impairment before the ejection fraction becomes abnormal [84–86]. Moreover, myocardial velocity tissue Doppler indices proved helpful in differentiating from control subjects patients with biopsy-proven cardiac amyloidosis with borderline conventional echocardiographic features and non-restrictive LV filling pattern [87]. Also the ratio of early transmitral flow velocity to early diastolic mitral annular velocity (E/E_m) has been suggested as a useful index of elevated LV filling pressure in cardiac amyloidosis [88]. Long-axis dysfunction might also be demonstrated by M-mode echocardiography in both the left [89] and the right ventricles [90], as well as by strain and strain rate imaging, that may also have potential for evaluating the prognosis in AL amyloidosis [75, 84, 85, 90–92]. Combined pulsed tissue Doppler and strain imaging may disclose early signs of infiltrative cardiac disease in both ventricles, even in the absence of myocardial wall thickening [93]. Moreover, the evaluation of systolic mechanical deformation by two-dimensional strain imaging via the speckle-tracking technique has been recently shown to differentiate cardiac amyloidosis from both asymmetric hypertrophic cardiomyopathy and secondary LV hypertrophy [75].

Also the myocardial velocity profile, derived from color-coded tissue Doppler imaging (TDI), can identify transmural heterogeneity, possibly differentiating cardiac amyloidosis from other causes of left ventricular hypertrophy. At comparable left ventricular wall thickness, myocardial velocity gradient during systole and early diastole is in fact depressed in cardiac amyloidosis when compared with hypertensive heart disease and hypertrophic cardiomyopathy [94]. Contrast echocardiography can also be used to recognize microvascular dysfunction in patients with cardiac amyloidosis [95], relying on the ultrasound detection of microbubble contrast agents that are confined to the intravascular space.

While echocardiography is an irreplaceable tool for the diagnosis and evaluation of cardiac amyloid disease, only a few reports describe the use of ultrasound scan for imaging amyloid deposits localized outside the heart, such as enlargement and increased echogenicity of the thyroid gland in patients with amyloid goiter [96] or hypoechogenic nodular plicae in the bowel of patients with gastrointestinal amyloidosis [97]. Ultrasonography has been used to study periarticular changes in patients with dialysis-related amyloidosis. It has been shown that patients with β_2-microglobulin amyloidosis have increased diameter of supraspinatus tendon, greater cross-sectional area of the long head of biceps tendon, and increased thickness of the rotator cuffs and may present echogenic pads between the muscle groups of the rotator cuffs [98, 99]. These findings indicate that shoulder ultrasound might have a role in the diagnosis and, possibly, in the follow-up of patients with dialysis-related amyloidosis.

Computed Tomography

Computed tomography (CT) imaging is of limited value in systemic amyloidosis mainly because of low specificity. Computed tomography was used to evaluate soft tissue [100], intestinal [97], and lymph node involvement [101]. The clinical usefulness of CT imaging is probably higher in localized amyloidosis. Several cases of orbital amyloidosis detected by CT scans were reported [102]. Localizations to the nasopharynx [103] and larynx [104, 105] have also been identified by CT. However, these findings were not specific and the final biopsy results were often unforeseen at the time of the CT scan. Nevertheless, CT imaging can be useful in the follow-up of localized amyloidosis.

One of the most important applications of CT in amyloidosis is the imaging of amyloid localized to the lungs and airways. In patients with respiratory tract amyloidosis standard chest radiography findings are usually non-specific and consist of a reticular pattern due to interlobular septal thickening, nodules, or postobstructive features such as atelectasias and consolidation [106]. Reticular patterns are consistent with systemic involvement. Pleural effusions are common in systemic amyloidosis, but are usually secondary to heart failure and nephrotic syndrome due to cardiac and renal involvement. However, pleural amyloid infiltration can be responsible for persistent effusion. Computed tomography recognizes three distinct patterns of localizations to the respiratory system: (1) tracheobronchial amyloidosis, (2) nodular parenchymal amyloidosis, and (3) diffuse alveolar septal amyloidosis. Tracheobronchial amyloidosis appears as focal or diffuse submucosal deposits resulting in nodules, plaques, or circumferential thickening often with luminal narrowing [106, 107]. Localization to segmental airways can result in collapse, consolidation, bronchiectasias, and hyperinflation [106]. In nodular parenchymal amyloidosis (Fig. 2-3), nodules are well defined, can be single or multiple with an extremely variable diameter, are usually subpleural in distribution, and often contain calcifications [108–110]. Due to non-specific appearance, amyloid pulmonary nodules are often interpreted as neoplasia [109]. Diffuse alveolar septal amyloidosis is a less common form of pulmonary involvement, but it is often associated with systemic amyloidosis. It manifests with widespread amyloid deposition involving small vessels and

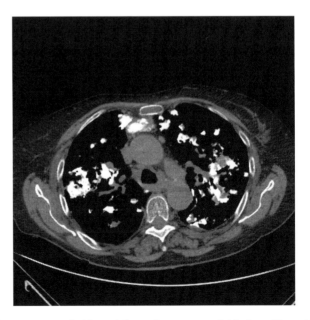

Fig. 2-3. CT appearance of AL nodular pulmonary amyloidosis, with multiple bilateral calcified amyloid nodules of variable diameter.

the interstitium, with reticular opacities, interlobular septal thickening, micronodules, and, less frequently, ground-glass opacification, traction bronchiectasias, and honeycombing at high-resolution CT [109]. Diffuse amyloidosis is sometimes accompanied by mediastinal lymphadenopathy [108].

In β_2-microglobulin amyloidosis, destructive arthropathy, spondylarthropathy, and periarticular cystic bone lesions can be demonstrated by plain X-ray and CT [111].

As to cardiac amyloidosis, ECG-gated enhanced multislice computed tomography can visualize wall thickening with partial fibrotic changes [112].

Magnetic Resonance Imaging

In systemic amyloidoses, magnetic resonance imaging (MRI) is mainly used in evaluating cardiac morphology and function (Fig. 2-4). Cardiac MRI in patients with advanced cardiac amyloidosis shows an unusual pattern characterized by global subendocardial late gadolinium enhancement and associated abnormal myocardial and blood pool gadolinium kinetics [113–117]. These abnormalities are common but not universally present in cardiac amyloidosis, probably due to expansion of infiltrated myocardial interstitium in association with impaired segmental and global

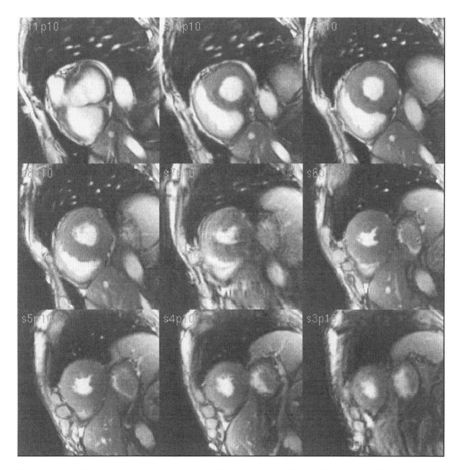

Fig. 2-4. Cardiac magnetic resonance imaging from a patient with cardiac AL amyloidosis. Transverse sections of the right and left ventricular cavities showing increased wall thickness and global subendocardial late gadolinium enhancement.

contractility [116]. Amyloid and collagenous fiber deposition was correlated with late enhancement that was shown to be associated with fibrosis due to ischemia of cardiomyocytes by small vessel amyloid deposition [118]. In patients with endomyocardial biopsy-proven cardiac amyloidosis, late gadolinium enhancement shows good sensitivity (80%) and excellent specificity (94%) [119], being strongly correlated with heart failure severity as assessed by brain natriuretic peptide [120]. Magnetic resonance relaxometry, measuring T_1 and T_2 relaxation times of the left ventricular myocardium, might improve the diagnostic reliability of this technique [121], and tissue characterization of the myocardium by T_1 quantification predicts survival [122].

A few reports describe the clinical use of magnetic resonance in imaging extracardiac localizations in systemic amyloidosis. In β_2-microglobulin amyloidosis MRI can show increased thickness of the supraspinatus tendon, capsular thickening at the hip, and osseous lesions [111, 123]. It has been suggested that MRI can detect early lesions in asymptomatic patients with dialysis-related amyloidosis [123]. In a patient with AL amyloidosis and liver involvement, who underwent MRI with an oral manganese-containing contrast agent, focal areas without contrast uptake and no bile excretion were detected [124]. These observations correlated with liver biopsy findings, such as atrophy of the hepatocytes, amyloid deposits in the portal veins, and compression of bile ducts [124]. Magnetic resonance imaging proved useful in detecting localized amyloid deposits in the nasopharynx [103], spine [125], larynx [105], urethra [126], and seminal vesicles [127]. Enhanced T_2 relaxation and hypointensity on T_2-weighted MR are considered peculiar characteristics of amyloid masses.

Conclusion

A wide armamentarium of imaging techniques has been developed for amyloidosis. Clinical practice will select those tools that will prove helpful in the management of this disease based on efficacy and availability.

Imaging techniques can provide not only anatomical but also functional information, particularly in evaluating cardiac amyloidosis. Functional imaging of cardiac involvement can now be combined with biochemical assessment of heart dysfunction with cardiac troponins and natriuretic peptides [128, 129]. This is very relevant since cardiac involvement predicts prognosis and affects treatment strategy.

Moreover, the imaging of amyloid deposits and the biochemical assessment of organ dysfunction can now be correlated with reliable measurement of the circulating precursors, such as FLC in AL and SAA in AA amyloidosis. This has the potential of answering questions on the pathogenesis of amyloidosis. One of the most important and still open issues in the field of amyloidosis is the mechanism of organ damage. Observations with SAP scintigraphy demonstrated that amyloid load is not always proportional to organ dysfunction [11]. Subsequent clinical observations suggested that the concentration of the amyloid precursor has a direct impact on biochemical indices of cardiac dysfunction and prognosis, independently from amyloid load [130]. Studies are warranted in correlating the extent of disease activity, amyloid load, biomarkers, and indices of myocardial function that can be derived from several functional imaging techniques.

References

1. Glaudemans AW, Slart RH, Zeebregts CJ, et al. Nuclear imaging in cardiac amyloidosis. Eur J Nucl Med Mol Imaging 2009;36:702–14.

2. Merlini G, Bellotti V. Molecular mechanisms of amyloidosis. N Engl J Med. 2003;349:583–96.
3. Hawkins P, Wootton R, Pepys M. Metabolic studies of radioiodinated serum amyloid P component in normal subjects and patients with systemic amyloidosis. J Clin Invest. 1990;86:1862–9.
4. Hawkins P, Lavender J, Pepys M. Evaluation of systemic amyloidosis by scintigraphy with 123I-labeled serum amyloid P component. N Engl J Med. 1990;323:508–13.
5. Hazenberg B, van Rijswijk M, Lub-de Hooge M, et al. Diagnostic performance and prognostic value of extravascular retention of 123I-labeled serum amyloid P component in systemic amyloidosis. J Nucl Med. 2007;48:865–72.
6. Hawkins P, Myers M, Lavender J, Pepys M. Diagnostic radionuclide imaging of amyloid: biological targeting by circulating human serum amyloid P component. Lancet 1988;1:1413–8.
7. Hachulla E, Maulin L, Deveaux M, et al. Prospective and serial study of primary amyloidosis with serum amyloid P component scintigraphy: from diagnosis to prognosis. Am J Med. 1996;101:77–87.
8. Hawkins P, Aprile C, Capri G, et al. Scintigraphic imaging and turnover studies with iodine-131 labelled serum amyloid P component in systemic amyloidosis. Eur J Nucl Med. 1998;25:701–8.
9. Nelson S, Hawkins P, Richardson S, et al. Imaging of haemodialysis-associated amyloidosis with 123I-serum amyloid P component. Lancet 1991;338:335–9.
10. Tan S, Baillod R, Brown E, et al. Clinical, radiological and serum amyloid P component scintigraphic features of beta2-microglobulin amyloidosis associated with continuous ambulatory peritoneal dialysis. Nephrol Dial Transplant. 1999;14:1467–71.
11. Hazenberg B, van Rijswijk M, Piers D, et al. Diagnostic performance of 123I-labeled serum amyloid P component scintigraphy in patients with amyloidosis. Am J Med. 2006;119:355.e15–24.
12. Maulin L, Hachulla E, Deveaux M, et al. 'Localized amyloidosis': 123I-labelled SAP component scintigraphy and labial salivary gland biopsy. QJM 1997;90:45–50.
13. Gertz M, Comenzo R, Falk R, et al. Definition of organ involvement and treatment response in immunoglobulin light chain amyloidosis (AL): a consensus opinion from the 10th International Symposium on Amyloid and Amyloidosis, Tours, France, 18–22 Apr 2004. Am J Hematol. 2005;79:319–28.
14. Hawkins P. Serum amyloid P component scintigraphy for diagnosis and monitoring amyloidosis. Curr Opin Nephrol Hypertens. 2002;11:649–55.
15. Lachmann H, Goodman H, Gilbertson J, et al. Natural history and outcome in systemic AA amyloidosis. N Engl J Med. 2007;356:2361–71.
16. Lachmann H, Gallimore R, Gillmore J, et al. Outcome in systemic AL amyloidosis in relation to changes in concentration of circulating free immunoglobulin light chains following chemotherapy. Br J Haematol. 2003;122:78–84.
17. Rydh A, Suhr O, Hietala S, Ahlström K, Pepys M, Hawkins P. Serum amyloid P component scintigraphy in familial amyloid polyneuropathy: regression of visceral amyloid following liver transplantation. Eur J Nucl Med. 1998;25:709–13.
18. Elliott PM, Mahon NG, Matsumura Y, Hawkins PN, Gillmore JD, McKenna WJ. Tissue Doppler features of cardiac amyloidosis. Clin Cardiol. 2000;23:701.
19. Gillmore J, Stangou A, Tennent G, et al. Clinical and biochemical outcome of hepatorenal transplantation for hereditary systemic amyloidosis associated with apolipoprotein AI Gly26Arg. Transplantation 2001;71:986–92.
20. Tan S, Irish A, Winearls C, et al. Long term effect of renal transplantation on dialysis-related amyloid deposits and symptomatology. Kidney Int. 1996;50:282–9.
21. Cardoso I, Pereira P, Damas A, Saraiva M. Aprotinin binding to amyloid fibrils. Eur J Biochem. 2000;267:2307–11.
22. Aprile C, Marinone G, Saponaro R, Bonino C, Merlini G. Cardiac and pleuropulmonary AL amyloid imaging with technetium-99m labelled aprotinin. Eur J Nucl Med. 1995;22:1393–401.

23. Merlini G, Palladini G, Obici L, et al. Accuracy of 99mTc-aprotinin scintigraphy for the detection of myocardial amyloidosis: long-term follow-up of 78 patients. Amyloid: J Protein Folding Disord. 2001;8:174–5.

24. Aprile C, Merlini G, Saponaro R, Palladini G, Cannizzaro G. 99mTc-aprotinin scintigraphic detection of myocardial amyloidosis: long-term follow-up of 78 patients. Eur J Nucl Med. 2001;28:OS413.

25. Schaadt B, Hendel H, Gimsing P, Jønsson V, Pedersen H, Hesse B. 99mTc-aprotinin scintigraphy in amyloidosis. J Nucl Med. 2003;44:177–83.

26. Han S, Chong V, Murray T, et al. Preliminary experience of 99mTc-aprotinin scintigraphy in amyloidosis. Eur J Haematol. 2007;79:494–500.

27. Kula RW, Engel WK, Line BR. Scanning for soft-tissue amyloid. Lancet 1977;1:92–3.

28. Falk R, Lee V, Rubinow A, Hood WJ, Cohen A. Sensitivity of technetium-99m-pyrophosphate scintigraphy in diagnosing cardiac amyloidosis. Am J Cardiol. 1983;51:826–30.

29. Falk R, Lee V, Rubinow A, Skinner M, Cohen A. Cardiac technetium-99m pyrophosphate scintigraphy in familial amyloidosis. Am J Cardiol. 1984;54:1150–1.

30. Gertz M, Brown M, Hauser M, Kyle R. Utility of technetium Tc 99m pyrophosphate bone scanning in cardiac amyloidosis. Arch Intern Med. 1987;147:1039–44.

31. Fournier C, Grimon G, Rinaldi J, et al. Usefulness of technetium-99m pyrophosphate myocardial scintigraphy in amyloid polyneuropathy and correlation with echocardiography. Am J Cardiol. 1993;72:854–7.

32. Casset-Senon D, Secchi V, Arbeille P, Cosnay P. Localization of myocardial amyloid deposits in cardiac amyloidosis by Tc-99m pyrophosphate myocardial SPECT: implication for medical treatment. Clin Nucl Med. 2005;30:496–7.

33. Ak I, Vardareli E, Erdinc O, Kasapoglu E, Ata N. Myocardial Tc-99m MDP uptake on a bone scan in senile systemic amyloidosis with cardiac involvement. Clin Nucl Med. 2000;25:826–7.

34. Perugini E, Guidalotti PL, Salvi F, et al. Noninvasive etiologic diagnosis of cardiac amyloidosis using 99mTc-3,3-diphosphono-1,2-propanodicarboxylic acid scintigraphy. J Am Coll Cardiol. 2005;46:1076–84.

35. Puille M, Altland K, Linke RP, et al. 99mTc-DPD scintigraphy in transthyretin-related familial amyloidotic polyneuropathy. Eur J Nucl Med Mol Imaging 2002;29:376–9.

36. Eriksson P, Backman C, Bjerle P, Eriksson A, Holm S, Olofsson BO. Non-invasive assessment of the presence and severity of cardiac amyloidosis. A study in familial amyloidosis with polyneuropathy by cross sectional echocardiography and technetium-99m pyrophosphate scintigraphy. Br Heart J. 1984;52:321–6.

37. Lee VW, Caldarone AG, Falk RH, Rubinow A, Cohen AS. Amyloidosis of heart and liver: comparison of Tc-99m pyrophosphate and Tc-99m methylene diphosphonate for detection. Radiology 1983;148:239–42.

38. Hartmann A, Frenkel J, Hopf R, et al. Is technetium-99 m-pyrophosphate scintigraphy valuable in the diagnosis of cardiac amyloidosis? Int J Card Imaging. 1990;5:227–31.

39. Janssen S, Piers D, van Rijswijk M, Meijer S, Mandema E. Soft-tissue uptake of 99mTc-diphosphonate and 99mTc-pyrophosphate in amyloidosis. Eur J Nucl Med. 1990;16:663–70.

40. Worsley D, Lentle B. Uptake of technetium-99m MDP in primary amyloidosis with a review of the mechanisms of soft tissue localization of bone seeking radiopharmaceuticals. J Nucl Med. 1993;34:1612–5.

41. Sty J, Starshak R. Tc-99m MDP scrotal image. Testicular amyloidosis. Clin Nucl Med. 1983;8:142.

42. Lee V, Caldarone A, Falk R, Rubinow A, Cohen A. Amyloidosis of heart and liver: comparison of Tc-99m pyrophosphate and Tc-99m methylene diphosphonate for detection. Radiology. 1983;148:239–42.

43. Kanoh T, Uchino H, Yamamoto I, Torizuka K. Soft-tissue uptake of technetium-99m MDP in multiple myeloma. Clin Nucl Med. 1986;11:878–9.

44. Nishihara M, Oda J, Kamura T, Kimura M, Odano I, Sakai K. SPECT imaging in a case of primary respiratory tract amyloidosis. Clin Nucl Med. 1993;18:675–8.

45. Yoshida S, Suematsu T, Koizumi T, et al. Demonstration of primary tracheobronchial amyloidosis by 99mTc-HMDP bone SPECT. Ann Nucl Med. 1993;7:269–72.

46. Nakata T, Shimamoto K, Yonekura S, et al. Cardiac sympathetic denervation in transthyretin-related familial amyloidotic polyneuropathy: detection with iodine-123-MIBG. J Nucl Med. 1995;36:1040–2.

47. Tanaka M, Hongo M, Kinoshita O, et al. Iodine-123 metaiodobenzylguanidine scintigraphic assessment of myocardial sympathetic innervation in patients with familial amyloid polyneuropathy. J Am Coll Cardiol. 1997;29:168–74.

48. Delahaye N, Dinanian S, Slama MS, et al. Cardiac sympathetic denervation in familial amyloid polyneuropathy assessed by iodine-123 metaiodobenzylguanidine scintigraphy and heart rate variability. Eur J Nucl Med. 1999;26:416–24.

49. Hongo M, Urushibata K, Kai R, et al. Iodine-123 metaiodobenzylguanidine scintigraphic analysis of myocardial sympathetic innervation in patients with AL (primary) amyloidosis. Am Heart J. 2002;144:122–9.

50. Ohta H, Endo K, Kanoh T, Konishi J, Kotoura H. Technetium-99m (V) DMSA uptake in amyloidosis. J Nucl Med. 1989;30:2049–52.

51. Yukihiro M, Tateno M, Hirano T, et al. Pentavalent technetium-99m dimercaptosuccinic acid uptake in primary amyloidosis: comparison with autopsy findings. Radiat Med. 1997;15:317–20.

52. Ohta H, Okada T, Furukawa Y, et al. Tc-99m(V) DMSA uptake in cardiac amyloidosis. Clin Nucl Med. 1991;16:673–5.

53. Ketteler M, Koch K, Floege J. Imaging techniques in the diagnosis of dialysis-related amyloidosis. Semin Dial. 2001;14:90–3.

54. Floege J, Schäffer J, Koch K. Scintigraphic methods to detect beta2-microglobulin associated amyloidosis (Abeta2-microglobulin amyloidosis). Nephrol Dial Transplant. 2001;16 Suppl 4:12–6.

55. Floege J, Nonnast-Daniel B, Gielow P, et al. Specific imaging of dialysis-related amyloid deposits using 131I-beta-2-microglobulin. Nephron 1989;51:444–7.

56. Linke R, Schäeffer J, Gielow P, et al. Production of recombinant human beta2-microglobulin for scintigraphic diagnosis of amyloidosis in uremia and hemodialysis. Eur J Biochem. 2000;267:627–33.

57. Yen T, Tzen K, Chen K, Tsai C. The value of gallium-67 and thallium-201 whole-body and single-photon emission tomography images in dialysis-related beta 2-microglobulin amyloid. Eur J Nucl Med. 2000;27:56–61.

58. Hrncic R, Wall J, Wolfenbarger D, et al. Antibody-mediated resolution of light chain-associated amyloid deposits. Am J Pathol. 2000;157:1239–46.

59. Leeson CP, Myerson SG, Walls GB, Neubauer S, Ormerod OJ. Atrial pathology in cardiac amyloidosis: evidence from ECG and cardiovascular magnetic resonance. Eur Heart J. 2006;27:1670.

60. Montes J, López L, Chamorro J, Galván R. Cardiac gallium uptake in amyloidosis. Eur J Nucl Med. 1984;9:438.

61. Li C, Rabinovitch M, Juni J, et al. Scintigraphic characterization of amyloid cardiomyopathy. Clin Nucl Med. 1985;10:156–9.

62. Lekakis J, Nanas J, Moustafellou C, et al. Cardiac amyloidosis detected by indium-111 antimyosin imaging. Am Heart J. 1992;124:1630–1.

63. Lekakis J, Dimopoulos M, Nanas J, et al. Antimyosin scintigraphy for detection of cardiac amyloidosis. Am J Cardiol. 1997;80:963–5.

64. Klein AL, Cohen GI. Doppler echocardiographic assessment of constrictive pericarditis, cardiac amyloidosis, and cardiac tamponade. Cleve Clin J Med. 1992;59:278–90.

65. Siqueira-Filho AG, Cunha CL, Tajik AJ, Seward JB, Schattenberg TT, Giuliani ER. M-mode and two-dimensional echocardiographic features in cardiac amyloidosis. Circulation 1981;63:188–96.

66. Klein AL, Hatle LK, Taliercio CP, et al. Serial Doppler echocardiographic follow-up of left ventricular diastolic function in cardiac amyloidosis. J Am Coll Cardiol. 1990;16:1135–41.

67. Child JS, Levisman JA, Abbasi AS, MacAlpin RN. Echocardiographic manifestations of infiltrative cardiomyopathy. A report of seven cases due to amyloid. Chest 1976;70: 726–31.

68. Carroll JD, Gaasch WH, McAdam KP. Amyloid cardiomyopathy: characterization by a distinctive voltage/mass relation. Am J Cardiol. 1982;49:9–13.

69. Koyama J, Ray-Sequin PA, Falk RH. Prognostic significance of ultrasound myocardial tissue characterization in patients with cardiac amyloidosis. Circulation 2002;106: 556–61.

70. Ganau A, Devereux RB, Roman MJ, et al. Patterns of left ventricular hypertrophy and geometric remodeling in essential hypertension. J Am Coll Cardiol. 1992;19:1550–8.

71. Dubrey SW, Cha K, Anderson J, et al. The clinical features of immunoglobulin light-chain (AL) amyloidosis with heart involvement. QJM 1998;91:141–57.

72. Sedlis SP, Saffitz JE, Schwob VS, Jaffe AS. Cardiac amyloidosis simulating hypertrophic cardiomyopathy. Am J Cardiol. 1984;53:969–70.

73. Hemmingson LO, Eriksson P. Cardiac amyloidosis mimicking hypertrophic cardiomyopathy. Acta Med Scand. 1986;219:421–3.

74. Eriksson P, Backman C, Eriksson A, Eriksson S, Karp K, Olofsson BO. Differentiation of cardiac amyloidosis and hypertrophic cardiomyopathy. A comparison of familial amyloidosis with polyneuropathy and hypertrophic cardiomyopathy by electrocardiography and echocardiography. Acta Med Scand. 1987;221:39–46.

75. Sun JP, Stewart WJ, Yang XS, et al. Differentiation of hypertrophic cardiomyopathy and cardiac amyloidosis from other causes of ventricular wall thickening by two-dimensional strain imaging echocardiography. Am J Cardiol. 2009;103:411–5.

76. Klein AL, Hatle LK, Burstow DJ, et al. Doppler characterization of left ventricular diastolic function in cardiac amyloidosis. J Am Coll Cardiol. 1989;13:1017–26.

77. Abdalla I, Murray RD, Lee JC, Stewart WJ, Tajik AJ, Klein AL. Duration of pulmonary venous atrial reversal flow velocity and mitral inflow a wave: new measure of severity of cardiac amyloidosis. J Am Soc Echocardiogr. 1998;11:1125–33.

78. Modesto KM, Dispenzieri A, Cauduro SA, et al. Left atrial myopathy in cardiac amyloidosis: implications of novel echocardiographic techniques. Eur Heart J. 2005;26:173–9.

79. Dubrey S, Pollak A, Skinner M, Falk RH. Atrial thrombi occurring during sinus rhythm in cardiac amyloidosis: evidence for atrial electromechanical dissociation. Br Heart J. 1995;74:541–4.

80. Santarone M, Corrado G, Tagliagambe LM, et al. Atrial thrombosis in cardiac amyloidosis: diagnostic contribution of transesophageal echocardiography. J Am Soc Echocardiogr. 1999;12:533–6.

81. Plehn JF, Southworth J, Cornwell GG, 3rd. Brief report: atrial systolic failure in primary amyloidosis. N Engl J Med. 1992;327:1570–3.

82. Moyssakis I, Triposkiadis F, Pantazopoulos NJ, Kyriakidis M, Nihoyannopoulos P. Left atrial systolic function in primary and familial amyloidosis: assessment from left atrial volume change. Clin Cardiol. 2004;27:528–32.

83. Murphy L, Falk RH. Left atrial kinetic energy in AL amyloidosis: can it detect early dysfunction? Am J Cardiol. 2000;86:244–6.

84. Koyama J, Ray-Sequin PA, Davidoff R, Falk RH. Usefulness of pulsed tissue Doppler imaging for evaluating systolic and diastolic left ventricular function in patients with AL (primary) amyloidosis. Am J Cardiol. 2002;89:1067–71.

85. Koyama J, Davidoff R, Falk RH. Longitudinal myocardial velocity gradient derived from pulsed Doppler tissue imaging in AL amyloidosis: a sensitive indicator of systolic and diastolic dysfunction. J Am Soc Echocardiogr. 2004;17:36–44.

86. Bellavia D, Abraham TP, Pellikka PA, et al. Detection of left ventricular systolic dysfunction in cardiac amyloidosis with strain rate echocardiography. J Am Soc Echocardiogr. 2007;20:1194–202.

87. Palka P, Lange A, Donnelly JE, Scalia G, Burstow DJ, Nihoyannopoulos P. Doppler tissue echocardiographic features of cardiac amyloidosis. J Am Soc Echocardiogr. 2002;15:1353–60.

88. Innelli P, Galderisi M, Catalano L, et al. Detection of increased left ventricular filling pressure by pulsed tissue Doppler in cardiac amyloidosis. J Cardiovasc Med (Hagerstown). 2006;7:742–7.

89. Perugini E, Rapezzi C, Reggiani LB, Poole-Wilson P, Branzi A, Henein MY. Comparison of ventricular long-axis function in patients with cardiac amyloidosis versus idiopathic restrictive cardiomyopathy. Am J Cardiol. 2005;95:146–9.

90. Ghio S, Perlini S, Palladini G, et al. Importance of the echocardiographic evaluation of right ventricular function in patients with AL amyloidosis. Eur J Heart Fail. 2007;9: 808–13.

91. Koyama J, Ray-Sequin PA, Falk RH. Longitudinal myocardial function assessed by tissue velocity, strain, and strain rate tissue Doppler echocardiography in patients with AL (primary) cardiac amyloidosis. Circulation 2003;107:2446–52.

92. Al-Zahrani GB, Bellavia D, Pellikka PA, et al. Doppler myocardial imaging compared to standard 2-dimensional and Doppler echocardiography for assessment of diastolic function in patients with systemic amyloidosis. J Am Soc Echocardiogr. 2008;22(3):290–8.

93. Lindqvist P, Olofsson BO, Backman C, Suhr O, Waldenstrom A. Pulsed tissue Doppler and strain imaging discloses early signs of infiltrative cardiac disease: a study on patients with familial amyloidotic polyneuropathy. Eur J Echocardiogr. 2006;7:22–30.

94. Oki T, Tanaka H, Yamada H, et al. Diagnosis of cardiac amyloidosis based on the myocardial velocity profile in the hypertrophied left ventricular wall. Am J Cardiol. 2004;93:864–9.

95. Abdelmoneim SS, Bernier M, Bellavia D, et al. Myocardial contrast echocardiography in biopsy-proven primary cardiac amyloidosis. Eur J Echocardiogr. 2008;9:338–41.

96. Siddiqui M, Gertz M, Dean D. Amyloid goiter as a manifestation of primary systemic amyloidosis. Thyroid 2007;17:77–80.

97. Kala Z, Válek V, Kysela P. Amyloidosis of the small intestine. Eur J Radiol. 2007;63:105–9.

98. Kantor G, Kasick J, Bergfeld W, McMahon J, Krebs J. Epidermolysis bullosa of the Weber–Cockayne type with macular amyloidosis. Cleve Clin Q. 1985;52:425–8.

99. Hayashi T, Yamanaka T, Fujinuma S, et al. Left ventricular filling disturbances in cardiac amyloidosis: a study of atrial sound and diastolic inflow velocities. J Cardiol. 1992;22:141–9.

100. Asaumi J, Yanagi Y, Hisatomi M, Konouchi H, Kishi K. CT and MR imaging of localized amyloidosis. Eur J Radiol. 2001;39:83–7.

101. Takebayashi S, Ono Y, Sakai F, Tamura S, Unayama S. Computed tomography of amyloidosis involving retroperitoneal lymph nodes mimicking lymphoma. J Comput Assist Tomogr. 1984;8:1025–7.

102. Murdoch I, Sullivan T, Moseley I, et al. Primary localised amyloidosis of the orbit. Br J Ophthalmol. 1996;80:1083–6.

103. Gean-Marton A, Kirsch C, Vezina L, Weber A. Focal amyloidosis of the head and neck: evaluation with CT and MR imaging. Radiology 1991;181:521–5.

104. Kennedy T, Patel N. Surgical management of localized amyloidosis. Laryngoscope 2000;110:918–23.

105. Aydin O, Ustündağ E, Işeri M, Ozkarakaş H, Oğuz A. Laryngeal amyloidosis with laryngocele. J Laryngol Otol. 1999;113:361–3.

106. Aylwin A, Gishen P, Copley S. Imaging appearance of thoracic amyloidosis. J Thorac Imaging 2005;20:41–6.

107. Kirchner J, Jacobi V, Kardos P, Kollath J. CT findings in extensive tracheobronchial amyloidosis. Eur Radiol. 1998;8:352–4.

108. Utz J, Swensen S, Gertz M. Pulmonary amyloidosis. The Mayo Clinic experience from 1980 to 1993. Ann Intern Med. 1996;124:407–13.

109. Pickford H, Swensen S, Utz J. Thoracic cross-sectional imaging of amyloidosis. AJR Am J Roentgenol. 1997;168:351–5.

110. Rubinow A, Celli B, Cohen A, Rigden B, Brody J. Localized amyloidosis of the lower respiratory tract. Am Rev Respir Dis. 1978;118:603–11.

111. Schaeffer J, Floege J, Koch K. Diagnostic aspects of beta 2-microglobulin amyloidosis. Nephrol Dial Transplant. 1996;11 Suppl 2:144–46.

112. Mikami Y, Funabashi N, Kijima T, et al. Focal fibrosis in the left ventricle of subjects with cardiac amyloidosis evaluated by multislice computed tomography. Int J Cardiol. 2007;122:72–5.

113. Maceira AM, Joshi J, Prasad SK, et al. Cardiovascular magnetic resonance in cardiac amyloidosis. Circulation 2005;111:186–93.

114. Kwong RY, Falk RH. Cardiovascular magnetic resonance in cardiac amyloidosis. Circulation 2005;111:122–4.

115. Thomson LE. Cardiovascular magnetic resonance in clinically suspected cardiac amyloidosis: diagnostic value of a typical pattern of late gadolinium enhancement. J Am Coll Cardiol. 2008;51:1031–2.

116. Perugini E, Rapezzi C, Piva T, et al. Non-invasive evaluation of the myocardial substrate of cardiac amyloidosis by gadolinium cardiac magnetic resonance. Heart 2006;92:343–9.

117. Fattori R, Rocchi G, Celletti F, Bertaccini P, Rapezzi C, Gavelli G. Contribution of magnetic resonance imaging in the differential diagnosis of cardiac amyloidosis and symmetric hypertrophic cardiomyopathy. Am Heart J. 1998;136:824–30.

118. Hosch W, Kristen AV, Libicher M, et al. Late enhancement in cardiac amyloidosis: correlation of MRI enhancement pattern with histopathological findings. Amyloid. 2008;15:196–204.

119. Vogelsberg H, Mahrholdt H, Deluigi CC, et al. Cardiovascular magnetic resonance in clinically suspected cardiac amyloidosis: noninvasive imaging compared to endomyocardial biopsy. J Am Coll Cardiol. 2008;51:1022–30.

120. Ruberg FL, Appelbaum E, Davidoff R, et al. Diagnostic and prognostic utility of cardiovascular magnetic resonance imaging in light-chain cardiac amyloidosis. Am J Cardiol. 2009;103:544–9.

121. Hosch W, Bock M, Libicher M, et al. MR-relaxometry of myocardial tissue: significant elevation of T1 and T2 relaxation times in cardiac amyloidosis. Invest Radiol. 2007;42:636–42.

122. Maceira AM, Prasad SK, Hawkins PN, Roughton M, Pennell DJ. Cardiovascular magnetic resonance and prognosis in cardiac amyloidosis. J Cardiovasc Magn Reson. 2008;10:54.

123. Escobedo E, Hunter J, Zink-Brody G, Andress D. Magnetic resonance imaging of dialysis-related amyloidosis of the shoulder and hip. Skeletal Radiol. 1996;25:41–8.

124. Møller J, Santoni-Rugiu E, Chabanova E, Løgager V, Hansen A, Thomsen H. Magnetic resonance imaging with liver-specific contrast agent in primary amyloidosis and intrahepatic cholestasis. Acta Radiol. 2007;48:145–9.

125. Mullins K, Meyers S, Kazee A, Powers J, Maurer P. Primary solitary amyloidosis of the spine: a case report and review of the literature. Surg Neurol. 1997;48:405–8.

126. Ichioka K, Utsunomiya N, Ueda N, Matsui Y, Yoshimura K, Terai A. Primary localized amyloidosis of urethra: magnetic resonance imaging findings. Urology 2004;64:376–8.

127. Furuya S, Masumori N, Furuya R, Tsukamoto T, Isomura H, Tamakawa M. Characterization of localized seminal vesicle amyloidosis causing hemospermia: an analysis using immunohistochemistry and magnetic resonance imaging. J Urol. 2005;173:1273–7.

128. Palladini G, Campana C, Klersy C, et al. Serum N-terminal pro-brain natriuretic peptide is a sensitive marker of myocardial dysfunction in AL amyloidosis. Circulation 2003;107:2440–5.

129. Dispenzieri A, Gertz M, Kyle R, et al. Serum cardiac troponins and N-terminal pro-brain natriuretic peptide: a staging system for primary systemic amyloidosis. J Clin Oncol. 2004;22:3751–7.

130. Palladini G, Lavatelli F, Russo P, et al. Circulating amyloidogenic free light chains and serum N-terminal natriuretic peptide type B decrease simultaneously in association with improvement of survival in AL. Blood 2006;107:3854–8.

Chapter 3

Diagnosis and Classification

Gilles Grateau and Katia Stankovic

Abstract A high degree of clinical suspicion in the context of a great diversity of clinical symptoms remains essential to make the diagnosis of amyloidosis that still relies on tissue biopsy. Standard tissue staining should be completed with Congo red as this stain gives a specific "apple-green birefringence" for amyloid under polarization. Identifying the type of amyloidosis is crucial to determine clinical management, prognosis, and treatment and thus explains that the actual nomenclature of amyloid disorders is based on the biochemical nature of amyloid. This typing requires a confrontation of clinical data to the results of some crucial blood tests such as the measure of the acute phase response and the search for a monoclonal component, histology, and genetics. Standard histological analysis is enriched with immunohistochemistry which analyses the fixation by amyloid of a panel of antibodies directed against most of the common human amyloid proteins. Rarely, sophisticated biochemical methods help to establish the true nature of the deposits. Once the steps have been cleared the disease can be classified as localized or multisystemic and its nature established. The main categories of multisystemic amylosis are the immunoglobulinic variety (AL, A for amyloid and L for light chain of immunoglobulin); amyloid associated with inflammation (AA, A for associated); and the transythyretin amyloidosis (ATTR, TTR for transthyretin) that consists in two varieties, the common "senile" and the rare hereditary.

Keywords Biopsy, Histology, Congo red, Polarization, Immunohistochemistry, Nomenclature, Biochemistry, Classification, Diagnosis, Immunofluorescence

During several centuries, amyloid has remained a simple curiosity for the pathologist and amyloidosis has been associated with a kind of fate and renunciation for the physician. That is no longer true as our knowledge of the nature, mechanisms, and treatment of amyloidoses has radically changed within two decades. The cornerstone of the modern management is the understanding that treatment of systemic amyloidoses depends on the molecular type of the amyloid protein, associated mechanisms, and eventually underlying disease. Amyloid deposits in humans can be derived from more than 25 different types of proteins and many more variants (Table 3-1) [1]. A limited number of them are involved in systemic amyloidoses, for which more and more efficient treatments exist, but directly depending on the type of the amyloidosis [2].

This renders early clinical diagnosis of amyloidosis mandatory and accurate classification of amyloid deposits imperative.

From: *Amyloidosis*, Contemporary Hematology,
Edited by: M.A. Gertz and S.V. Rajkumar, DOI 10.1007/978-1-60761-631-3_3,
© Springer Science+Business Media, LLC 2010

Table 3-1. Amyloid fibril proteins and their precursors in human.

Amyloid protein	Precursor	Systemic (S) or localized (L)	Syndrome or involved tissue
AA	AoSAA	S	Reactive, secondary to chronic inflammation
AL	Light chain of immunoglobulin	S, L	Primary or myeloma associated
AH	Heavy chain of immunoglobulin	S	
ATTR	Mutated TTR	S	Hereditary
	Wild-type TTR	S, L	senile
AApoAI	ApoAI	S	Hereditary
		L	Aorta, meniscus, vertebral discus
AApoAII	ApoAII	S	Hereditary
AApo AIV	ApoAIV	S	Aging
AGel	Gelsolin	S	Hereditary
AFib	Fibrinogen Aα chain	S	Hereditary
ALys	Lysozyme	S	Hereditary
Aβ2 M	β2-Microglobulin	S	Associated with dialysis
ACys	Cystatin C	S	Hereditary
Aβ	Aβ protein precursor AβPP	L	Alzheimer's disease, aging
Abri[a]	ABriPP	L	Hereditary dementia, British
ADan	ADanPP	L	Hereditary dementia, Danish
APrP	Prion protein	L	Spongiform encephalopathies
ACal	Procalcitonin	L	C-cell thyroid cancer
AIAPP	Islet amyloid polypeptide	L	Langerhans' islets, insulinoma
AANF	Atrial natriuretic peptide	L	Cardiac atria
APro	Prolactin	L	Aging hypophyse, prolactinoma
AMed	Lactadherin	L	Senile aortic media
AIns	Insulin	L	Iatrogenic
Aker	Keratoepithelin	L	Hereditary corneal dystrophies
ALac	Lactoferrin	L	Cornea
AOaap	Odontogenic ameloblast-associated protein	L	Odontogenic tumor
ASemI	Semenogline I	L	Vesicula seminalis
		L	
ATau	Tau	L	Alzheimer's disease, fronto-temporal dementia, senile brain

[a]ABriPP and ADanPP are derived from the same gene

The Current Nomenclature of Amyloidoses

The increasing knowledge of the exact biochemical nature of amyloid disorders has made a logical, easily understood, and possible to be enriched nomenclature absolutely necessary. In fact, in order to avoid a mix of clinical and histochemically based designation, the International Society of Amyloidosis has set up a nomenclature based on the nature of the main protein that constitutes the amyloid fibril. Thus, the fibril protein, which varies according to the type of amyloidosis, is always designated protein A plus a suffix which is an abbreviation of the name of the precursor protein. The fibril proteins involved in the main forms of systemic amyloidosis are designed as follows: AL is the protein derived from immunoglobulin light (L) chains; AA the fibril protein derived from the acute phase protein SAA; and ATTR the fibril protein derived from the plasma protein transthyretin, formerly called prealbumin. This biochemical nomenclature also allows more detailed designations for specific mutations. Thus ATTRV30M is the name of the most common mutant amyloid protein of transthyretin nature in Europe where the normal valine residue at position 30 has been substituted with methionine. In this nomenclature the amyloid disorder itself is simply denoted by adding the term amyloidosis. Thus AA amyloidosis is the disease created by the deposition of AA fibril protein in tissues. This term has favorably replaced secondary or reactive amyloidosis. Likewise AL amyloidosis should be used for the former primary and myeloma-associated forms. The flexibility of this nomenclature allows to characterize further an amyloidosis by clinical data. A localized form of AL amyloidosis is thus designated as localized AL amyloidosis and the systemic form as systemic AL amyloidosis; when myeloma is defined in association with AL amyloidosis this form is denoted as myeloma-associated AL amyloidosis. Lastly there are two forms of ATTR amyloidosis: one is genetic and the second one is linked with ageing and usually called senile ATTR [1].

Clinical Diagnosis—Amyloidosis as a Great Masquerader

A constant complaint of patients with rare diseases is the long delay between the first symptom and the clinical diagnosis made by physicians. This is also true for amyloidosis and can be explained in part by the great number of organs and systems that can be affected by amyloid deposits leading to a large variety of symptoms, none of them being specific of the disease.

Virtually all organs can be affected by amyloidosis. We will only recall the main symptoms of systemic and localized amyloidoses, except for the central nervous system and amyloid associated with hormonal polypeptides.

Renal abnormalities are the most frequent but also the least specific signs. Proteinuria is the principal mode of discovery of systemic amyloidosis. Persistent nephrotic syndrome accompanied with advanced renal failure and enlarged kidneys can be considered as suggestive of amyloidosis. Cardiac involvement gives relatively consistent signs including heart failure, arrhythmia, or conduction disturbances. Other signs which are less common include angina pectoris, systemic arterial emboli, pericarditis, mitral regurgitation, and right ventricular rupture. Cough, hemoptysis, and dyspnea can also reveal the various types of respiratory tract lesions: bronchial, mediastinal, and parenchymatous. Hepatic enlargement is common but complications such as portal hypertension, ascites, jaundice, liver rupture are rare. Splenic enlargement is also common, hyposplenism and splenic rupture are rare. There are many digestive tract symptoms, reflecting the different levels of anatomical lesions: dysphagia, abdominal pain, vomiting, hemorrhage, diarrhea, pseudo-obstruction or true occlusion, perforation, and intestinal infarction. Nerve involvement is essentially a sensory and motor polyneuropathy starting in the lower limbs. Cranial nerves are rarely affected. Amyloidosis is an established cause of the carpal canal syndrome. Muscle involvement with pseudohypertrophy and functional impairment is uncommon.

Skin lesions are highly polymorphic: common lesions are petechiae, purpura and ecchymoses, papules, nodules, and plaques; uncommon lesions are scleroderma-like diffuse infiltration, bullous lesions, onychodystrophy, and alopecia. Joint amyloidosis can present as a symmetric polyarthropathy involving shoulders with the classic shoulder pad sign, wrists, hands, and knees. Rarely, it may present as a polymyalgia rheumatica. Spinal cord lesions are uncommon. Fractures secondary to destructive bone lesions have been reported. Pain and hematuria can be signs of ureteral and bladder amyloidosis. Rarely, amyloid deposits target the eye involving the eyelid, the conjunctiva, the cornea, and/or the orbit. Vitreous deposits can mimic uveitis. Dysphonia is characteristic of laryngeal amyloidosis.

The least specific but frequent signs in severe forms of the disease are general signs such as fatigue and weight loss.

In fact, the diagnosis must be considered when there is a combination of nonspecific signs or when a sign is present in a clinical context compatible with the existence of amyloidosis. The most important context to consider is chronic inflammation. In this setting, the routine search for proteinuria is mandatory to detect AA amyloidosis and an inquiry of the family medical history directs toward a genetic form. AL amyloidosis is difficult to diagnose because it has the highest degree of variety of clinical symptoms and because the context of a plasmacytic disease is not apparent, except the uncommon cases where a monoclonal component is already known.

How to Make the Diagnosis of Amyloidosis?

The Different Types of Biopsy

The diagnosis of systemic amyloidosis still relies on a biopsy showing amyloid deposits. Two strategies are possible for the biopsy. First, it can be taken from a clinically involved organ. Second, it can be taken from a clinically uninvolved organ which is known to frequently contain amyloid deposits in the systemic forms. In general, biopsy of a clinically involved organ is performed as a second-line technique, and the second strategy should be favored. This implies, however, that the diagnosis of amyloidosis has been suspected on clinical signs.

Nowadays, three first-line types of biopsy are commonly performed: (1) biopsy of the gastrointestinal tract: rectal or gastroduodenal; (2) labial salivary gland (LSG) biopsy; and (3) subcutaneous abdominal fat aspiration biopsy (AFA).

Gastrointestinal Biopsy

Rectal biopsy was introduced in the 1960s by the Tel-Hashomer Hospital group in Israel for the diagnosis of AA amyloidosis [3]. Rectal biopsy is performed during a proctoscopy or sigmoidoscopy and is not painful, and the risk of hemorrhage is low; however, sigmoidoscopy is unpleasant. Many other series have found good sensitivity of this technique for the diagnosis of systemic AA, AL, and ATTR amyloidoses [4].

Since all gastrointestinal vessels are involved, amyloid deposits can also be found in gastric or duodenal biopsy obtained during endoscopy. Some data suggest that gastroduodenal biopsy could be as informative as rectal biopsy [5, 6].

Whatever the place, amyloid may be present as vascular and interstitial deposits and can affect all the layers of the gastrointestinal wall. It is found more commonly in submucosa than in muscularis mucosae or mucosa, therefore biopsies should be deep enough to provide the highest level of sensitivity [7, 8].

Labial Salivary Gland Biopsy

Accessory salivary glands are situated in the labial mucosa and their biopsies do not require special endoscopic equipment. Labial salivary gland biopsy has replaced the older gingival biopsy that was unpleasant and its sensitivity very variable. The development of labial salivary gland biopsy was inspired by some isolated cases of amyloidosis revealed by a sicca syndrome and salivary gland infiltration [9]. The current technique is simple with a short incision and may require no suture. LSG biopsy can be used for the diagnosis of AL, AA, and ATTR amyloidoses [10, 11].

Abdominal Fat Aspiration

Subcutaneous abdominal fat aspiration biopsy (AFA) as a diagnostic tool of systemic amyloidosis has been introduced in 1973 by Per Westermark and has been validated subsequently by many different investigators. Using a disposable syringe and a needle with an internal diameter of 0.7–1.2 mm, subcutaneous adipose tissue is aspirated and smeared onto a glass slide, air dried, and stained with Congo red. This procedure, which is not stricto sensu a biopsy, but rather an aspiration, requires only minimal local anesthesia of the periombilical subcutaneous tissue which is the preferential site [12]. AFA is thus simple, does not require specific equipment, bears a negligible risk of complications, and mainly has no risk of serious bleeding. However, the sample should not contain fat droplets only, as amyloid is located in the surrounding tissue. Studies with biopsies from organ and tissue at distant sites as gold standard reported that sensitivity of AFA ranged from 35 to 84 [8]. Most types of amyloid can be diagnosed by AFA, including AL, AA, and hereditary forms [8].

How to Choose Between These Three Techniques?

There is no study rigorously comparing these three techniques. In particular, in series evaluating AFA, the gold standard biopsy varies from one series to the other. Only two series compare LSG biopsy with AFA; however, the first one relies on a selected population of people over 80 years [13]. In the second study, the gold standard is renal biopsy, which is compared to rectal, labial, and subcutaneous fat biopsy (not AFA) and suggests that rectal and LSG biopsies have a higher sensitivity to disclose amyloid deposits than subcutaneous fat biopsy [14]. Another series compares gastroduodenal and renal biopsies to AFA in Japanese patients with rheumatoid arthritis and suggests that gastroduodenal biopsy is more sensitive than AFA [6]. Conversely, in the largest series of 162 patients, AFA was compared with at least one biopsy from another site. In this series the specificity of AFA is 100 and the sensitivity is 93 when three smears were thoroughly examined [15]. This last result comes from a tertiary center which is experienced in AFA and explains why it has good results compared to other studies. It is thus difficult to express general recommendations with these methods. All these methods are efficient when they are used by experienced hands.

Liver Biopsy

Vascular involvement is constant in amyloidosis and leads to various bleeding manifestations [16]. It is thus usually considered that liver and kidney biopsies in patients with amyloidosis have a greater risk of bleeding complications. Spontaneous hemorrhagic rupture of the liver may occur in AL and ALys amyloidoses [17, 18]. Fatal accidents have been formerly described with transparietal liver biopsy in AL patients who had probably major hemostasis disorders such as acquired factor X deficiency. Liver biopsy probably increases moderately the risk of bleeding in patients with amyloidosis and no overt disorder of the coagulation as in other liver disorders with small vessel involvement such as sickle cell disease [19]. Experience with fine-needle or transjugular liver biopsy to decrease this potential risk is limited [20]. Moreover the majority of the patients undergoing liver biopsy are rather suspected of having neoplastic disease rather than amyloidosis, and special precautions are thus generally not taken.

Kidney Biopsy

Renal involvement is common in AL, AA, and most familial forms of amyloidosis and kidney biopsy therefore is an important diagnostic tool. In addition, tissue obtained from kidney biopsy is ideal for amyloid subtyping [21]. Kidney biopsy remains often indispensable in case of suspicion of amyloidosis and other types of renal involvement in systemic disease. Although the risk of moderate bleeding has been suggested by some series, it seems that in the absence of a hemostatic disorder and/or uncontrolled hypertension, bleeding risk during kidney biopsy is not increased in patients with systemic amyloidosis [22, 23].

Other Sites

Heart Biopsy
In rare cases of isolated cardiac symptoms, endomyocardial biopsy alone allows the diagnosis of amyloidosis [24]. Current statement with endomyocardial biopsy does not highlight a specific risk for amyloidosis except of the hemorrhagic nature [25].

Nerve Biopsy
Neuronal amyloid deposits are patchy, and thus sural nerve biopsy is not very sensitive [26]. Moreover, it is not a simple procedure; bears a risk of long-lasting discomfort, sensory deficit, infection, and wound dehiscence; and should be performed only in cases that cannot be diagnosed by other means [27].

Bone Marrow Biopsy
Bone marrow biopsy is performed in cases of AL amyloidosis to disclose plasma cell dyscrasia. It reveals vascular or interstitial amyloid deposits in more than 50 of the cases and allows immunochemistry [28, 29]. Amyloid deposits may also be found in AA amyloidosis and incidentally in ATTR amyloidosis [30, 31].

Stains and Their Pitfalls

Amyloid deposits may be apparent, although not constantly, with standard stains such as hematoxylin eosin (HE) without or with safran (HES), yielding a monomorphous pale eosinophilic pattern. Conversely, Masson trichrome and Gieson's elastica stain are not able to reveal amyloid [8, 32].

It has been shown in the past that several molecules offer specific staining of amyloid deposits. Among them thioflavin S and T dyes are sensitive stains for amyloid deposition and have been used for a long time. An intensive fluorescent reaction is observed when thioflavin binds amyloid fibril. However, these methods are not specific for amyloid. They are at the most helpful in screening, and positive results should always be confirmed by more specific methods [33].

Congo red still reigns as the "king of dyes" in the diagnosis of amyloid [34]. The old Bennhold technique has been significantly modified by Puchtler and provides a better specificity [35]. Others used a slightly modified method by Romhányi [36]. Moreover, following Congo red staining, amyloid gives an "apple-green birefringence" under polarization which is specific for amyloid and definitely distinguishes amyloid from collagen. Rather than showing "apple-green birefringence in polarized light" as usually reported, some authors have recently proposed that more accurately the phenomenon should be said to show "anomalous colors" [37].

It is important to mention that Puchtler's Congo red in conjunction with polarization microscopy is highly specific but of limited sensitivity. Small and scattered deposits can be missed. To increase the sensitivity one can use thicker tissue sections (5–10 μm instead of 2–5 μm) and/or apply fluorescence microscopy on Congo red-stained sections so that amyloid yields a yellow–orange fluorescence [38]. This is, however, not specific and does not allow to free from the polarization phenomenon.

Coupling Congo red with immunohistochemistry using antibodies directed against amyloid proteins may also increase sensitivity but cannot be considered as an appropriate technique for routine detection, as it implies to know the nature of amyloid deposits to choose the antibody or to use a panel of antibodies against various proteins [39].

All forms of amyloid contain amyloid P component, and antisera against serum amyloid P component may help first to establish the nature of some deposits of undetermined status after staining with Congo red and second to provide a suitable positive control for immunohistochemical studies [21].

Electron Microscopy

Electron microscopy exhibits, as X-ray diffraction, the fibrillar nature of amyloid. On electron microscopy, amyloid consists of rigid, non-branching microfibrils of indefinite length, a mean diameter of 1 Å, and a central electron-lucent core. These characteristics differentiate them from other types of microfibrils which underline other varieties of extracellular deposits, particularly those derivating from immunoglobulins [40]. In routine practice, there is no place for the use of standard electron microscopy for the diagnosis of amyloidosis.

How to Establish the Type of Amyloidosis?

Establishing the type of amyloidosis has become a central issue as the current treatment of systemic amyloidosis directly depends on the molecular type of the amyloid protein.

This crucial step requires a rigorous strategy aiming at collecting a series of arguments to eventually retain one type of amyloidosis.

Clinical Arguments

The type of amyloidosis is sometimes obvious due to relatively suggestive combinations of arguments. In fact, AL amyloidosis, which comprises the greatest variety of symptoms, is strongly supported when several of the following organs are involved:

heart, skin, peripheral nerve, carpal tunnel syndrome, tongue with macroglossia, joints, and factor X deficiency [28]. In these settings, the added value of a monoclonal component renders the diagnosis of AL quite sure. Virtually all patients have a detectable monoclonal light chain in the serum or urine shown by immunofixation or an elevation of the immunoglobulin free light chain level revealed by nephelometry. The association of both techniques is still recommended to enhance the sensitivity and thus, the combination of immunofixation of both serum and urine with the serum free light chain concentration has a 100 sensitivity [41, 42]. Bone marrow examination will demonstrate clonal plasma cells as the source of the light chain production [29].

Of utmost importance for the diagnosis of AA amyloidosis is the existence of a disease known to lead to this complication. Usually it is a longstanding inflammatory disease with marked and constant acute phase response routinely evaluated by the measurement of blood serum amyloid A (SAA) or C-reactive protein (CRP) [43]. However, when the underlying disease is a cancer, it may be previously undiagnosed and discovered only at the same time as the amyloidosis [44]. There are also some cases of AA amyloidosis with no evidence of underlying inflammatory disorder [45].

A history of familial disease with a dominant mode of inheritance should be investigated in every patient with amyloidosis, mainly when there is a peripheral neuropathy, but also in the case of renal, cardiac, hepatic, cutaneous, or ocular disease.

In fact, it may be more difficult to distinguish the main forms of multisystemic amyloidosis. Several organs can be frequently affected in two different types of systemic amyloidosis: kidney, liver, gastrointestinal tract, and spleen may be involved in AL and AA amyloidoses; heart, peripheral nerve, gastrointestinal tract, and kidney in AL and ATTR amyloidoses. Patients with non-TTR hereditary amyloidosis have commonly renal involvement that can result from the deposition of apolipoprotein AI or AII, lysozyme, or fibrinogen αA chain [46]. Clinically, the syndrome is indistinguishable from AL amyloidosis.

Histology

Conventional morphology of amyloid deposits does not bring many arguments for the typing of amyloid deposits, although subtle differences have been emphasized in the past such as a difference between AA and AL amyloidosis with respect to the site where amyloid fibrils are deposited [47]. AA fibrils were proposed to be seen most commonly in association with reticular fibrils, while fibrils associated with primary and most other amyloid forms were proposed to accumulate in association with collagen fibers. The difficulty with this classification has made it obsolete and it is no longer used. It is in fact difficult to determine an amyloid type based on pattern of distribution in the disease, particularly in the early stages, i.e., at the time point when the determination of type is of greatest importance. One exception could be the pure glomerular pattern which is characteristic of AFib amyloidosis in the kidney [48].

Immunohistochemistry

Important studies to classify the type of amyloid would include immunohistochemical staining of tissues with appropriate commercially available antisera directed against amyloid proteins. Besides immunohistochemistry, the potassium permanganate method helps to characterize amyloid proteins [49]. The sensitivity of amyloid proteins to permanganate, as shown by loss of Congo red affinity and altered birefringence, is specific to AA and Aβ2 M amyloids, whereas AL and ATTR amyloids are resistant to such treatment. This method is most of the time well correlated with immunochemistry, but its interpretation is sometimes difficult especially when amyloid deposits are thick or extensive and the sensitivity to permanganate incomplete. Practically, the permanganate method permitted distinction between AA and AL amyloidosis, but it is now supplanted by immunohistochemistry [50].

Immunohistochemical diagnosis of amyloidosis is a particular and demanding domain and is still far from being codified when considering the surprisingly wide range of success in immunohistochemical amyloid typing, ranging from 38 to 87 in recently published series [32]. Its principles and pitfalls have been recently highlighted [21, 32, 51, 52].

The first and crucial question for the pathologist is to recognize AL amyloidosis. This should no more be a diagnosis by default being hold when amyloid deposits are not reactive with antibodies raised against AA protein. Diagnosing AL requires the reaction of amyloid deposits with antibodies directed either against kappa or lambda chains of immunoglobulin. It must be first emphasized that results of immunohistochemical staining frequently are better on frozen tissue samples and this is especially true for anti-light chains of immunoglobulins. Therefore, immunofluorescence is the technique of choice for typing amyloid derived from immunoglobulin light (and exceptionally heavy) chains. Second, due to intrinsic variability of the light chain of immunoglobulin, standard antibodies may not recognize light chain epitopes in the deposits. Third, commercially available anti-light chain antibodies lack specificity, that is, they do not necessarily reveal a predominant immunostaining of one light chain type. Fourth, they may also cross-react with AA fibrils due to the "sticky" nature of this material [51, 53].

Conversely, immunohistochemical diagnosis with anti-AA and anti-TTR antibodies is more reliable with immunoperoxydase method, even in fixed tissues [21].

Due to the recent recognition of the diversity of hereditary amyloidoses, the discrimination between AL and these varieties has become the main diagnostic problem (Table 3-2). In one series of 350 patients from a reference center with a presumptive diagnosis of AL amyloidosis and the absence of a family history, 10 of patients were shown to have genetic amyloidosis, mainly AFib and ATTR [54]. Twenty four percent of these patients also had a low-grade monoclonal gammopathy which was particularly misleading. In another series the association of both a monoclonal gammopathy and a mutation in an amyloid protein was found in some patients [55]. In fact the diagnosis is difficult mainly in two clinical presentations. The first one is isolated renal amyloidosis with no familial history. This syndrome is associated with virtually all types of amyloidosis, including a recently discovered novel type with leukocyte chemotactic factor 2 as amyloid protein [56]. The most frequent hereditary type which can be mistaken with AL is AFib. In most cases, however, a renal biopsy is performed and the specific glomerular pattern should evoke the diagnosis which can be further supported by immunohistochemistry with anti-fibrinogen Aα chain antibodies and confirmed by genetic analysis [48].

The second presentation which may raise diagnostic problems is peripheral neuropathy or cardiopathy or both organs involvement. This syndrome may be associated with AL as well as ATTR amyloidosis. Amyloid cardiopathy may be encountered both in the hereditary form and in the senile form of ATTR amyloidosis [57–59]. In fact ATTR is probably the third most prevalent amyloid in surgical pathology [60] and this form probably remains underdiagnosed in current practice.

Table 3-2. Main pitfalls in the diagnosis of AL amyloidosis.

Other amyloidoses mistaken for AL	AA	ATTR	AFib	ALys	AApoAI
Organ involvement	Kidney, liver, spleen, gut	Heart, nerve, carpal tunnel syndrome	Kidney	Kidney, digestive tract, skin	Kidney, heart, liver, skin, larynx, nerve
Diagnostic key	Anti-protein AA fixation in immunohistochemistry	Anti-TTR fixation in immunohistochemistry Genetic test	Pure glomerular pattern of the deposits Genetic test	Anti-lysozyme fixation in immunohistochemistry Genetic test	Anti-apoAI fixation in immunohistochemistry Genetic test

The main difficulty is when there is a monoclonal component in the plasma or urine supporting at first glance the diagnosis of AL

The greatest diagnosis difficulty is the case of patients with both a monoclonal component and a mutation in the TTR or in the fibrinogen Aα chain. When this combination is present, patients usually have a genetic amyloidosis [54], but the presence of a mutation within the sequence of an amyloidogenic protein does not necessarily indicate that the amyloid in the patient is derived from that mutated protein. Immunohistochemistry is here crucial to determine the actual nature of the deposits. In fact, patients with proven AL amyloidosis, who also had mutations in one of the amyloidogenic proteins, were thus recently reported [61, 62]. In some of these cases, immunohistochemistry may suggest that both κ chains and TTR are deposited in tissues [63]. Co-deposition of more than one amyloid protein, even without an immunoglobulin light chain, has been reported either in different compartments of an organ or at the same site [21, 64].

Distinguishing AL from AA is currently considered to be easier. However, examples of AL diagnosed in a clinical setting suggestive of AA amyloidosis have been demonstrated [65]. Moreover some inflammatory diseases can be associated with a monoclonal component and complicated with AA amyloidosis [66] or AL amyloidosis [67]. A recent study of amyloid typing on kidney biopsy suggests that immunofluorescence staining for immunoglobulin light chains alone is not sufficient to distinguish AL from AA and consequently supports amyloid A immunostain on a routine basis to avoid misclassification [51].

It is likely that using a panel of anti-light chain antibodies in immunofluorescence on frozen samples coupled with anti-AA and anti-TTR antibodies on a routine basis would greatly improve the determination of the nature of amyloid deposits [21]. Other antibodies would be kept for expert laboratories.

More sophisticated techniques of immunohistochemistry have been used to improve the accuracy of the diagnosis such as immunolabeling of amyloid fibrils by colloidal gold particles in different types of biopsy including nerve biopsy [68] or immunoelectron microscopy [69].

Beyond Immunohistochemistry

When immunohistochemical determination of the chemical type of amyloid remains inconclusive, other methods are needed, particularly to show the presence of light chain of immunoglobulin. Several techniques have been proposed by different authors to go beyond immunohistochemistry and its pitfalls. None of them is routinely used nowadays.

A first group of methods consists in partially purifying the material obtained from amyloid-rich tissue sample even of very small size as obtained by standard biopsy including AFA. The obtained material is then forwarded to enzyme-linked immunosorbent assays [70]. Some authors have refined the method to measure the amount of the amyloid A protein in patients with rheumatoid arthritis-associated amyloidosis and showed it was correlated to the extension of amyloid evaluated with Congo red staining [71]. After isolation, the protein may also be placed on gel electrophoresis and subjected to Western blot [72]. These methods need appropriate specific antibodies often monoclonal and private.

By essence biochemical typing is the gold standard to determine the nature of a protein. Most of the amyloid proteins have been first characterized by extraction, purification, and sequencing following the discovery of the landmark method of Pras [73]. These experiments were carried on tissue samples of big size obtained usually from autopsy and containing large amounts of amyloid material and therefore inappropriate for routine diagnosis with samples obtained from biopsies. That is why biochemical typing of amyloid proteins extracted from routine frozen and formalin-fixed, paraffin-embedded specimens has been developed for several years [74, 75].

More recently, besides its use in research, the application of proteomics techniques for amyloid typing has been reported. These very delicate procedures require lesser amounts of material for study, but a more complex preparation for the mass spectrometry sequence. While such studies are feasible in paraffin-embedded biopsies, fresh, unfixed tissue is also here preferable [76, 77]. Merger of laser capture microdissection and mass spectrometry allow to consider the power to extract minute amount of amyloid deposits [78].

These sophisticated and consuming techniques are available only in highly specialized research laboratories and have not yet been validated for routine diagnosis of amyloid.

Genetic Tools

Although some mutations may be shown at the protein level, namely from the plasma precursor of amyloid protein [79], the mainstay of diagnosing the hereditary amyloidosis is DNA testing. The choice of the gene to sequence is guided by the clinical presentation and when available by the results of histology and immunohistochemistry [55]. Full DNA sequencing usually demonstrates one of the known mutations. Occasionally, a new mutation will be found by direct DNA sequencing and correlation of disease and genetics will be needed. This may be difficult in case of reduced penetrance of some mutations and DNA testing results should always be compared to other data.

Is Amyloid Localized?

Some forms of AL amyloidosis are localized, and the light chain production is local and not part of a systemic plasma cell dyscrasia where the bone marrow produces most of the amyloid light chains [80]. Localized forms of amyloid might be suspected right away because of the organ involved. When deposits of amyloid are found in the urinary tract (bladder, urethra, and ureter), it is virtually always a localized process [81]. The other site is the respiratory tract where the commonest localized form involves the larynx and tracheobronchial tree [82, 83]. These localizations although not systemic may cause troublesome complications such as hemorrhage and dyspnea. Most cases of amyloid in the orbit and conjunctivae are localized and the latter may be mistaken for a lymphoma.

When amyloid deposits are found in one of these localizations, it seems reasonable to set up a minimal workup consisting in physical examination and routine blood tests—possibly completed if any doubt on another specific amyloid organ involvement—and a search for a blood monoclonal component with serum immunofixation and immunoglobulin light chain in blood. A long-term follow-up is nevertheless mandatory for both managing the local process and detecting potential emergence of a systemic process as this has been described in very rare cases [82]. AL amyloidosis localized to the skin deserves the same surveillance. Non-immunoglobulinic amyloid of various biochemical origin deposits in the atria of the heart, endocrine tumor, knee joint meniscus, intervertebral disk is localized, and the diagnosis of systemic amyloidosis should not be made in these cases.

References

1. Westermark P, Benson MD, Buxbaum JN, Cohen AS, Frangione B, Ikeda S, et al. A primer of amyloid nomenclature. Amyloid 2007;14:179–83.
2. Merlini G, Palladini G. Amyloidosis: is a cure possible? Ann Oncol. 2008;19 Suppl 4:iv63–6.
3. Gafni J, Sohar E. Rectal biopsy for the diagnosis of amyloidosis. Am J Med Sci. 1960;240:332–6.
4. Kyle RA, Spencer RJ, Dahlin DC. Value of rectal biopsy in the diagnosis of primary systemic amyloidosis. Am J Med Sci. 1966;251:501–6.
5. Kobayashi H, Tada S, Fuchigami T, Okuda Y, Takasugi K, Matsumoto T, et al. Secondary amyloidosis in patients with rheumatoid arthritis: diagnostic and prognostic value of gastroduodenal biopsy. Br J Rheumatol. 1996;35:44–9.
6. Kuroda T, Tanabe N, Sakatsume M, Nozawa S, Mitsuka T, Ishikawa H, et al. Comparison of gastroduodenal, renal and abdominal fat biopsies for diagnosing amyloidosis in rheumatoid arthritis. Clin Rheumatol. 2002;21:123–8.
7. Yamada M, Hatakeyama S, Tsukagoshi H. Gastrointestinal amyloid deposition in AL (primary or myeloma associated) and AA (secondary) amyloidosis: diagnostic value of gastric biopsy. Hum Pathol. 1985;16:1206–11.
8. Röcken C, Sletten K. Amyloid in surgical pathology. Virchows Arch. 2003;443:3–16.
9. Simon BG, Moputsopoulos HM. Primary amyloidosis resembling sicca syndrome. Arthritis Rheum. 1979;22:932–4.
10. Hachulla E, Janin A, Flipo RM, Saïle R, Facon T, Bataille D, et al. Labial salivary gland biopsy is a reliable test for the diagnosis of primary and secondary amyloidosis. Arthritis Rheum. 1993;36:691–7.
11. Lechapt-Zalcman E, Authier FJ, Creange A, Voisin MC, Gherardi RK. Labial salivary gland biopsy for diagnosis of amyloid polyneuropathy. Muscle Nerve 1999;22:105–7.
12. Westermark P, Stenkvist B. A new method for the diagnosis of systemic amyloidosis. Arch Int Med. 1973;132:522–3.
13. Dupond JL, de Wazières B, Saile R, Closs F, Viennet G, Kantelip B, et al. L'amylose systémique su sujet âgé: valeur diagnostique de l'examen de la graisse sous-cutanée abdominale et des glandes salivaires accessoires. Étude prospective chez 100 patients âgés. Rev Med Interne. 1995;16:314–7.
14. Fatihi E, Ramdani B, Fadel H, Hachim K, Zahiri K, Benghanem GM, et al. Prevalence of subcutaneous, labial, and rectal amyloidosis in patients with renal amyloidosis. Nephrologie 2000;21:19–21.
15. Van Gameren II, Hazenberg BP, Bijzet J, van Rijswijk MH. Diagnostic accuracy of subcutaneous abdominal fat tissue aspiration for detecting systemic amyloidosis and its utility in clinical practice. Arthritis Rheum. 2006;54:2015–21.
16. Yood RA, Skinner M, Rubinow A, Talarico L, Cohen AS Bleeding manifestations in 100 patients with amyloidosis. J Am Med Assoc. 1983;249:1322–4.
17. Naito KS, Ichiyama T, Kawakami S, Kadoya M, Tabata T, Matsuda M, et al. AL amyloidosis with spontaneous hepatic rupture: successful treatment by transcatheter hepatic artery embolization. Amyloid 2008;15:137–9.
18. Loss M, Ng WS, Karim RZ, Strasser SI, Koorey DJ, Gallagher PJ, et al. Hereditary lysozyme amyloidosis: spontaneous hepatic rupture (15 years apart) in mother and daughter. Role of emergency liver transplantation. Liver Transplant. 2006;12:1152–5.
19. Zakaria N, Knisely A, Portmann B, Mieli-Vergani G, Wendon J, Arya R, et al. Acute sickle cell hepatopathy represents a potential contraindication for percutaneous liver biopsy. Blood 2003;101:101–3.
20. Srinivasan R, Nijhawan R, Gautam U, Bambery P. Potassium permanganate resistant amyloid in fineneedle aspirate of the liver. Diagn Cytopathol. 1994;10:383–4.
21. Kebbel A, Röcken C. Immunohistochemical classification of amyloid in surgical pathology revisited. Am J Surg Pathol. 2006;30:673–83.
22. Eiro M, Katoh T, Watanabe T Risk factors for bleeding complications in percutaneous renal biopsy. Clin Exp Nephrol. 2005;9:40–5.

23. Soares SM, Fervenza FC, Lager DJ, Gertz MA, Cosio FG, Leung N. Bleeding complications after transcutaneous kidney biopsy in patients with systemic amyloidosis: single-center experience in 101 patients. Am J Kidney Dis. 2008;52:1079–83.

24. Pellika PA, Holmes DR, Edwards WD, et al. Endomyocardial biopsy in 30 patients with primary amyloidosis and suspected cardiac involvement. Arch Intern Med. 1988;148:662–6.

25. Cooper LT, Baughman KL, Feldman AM, Frustaci A, Jessup M, Kuhl U, et al. The role of endomyocardial biopsy in the management of cardiovascular disease: a scientific statement from the American Heart Association, the American College of Cardiology, and the European Society of Cardiology. Endorsed by the Heart Failure Society of America and the Heart Failure Association of the European Society of Cardiology. J Am Coll Cardiol. 2007;50:1914–31.

26. Simmons Z, Blaivas M, Aguilera AJ, Feldman EL, Bromberg MB, Towfighi J. Low diagnostic yield of sural nerve biopsy in patients with peripheral neuropathy and primary amyloidosis. J Neurol Sci. 1993;120:60–3.

27. Bevilacqua NJ, Rogers LC, Malik RA, Armstrong DG. Technique of the sural nerve biopsy. J Foot Ankle Surg. 2007;46:139–42.

28. Kyle RA, Gertz MA Primary systemic amyloidosis: clinical and laboratory features in 474 cases. Semin Hematol. 1995;32:45–59.

29. Swan N, Skinner M, O'Hara CJ. Bone marrow core biopsy specimens in AL (primary) amyloidosis: a morphologic and immunohistochemical study of 100 cases. Am J Clin Pathol. 2003;120:610–6.

30. Sungur C, Sungur A, Ruacan S, Ank N, Yasavul U, Turgan C, et al. Diagnostic value bonemarrow biopsy in patients with renal amyloidosis secondary to familial Mediterranean fever. Kidney Int. 1993;44:834–6.

31. Wong KF, Tam S, Kwong YL. Diagnosis of familial amyloidotic polyneuropathy by bone marrow biopsy. Br J Haematol. 2007;139:517.

32. Picken MM. New insights into systemic amyloidosis: the importance of diagnosis of specific type. Curr Opin Nephrol Hypertens. 2007;16:196–203.

33. Elghetany MT, Saleem A. Methods for staining amyloid in tissues: a review. Stain Technol. 1988;63:201–12.

34. Steensma DP. "Congo" red—out of Africa. Arch Pathol Lab Med. 2001;125:250–2.

35. Puchtler H, Sweat F, Levine M. On the binding of Congo red by amyloid. J Histochem Cytochem. 1962;10:355–64.

36. Bély M, Makovitzky J. Sensitivity and specificity of Congo red staining according to Romhányi. Comparison with Puchtler's or Bennhold's methods. Acta Histochem. 2006;108:175–80.

37. Howie AJ, Brewer DB, Howell D, Jones AP. Physical basis of colors seen in Congo red-stained amyloid in polarized light. Lab Invest. 2008;88:232–42.

38. Linke RP. Highly sensitive diagnosis of amyloid and various amyloid syndromes using Congo red fluorescence. Virchows Arch. 2000;436:439–48.

39. Linke RP, Gärtner HV, Michels H. High-sensitivity diagnosis of AA amyloidosis using Congo red and immunohistochemistry detects missed amyloid deposits. J Histochem Cytochem. 1995;43:863–9.

40. Picken MM. Immunoglobulin light and heavy chain amyloidosis AL/AH: renal pathology and differential diagnosis. Contrib Nephrol. 2007;153:135–55.

41. Abraham RS, Katzmann JA, Clark RJ, et al. Quantitative analysis of serum free light chains: a new marker for the diagnostic evaluation of primary systemic amyloidosis. Am J Clin Pathol. 2003;119:274–8.

42. Palladini G, Russo P, Bosoni T, Verga L, Sarais G, Lavatelli F, et al. Identification of amyloidogenic light chains requires the combination of serum-free light chain assay with immunofixation of serum and urine. Clin Chem. 2009 Jan 8 (Epub);55:499–504.

43. Lachmann HJ, Goodman HJB, Gilbertson JA, Gallimore JR, Sabin CA, Gillmore JD, et al. Natural history and outcome in systemic AA amyloidosis. N Engl J Med. 2007;356:2361–71.

44. Lachmann HJ, Gilbertson JA, Gillmore JD, Hawkins PN, Pepys MB. Unicentric Castleman's disease complicated by systemic AA amyloidosis: a curable disease. QJM. 2002;95:211–8.

45. Maury CPJ, Tornroth T, Wegelius O. Is amyloid A (AA) amyloidosis always secondary? Ann Rheum Dis. 1985;44:273–6.

46. Benson MD. Ostertag revisited: the inherited systemic amyloidoses without neuropathy. Amyloid 2005;12:75–87.

47. Missmahl HP. Reticulin and collagen as important factors for the localization of amyloid and the use of polarization microscopy as a tool in the detection of the composition of amyloid. Amyloidosis. In: Mandema E, Ruinen L, Scholten JH, Cohen AS, editors. Amsterdam: Excerpta Medica; 1968. p. 22–9.

48. Gillmore JD, Lachmann HJ, Rowczenio D, Gilbertson JA, Zeng CH, Liu ZH, et al. Diagnosis, pathogenesis, treatment, and prognosis of hereditary fibrinogen Aα-chain amyloidosis J Am Soc Nephrol. 2009;20:444–51.

49. Wright JR, Calkins E, Humphrey RC. Potassium permanganate reaction in amyloidosis: a histologic method to assist in differentiating forms of this disease. Lab Invest. 1977;36:274–81.

50. Janssen S, Elema JD, Van Rijswijik MH, Limburg PC, Meijer S, Mandema E. Classification of amyloidosis: immunohistochemistry versus the potassium permanganate method in 2 differentiating AA from AL amyloidosis. Appl Pathol. 1985;3:29–38.

51. Satoskar AA, Burdge K, Cowden DJ, Nadasdy GM, Hebert LA, Nadasdy T. Typing of amyloidosis in renal biopsies: diagnostic pitfalls. Arch Pathol Lab Med. 2007;1319:17–22.

52. Solomon A, Murphy CL, Westermark P. Unreliability of immunohistochemistry for typing amyloid deposits. Arch Pathol Lab Med. 2008;132:14.

53. Picken MM, Herrera GA. The burden of "sticky" amyloid: typing challenges. Arch Pathol Lab Med. 2007;131:850–1.

54. Lachmann HJ, Booth DR, Booth SE, Bybee A, Gilbertson JA, Gillmore JD, et al. Misdiagnosis of hereditary amyloidosis as AL (primary) amyloidosis. N Engl J Med. 2002;346:1786–91.

55. Comenzo RL, Zhou P, Fleisher M, et al. Seeking confidence in the diagnosis of systemic AL (Ig light chain) amyloidosis: patients can have both monoclonal gammopathies and hereditary amyloid proteins. Blood 2006;107:3489–91.

56. Benson MD, James S, Scott K, Liepnieks JJ, Kluve-Beckerman B. Leukocyte chemotactic factor 2: a novel renal amyloid protein. Kidney Int. 2008;74:218–22.

57. Benson MD, Kincaid JC. The molecular biology and clinical features of amyloid neuropathy. Muscle Nerve 2007;36:411–23.

58. Ng B, Connors LH, Davidoff R, Skinner M, Falk RH. Senile systemic amyloidosis presenting with heart failure: a comparison with light chain-associated amyloidosis. Arch Intern Med. 2005;165:1425–9.

59. Gertz MA, Kyle RA, Thibodeau SN. Familial amyloidosis: a study of 52 north American-born patients examined during a 30-year period. Mayo Clin Proc. 1992;67:428–40.

60. Eriksson M, Büttner J, Todorov T, Yumlu S, Schönland S, Hegenbart U, et al. Prevalence of germline mutations in the TTR gene in a consecutive series of surgical pathology specimens with ATTR amyloid. Am J Surg Pathol. 2009;33:58–65.

61. Landau H, Comenzo RL, Zhou P, Clark B, Teruya-Feldstein J, Wang S, Murphy CL, Solomon A AL amyloidosis in a patient with a T60A TTR mutation. Amyloid 2006;13 Suppl 1:40.

62. Wechalekar AD, Offer M, Gillmore JD, Hawkins PN, Lachmann HJ. Cardiac amyloidosis, a monoclonal gammopathy and a potentially misleading mutation. Nat Clin Pract Cardiovasc Med. 2009;6:128–33.

63. Bergström J, Patrosso MC, Colussi G, Salvadore M, Penco S, Lando G, et al. A novel type of familial transthyretin amyloidosis, ATTR Asn124Ser, with co-localization of kappa light chains. Amyloid 2007;14:141–5.

64. de Sousa MM, Vital C, Ostler D, Fernandes R, Pouget-Abadie J, Carles D, et al. Apolipoprotein AI and transthyretin as components of amyloid fibrils in a kindred with apoAI Leu178His amyloidosis. Am J Pathol. 2000;156:1911–7.

65. Kracker D, Litbarg N, Picken MM. Amyloidosis in ankylosing spondylitis: unexpected findings underscoring the importance of typing amyloid deposits. Amyloid 2006;13 Suppl 1:38A.

66. Quinton R, Siersema PD, Michiels JJ, Ten Kate FJWW. Renal AA amyloidosis in a patient with Bence Jones proteinuria and ankylosing spondylitis. J Clin Pathol. 1992;45:934–6.

67. Husby G, Williams RC, Tung KSK, Smith FE, Cronin RJ, Sletten K, et al. Immunologic studies in identical twins concordant for juvenile rheumatoid arthritis but discordant for monoclonal gammopathy and amyloidosis. J Lab Clin Med. 1988;111:307–14.

68. Adams D, Said G. Ultrastructural immunolabelling in acquired and hereditary amyloid neuropathies. J Neurol. 1996;243:63–7.

69. Arbustini E, Verga L, Concardi M, Palladini G, Obici L, Merlini G. Electron and immuno-electron microscopy of abdominal fat identifies and characterizes amyloid fibrils in suspected cardiac amyloidosis. Amyloid 2002;9:108–14.

70. Olsen KE, Sletten K, Westermark P. The use of subcutaneous fat tissue for amyloid typing by enzyme-linked immunosorbent assay. Am J Clin Pathol. 1999;111:355–62.

71. Hazenberg BPC, Limburg PC, Bijzet J, Vanrijswijk MH. A quantitative method for detecting deposits of amyloid A protein in aspirated fat tissue of patients with arthritis. Ann Rheum Dis. 1999;58:96–102.

72. Westermark P, Davey E, Lindbom K, Enqvist S. Subcutaneous fat tissue for diagnosis and studies of systemic amyloidosis. Acta Histochem. 2006;108:209–13.

73. Pras M, Schubert M, Zucker-Franklin D, Rimon A, Franklin EC. The characterization of soluble amyloid prepared in water. J Clin Invest. 1968;47:924–33.

74. Murphy CL, Eulitz M, Hrncic R, Sletten K, Westermark P, Williams T, et al. Chemical typing of amyloid protein contained in formalin–fixed paraffin-embedded biopsy specimens. Am J Clin Pathol. 2001;116:135–42.

75. Kaplan B, Martin BM, Livneh A, Pras M, Gallo GR. Biochemical subtyping of amyloid in formalin-fixed tissue samples confirms and supplements immunohistologic data. Am J Clin Pathol. 2004;121:794–800.

76. Murphy CL, Wang S, Williams T, Weiss DT, Solomon A. Characterization of systemic amyloid deposits by mass spectrometry. Methods Enzymol. 2006;412:48–62.

77. Lavatelli F, Perlman DH, Spencer B, Prokaeva T, McComb ME, Théberge R, et al. Amyloidogenic and associated proteins in systemic amyloidosis proteome of adipose tissue. Mol Cell Proteomics 2008;7:1570–83.

78. Gozal YM, Cheng D, Duong DM, Lah JJ, Levey AI, Peng J. Merger of laser capture microdissection and mass spectrometry: a window into the amyloid plaque proteome. Methods Enzymol. 2006;412:77–93.

79. Théberge R, Connors L, Skinner M, Skare J, Costello CE. Characterization of transthyretin mutants from serum using immunoprecipitation, HPLC/electrospray ionization and matrix-assisted laser desorption/ionization mass spectrometry. Anal Chem. 1999;71:452–9.

80. Hamidi Asl K, Liepnieks JJ, Nakamura M, Benson MD. Organ-specific (localized) synthesis of Ig light chain amyloid. J Immunol. 1999;162:5556–60.

81. Paccalin M, Hachulla E, Cazalet C, Tricot L, Carreiro M, Rubi M, et al. Localized amyloidosis: a survey of 35 French cases. Amyloid 2005;12:239–45.

82. Bartels H, Dikkers FG, van der Wal JE, Lokhorst HM, Hazenberg BP. Laryngeal amyloidosis: localized versus systemic disease and update on diagnosis and therapy. Ann Otol Rhinol Laryngol. 2004;113:741–8.

83. Berk JL, O'Regan A, Skinner M. Pulmonary and tracheobronchial amyloidosis. Semin Respir Crit Care Med. 2002;23:155–65.

Chapter 4

Pathogenesis of Systemic Amyloidoses

Francesca Lavatelli, Giovanni Palladini, and Giampaolo Merlini

Abstract Systemic amyloid diseases are complex entities, in which an intricate interplay between multiple factors is responsible for protein misfolding and deposition, with consequent cell and organ dysfunction. The chapter provides an overview of major past and recent advancements in the study of the molecular bases of protein misfolding diseases. Many questions are still open, notably the molecular mechanisms underlying tissue targeting and organ dysfunction remain elusive. However, the use of a multidisciplinary approach has allowed making important steps towards the clarification of the pathogenic mechanisms, opening the way for the study of new targeted therapies. It is now clear that interactions with the environment, along with inherent biochemical and biophysical properties, determine the fate of an amyloidogenic protein in vivo. During the years, the concept of a direct toxicity of protein aggregates has emerged, and the pathogenic role of fibrils and prefibrillar species and the pathways through which the damage occurs have been objects of intense investigation, leading to a deeper—although not yet complete—understanding of the molecular events behind organ dysfunction and to the development of new paradigms in the treatment of systemic amyloidosis.

Keywords Protein misfolding, Fibrils, Oligomers, Tissue targeting, Common constituents, Cytotoxicity

Introduction

The amyloidoses are a broad group of diseases in which specific proteins aggregate forming insoluble fibrils that deposit in tissues, leading to cell toxicity and organ dysfunction. A complex interplay between biochemical, genetic, environmental and other biological factors sustains the cascade of events that lead to amyloid deposition and pathology [1] (Fig. 4-1), and important steps towards the clarification of the pathogenesis of these diseases have been made by biochemical, biophysical and cell biology investigations on amyloidogenic proteins and affected tissues. However, many questions still remain to be addressed for a unifying description of the detailed mechanisms of amyloidoses, and there is a fervid activity among scientists to clarify the nodal pathogenetic points that could be targeted to prevent, stop or reverse the damage. Three crucial and partially overlapping processes must be described in this class of diseases: how the precursors lose their native structure and aggregate into amyloid fibrils in vivo, which factors determine the tissue targeting and how the presence of fibrils and aggregates damages cells and tissues, leading to organ dysfunction.

From: *Amyloidosis*, Contemporary Hematology,
Edited by: M.A. Gertz and S.V. Rajkumar, DOI 10.1007/978-1-60761-631-3_4,
© Springer Science+Business Media, LLC 2010

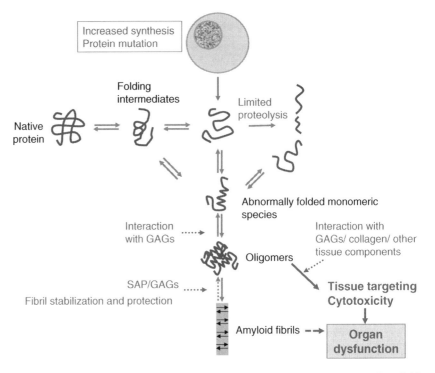

Fig. 4-1. Pathogenetic steps in the development of amyloid diseases. Intermediate folding states are populated during the acquisition of the native structure. The acquisition of an alternative (misfolded) structure or destabilization of the native structure, which is favoured by the presence of mutations (as in hereditary amyloidoses), proteolytic remodelling, physicochemical stimuli and interaction with other molecules or cell/tissue components (notably glycosaminoglycans and SAP), renders the protein prone to aggregation into oligomers and formation of amyloid fibrils. Organ dysfunction may result primarily from the cytotoxicity of the amyloid protein prefibrillar oligomers and, to a less extent, from the accumulation of amyloid deposits in the tissues.

In addressing the first point, the isolation of the protein components of natural amyloid fibrils and their chemical and physical characterization are key investigative tools. Besides allowing the identification of their protein constituent, fibrils from biopsy or autopsy specimens are a source of material for biochemical and biophysical in vitro studies and can reveal the presence of in vivo modifications relevant for protein destabilization and toxicity. The investigation of the molecular basis of tissue targeting requires the analysis of the interactions between the amyloidogenic protein and the tissue constituents: cells and matrix components. For dissecting the mechanisms of tissue damage, appropriate experimental models of toxicity must be designed, with sensitive assessment of the cell and tissue responses occurring as a reaction to the presence of amyloid proteins or fibrils.

Protein Misfolding and Aggregation

More than 25 different proteins are known to be causative agents of amyloid diseases in vivo [2] (see Table 4-1). The primary event behind the onset of amyloidoses is the loss of the soluble, native state of a protein, with acquisition of an alternative, predominantly β-sheet secondary conformation and consequent tendency to form aggregates

Table 4-1. Amyloid fibril proteins and their precursors causing the most clinically relevant amyloid diseases[a].

Precursor	Amyloid protein	Syndrome or involved tissues
Aβ protein precursor (AβPP)	Aβ	Alzheimer's disease sporadic, aging Hereditary cerebral amyloid angiopathy—Dutch type
Prion protein	APrP	CJD sporadic (iatrogenic), nv CJD Familial CJD, GSSD, FFI
ABriPP/ADanPP	ABri/ADan	British and Danish familial dementia
Cystatin C	ACys	Icelandic hereditary cerebral amyloid angiopathy
β2-microglobulin	Aβ2M	Chronic haemodialysis Joints
Immunoglobulin light chain	AL	Primary, myeloma associated
(Apo) serum AA	AA	Secondary, reactive to chronic inflammation, infections, neoplasia
Transthyretin Senile	ATTR	Prototypic FAP, approximately 100 variants reported Heart, vessels
Apolipoprotein A-I	AApoAI	Liver, kidney, heart according to variants, 12 reported Aortic
Apolipoprotein A-II	AApoAII	Kidney, heart
Gelsolin	AGel	Finnish hereditary amyloidosis
Lysozyme	ALys	Kidney, liver, spleen, lymph nodes
Fibrinogen Aαchain	AFib	Kidney (liver, heart)[b]

CJD: Creutzfeldt–Jakob's disease; nv: new variant; GSSD: Gerstmann–Sträussler–Scheinker's disease; FFI: fatal familial insomnia

[a]The following proteins may also cause amyloidosis: immunoglobulin heavy chain; (pro)calcitonin; islet amyloid polypeptide; atrial natriuretic factor; prolactin; insulin; lactadherin; kerato-epithelin; leukocyte chemotactic factor 2

[b]Rare, but severe

Modified from Westermark et al. [2].

and insoluble amyloid fibrils [3] (Fig. 4-1). Despite the heterogeneous structures and functions of the precursors, the fibrils are morphologically almost indistinguishable, although a certain degree of variability is disclosed by the accurate evaluation of the number of protofilaments assembled within the mature fibre, ranging from three protofilaments in the fibres deriving from apolipoprotein A-I (apoA-I) to six for fibres of different chemical composition [1, 4, 5]. Since the end of the 1990s, however, seminal studies have cast new light on the process of amyloid formation, showing that self-organization into amyloid fibrils is not a specific characteristic of the proteins known to be causative agents of this class of diseases, but may be regarded as a general property, common to most proteins when subjected to opportune conditions, configuring amyloid as a generic, primordial structure enabling proteins to self-organize [6–10].

This conformational conversion, in vivo, is a pathologic event closely related to the physiology of protein folding. The acquisition of the fully folded, so-called native state, is, in fact, a dynamic process that leads to the achievement of the energetically most stable structure under physiological conditions [3]. The hallmarks of amyloidogenic proteins are a native conformation that is thermodynamically less stable than the normal counterpart and a particularly high propensity for self-aggregation during the fluctuations between fully unfolded, locally unfolded and folded states, which naturally occur during the life of a protein. The exposure to various extracellular denaturing stimuli can cause transient unfolding of the polypeptide chain; this is usually reversible but may, in some instances, bring to surface normally hidden hydrophobic residues, thus making the protein prone to self-aggregation. Moreover, specific post-translational modifications, such as proteolytic cleavage, may be favoured by partial unfolding, thus destabilizing the protein to the point of preventing the reacquisition of the native structure.

According to the basic mechanisms of amyloid formation, amyloid proteins may be divided into four categories: (1) proteins with an intrinsic propensity for conformational fluctuations, which further increases with age. Transthyretin, with its ability to form amyloid deposits in elderly people even in its wild-type form, is one example of this category of amyloid-forming proteins; (2) proteins which, in spite of their susceptibility to partial denaturation and self-aggregation, do not normally form amyloid deposits due to their low serum concentration, but can generate deposits once a persistently high serum concentration is achieved, such as β2-microglobulin (b2-m) in patients undergoing long-term dialysis; (3) proteins in which the conversion to fibrils requires the presence of mutations. For instance, human lysozyme, which does not produce amyloid fibrils in its wild-type form, is the causative agent of an autosomal dominant hereditary disease transmitted when one of the amyloidogenic variants is present [11]. In certain proteins, the mutation may favour the proteolytic cleavage that releases a polypeptide fragment with high propensity for fibrillar aggregation; (4) proteins in which both mutations and increased concentration concur to amyloid formation, as in the case of immunoglobulin light chains in AL amyloidosis [12–14].

The extreme variability among immunoglobulin light chains complicates finding a single mechanistic explanation for their low stability, but specific features are known to be statistically linked to the development of amyloidosis. For example, λ light chains are more frequently amyloidogenic than κ light chains and, among λ light chains, those derived from some genes, as Vλ3r (λIII) [15] and Vλ6 [16–19], have a strong tendency to form fibrils. Moreover, a substantial proportion of the amyloid clones develop from B cells selected for improved antigen-binding properties, and pathogenic light chains show evidence of this selection [20].

Among the globular proteins associated with clinical amyloidosis, the systems characterized in more detail for their transition from a globular monomeric structure to the fibrillar state are probably human transthyretin, lysozyme and β2-microglobulin. In the hereditary forms, like ATTR and lysozyme amyloidosis, the acquisition of an amyloidogenic propensity is the consequence of DNA mutations. Even single amino acid substitutions, in fact, can cause the loss of intramolecular bonds, which, in the wild-type form, play a role in maintaining the stability of the globular structure. More than 100 different TTR mutations have been reported [21–23], and most of them are amyloidogenic. Transthyretin is a homotetrameric protein with approximately 60% β-sheet secondary structure. Four monomers associate non-covalently to form the tetrameric plasma transport protein which has binding sites for thyroxine in a central channel and surface receptors for RBP/vitamin A. According to the commonly accepted model, the presence of TTR mutations translates in the loss of cohesion between the four monomers constituting the tetramer, which dissociate into monomers that become then prone to aggregation.

During the years it has become clear, however, that the process of amyloid deposition in vivo is affected by a number of biological factors, which have to be taken into account during in vitro studies, to elucidate the real mechanisms behind amyloidoses. To initiate protein fibrillogenesis in vitro, in fact, it is necessary to adopt harsh conditions, such as buffer acidification or the use of other chemical or physical denaturants (as high temperature or addition of co-solvents), which are non-physiological and almost impossible to be reached at the site of amyloid deposition. In buffer solutions that reproduce physiological pH, ion strength and temperature, the proteins known to be amyloidogenic in vivo, either in the wild-type or mutated form, do not spontaneously convert into fibrils. These observations indicate that physiological factors, which are not generally present in the test tube, are required for amyloid formation [24].

The Fate of Misfolded Proteins Is Regulated by the Cellular Quality Control Mechanisms

A proper balance between protein synthesis, maturation and degradation is crucial for cell survival. Protein folding in the cell is a central process, carefully assisted, from transcription to secretion, by tightly regulated molecular machineries requiring energy consumption [25]. Proteins that do not attain a correctly folded state are targeted for degradation. However, amyloidogenic proteins, which are susceptible to extracellular misfolding, must escape the endoplasmic reticulum (ER) quality control mechanisms to be secreted. The role of the intracellular quality control system in dictating the fate of amyloidogenic proteins has been most thoroughly investigated in the case of transthyretin. In this form of amyloidosis, experimental models have shown that, in fact, ER quality control apparatus discriminates amyloidogenic variants compared to the wild type [26, 27], increasing their retention, albeit with an efficacy that depends on the mutation and on the type of tissue involved [28]. For example, certain transthyretin variants are scantly secreted by hepatocytes but less retained by choroid cells, therefore creating a low concentration of the variant in plasma, but a higher concentration in the cerebrospinal fluid, thus explaining its selective leptomeningeal deposition.

Differences in secretion efficiency, based on the chaperone content of the endoplasmic reticulum in various tissues, may be one of the factors that influence the tissue specificity, severity and age of onset of extracellular amyloid disease. Thus, enhancing the clearance of misfolded proteins through increased interaction with molecular chaperones is a possible therapeutic strategy for systemic amyloidoses. Clarification of these aspects is particularly important in the perspective of growing life expectancy and expansion of the aged population, since aging is expected to be associated with a progressive decrease in folding efficiency and a concomitant increase in misfolded products.

Detailed Chemical Analysis of Ex Vivo Fibrils and Precursors Discloses Features of Amyloidogenicity

The presence of post-translational modifications or proteolytic processing is now considered relevant in destabilizing the amyloidogenic precursor and leading to amyloid formation under physiological conditions. The biochemical detailed investigation of the amyloid fibrils and precursors has been crucial for characterizing all the deposited species and designing appropriate experimental models [14, 29–34]. Proteomics, centred on protein analysis by mass spectrometry, proved to be a particularly powerful tool for a global and sensitive dissection of these aspects and has been applied to the study of isolated fibrils, whole tissues and circulating precursors.

A very high degree of heterogeneity, in terms of charge properties and molecular weight, is present in deposited light chains and transthyretin in subcutaneous fat tissues from patients with, respectively, AL and ATTR amyloidoses [30]. The molecular weight heterogeneity is particularly pronounced in AL amyloidosis, where the deposits are constituted by tens of different species, consisting of N-terminal fragments of the precursor light chain, missing a progressively longer portion of constant region. The exact points of truncation in all species are unknown, but they are likely to reflect specific cleavage mechanisms or involvement of particular undetermined enzymes. In addition, in AL amyloidosis, the full-length light chain invariably constitutes a large percentage of the deposited proteins. Besides the presence of fragments, a high degree of charge heterogeneity has been described, which reflects the presence of possible post-translational chemical modifications, such as deamidation.

Truncation, often occurring between residues 46 and 55 of the protein, is also a prominent feature in some, but not all cases of transthyretin-related amyloidosis [30, 35–38]. In particular, considerable heterogeneity has been described within the population of ATTR patients carrying the Val30Met TTR mutation, suggesting a prominent role of individual factors in determining the processing and fate of the protein [36]. Occurrence of oxidation of specific transthyretin residues, such as tryptophan 41, is also a known phenomenon [30, 39].

Proteomics of isolated amyloid fibrils has also had an important role in defining a new model of disease in other forms of amyloidosis, such as those caused by the deposition of b2-m [40, 41] and apolipoprotein A-I [42]. Whatever the source of natural b2-m fibrils analysed so far, 25% or more of b2-m located in the deposits is invariably cleaved at the N-terminus, with formation of a truncated form of the protein (DN6 b2-m). Extensive investigation showed the total absence of this cleavage in free circulating b2-m of plasma, cerebrospinal fluid or excreted in urines. The presence of fragments of the precursors, instead, is a notorious phenomenon observed in urines of patients with AL amyloidosis [43, 44], while their presence in the circulation in vivo is less well defined.

The pathogenetic role of truncation and proteolytic remodelling is controversial. In some forms of systemic amyloidosis, such as apolipoprotein A-I amyloidosis, consistent experimental data indicate that the cleavages can favour amyloidogenesis [42] or even dictate the tissue targeting of amyloid deposition, as in the case of transthyretin amyloidosis [36]. In other amyloid pathologies, such as Alzheimer's disease, proteolytic cleavage of the APP precursor protein, leading to the formation of Aβ40/42, is universally accepted as necessary for fibril formation [45, 46]. In AL amyloidosis, its role is less well defined, and it may occur after fibrils are formed and deposited in tissues. Despite uncertainties on timing of the proteolytic event during in vivo fibrillogenesis, the way the amyloidogenic protein is processed is associated to the clinical phenotype, at least in some forms of amyloidosis as ATTR, where the presence of truncated species in Val30Met patients is related to a later clinical onset and cardiac involvement [36].

A proteomic approach has also been used for the characterization of circulating precursors. Sulphonation and cysteinylation of the thiol group on the cysteine 10 residue of serum transthyretin are common physiological modifications, which are able to modulate TTR stability under denaturing and non-denaturing conditions and may be involved in the pathogenesis of senile systemic amyloidosis, where fibrils are formed by wild-type TTR, and in certain variants, such as Phe33Cys, where an additional cysteine residue is available for conjugation [37, 47, 48].

Accumulating evidence, started from the chemical analysis of amyloid deposits in Alzheimer's and other neurodegenerative diseases, is also pointing to the role of metals, mainly copper, zinc and aluminium, in favouring the process of protein aggregation and toxicity, since these elements have been found in large amounts in association with the deposited proteins [49–51].

Common Constituents: Role in Fibril Formation and Tissue Targeting

Besides being determined by intrinsic chemical properties, protein folding and behaviour in vivo can be deeply influenced by the interaction with other proteins or cells and tissue components.

In addition to the main amyloidogenic protein, amyloid contains a variety of common constituents, irrespectively of the tissue and disease type (Fig. 4-1). One of these ubiquitous molecules is serum amyloid P component (SAP), a glycoprotein with a specific binding site for the common conformation of amyloid, located on the B surface of the pentameric form (pentraxin) of the protein. The common conformational motif of amyloid, which is recognized with high affinity by SAP, has not been identified, but it is presumed to be present in all types of amyloid fibrils. In Alzheimer's disease, SAP binding to Aβ protein has been suggested to occur in a calcium-dependent manner [52]. Serum amyloid P protects fibrils from several proteases and from the activity of phagocytic cells [53, 54]. However, in the clinical setting, it has been demonstrated that amyloid deposits can be reabsorbed if the supply of the amyloidogenic protein is reduced or abolished, despite the presence of SAP.

Additionally, other molecules, such as apolipoprotein E, whose role in the disease pathogenesis is not completely defined, are common amyloid components [55, 56]. In b2-m and reactive amyloidosis (AA), association between fibrils and various forms of metalloproteinases (MMP-1, MMP-2 and MMP3) was observed by immunohistochemistry [57].

Histopathology has always highlighted the ubiquitous presence of glycosaminoglycans (GAGs), particularly heparan sulphate proteoglycans (HSPG), in all the natural amyloid deposits [58], and they are thought to have an important role in their genesis and stabilization. Heparan sulphate, in particular, has an active role in amyloid formation rather than passively accumulating in amyloid deposits [59a–59b]. One of the hypothesized roles of proteoglycans is to act as a structural scaffold which facilitates the adhesion and orientation of the first nuclei of aggregated amyloid protein, thus promoting the formation of oligomers. In vitro studies show that heparin and its analogues accelerate the kinetics of fibrillar aggregation of peptides in different types of amyloid diseases, such as Alzheimer's disease, prion diseases, serum amyloid A (SAA), b2-m and gelsolin amyloidoses [60–67b]. The intimate spatial association between sulphated proteoglycans and amyloid fibrils has also been demonstrated by direct visualization with electron microscopy [68]. Since different types of proteoglycans, which vary for chemical and structural composition, characterize different tissues, they are one of the factors that may play a role in directing the localization of amyloid deposits in target organs. The critical function of the glycosaminoglycan heparan sulphate in the genesis of amyloid deposits has been demonstrated in cell culture models [69] and in a transgenic experimental model in which the fragmentation of heparan sulphate by heparanase over-expression resulted in protection from reactive amyloidosis (AA amyloidosis) [70]. The observation that use of heparan sulphate analogues could arrest the progression of amyloid deposits in vivo [71] and the identification of specific binding sites for heparan sulphate on serum SAA [72] leads to the design of specific drugs to inhibit polymerization of amyloid fibrils and deposition of the fibrils in tissues [73]. One of these drugs, eprodisate, proved to be capable of delaying progression of renal damage in patients with AA amyloidosis [73].

Studies carried out in vitro have demonstrated that surfaces have an aggregation-inducing action and a direct role on the kinetics of aggregation [74–76]. In the connective tissue, where amyloid deposits preferentially form, fibrous proteins could mimic the ordered hydrophilic surfaces offered by synthetic polymers or by the polymeric structure of minerals like mica. A particularly important role in working as a scaffold for the growing amyloid fibrils, inferred by histological and imaging studies, has been postulated for collagen. A close spatial interaction of natural fibres of b2-m and collagen was observed by atomic force microscopy [77], while fibrils from amyloidogenic immunoglobulin light chains were shown to be growing on collagen, upon incubation of the precursor with nascent collagen fibrils [78]. The interaction between collagen and amyloidogenic proteins has been thoroughly investigated in the case of b2-m. In vitro studies showed that, in a physiologic-like environment, collagen is a potent promoter of b2-m fibrillogenesis [77], and that the interaction of b2-m with collagen I and III, which are highly represented in bones and ligaments that are natural target of the disease, is effective in generating amyloid fibrils under conditions comparable with the biological setting, providing additional clues to the mechanism of organ targeting.

Additional important surfaces for the promotion of protein fibrillation are lipid membranes, which can interact with amyloidogenic proteins, including recombinant light chains, accelerating fibril growth in a manner dependent on membrane composition [79]. Cellular membranes are considered one of the possible preferential sites for initiating amyloid aggregation.

The observation that amyloid deposition occurs in the extracellular space prompted further studies on the pathogenetic role of this compartment, leading to the development of novel mechanistic hypotheses to integrate the process of assembly forming in its biological environment, such as the theory of the effect of macromolecular crowding in increasing the propensity for fibrillogenesis [24]. The direct consequence of macromolecular crowding, a situation in which biopolymers occupy a high percentage of the available space, is that little space is left for additional macromolecules, which reduce their configurational entropy and therefore increase their free energy, favouring aggregation. In the interstitial space where amyloid accumulates, macromolecular crowding is determined mainly by the ubiquitous presence of fibrous proteins, glycosaminoglycans and proteoglycans, which, in addition to directly interacting with precursor proteins and oligomers as previously described, may favour amyloidogenesis through a pure 'excluded volume' mechanism.

All the above-described biological factors that contribute to the onset and perpetuation of protein aggregation and deposition, and which differ between individuals, may play a role in the biological variability of amyloid diseases, explaining why the timescale and pattern of amyloid deposition are so variable in vivo.

Misfolded Proteins Cause Cytotoxicity and Tissue Dysfunction

Protein misfolding and amyloid deposition are associated with cellular damage and tissue injury, which, in systemic amyloidoses, ultimately lead to failure of vital organs and to the patient death [1] (Fig. 4-1). A universally accepted theory to explain the mechanisms of damage does not exist, but various pathogenetic hypotheses are supported by numerous experimental and clinical observations. As different proteins can generate similar fibrils, via an early oligomerization phase, it is expected that also common mechanisms of toxicity occur in the various forms of amyloidoses, possibly with some stereotyped reactions in diverse tissues.

The deposition of large amounts of fibrillar material can subvert the tissue architecture and consequently cause organ dysfunction [1, 80]. However, the simple explanation of a physical, mechanical substitution of parenchymal tissue by amyloid deposits seems to be insufficient. Other observations indicate that amyloid fibrils can interact with local receptors, such as RAGE [81, 82], or, as observed in the cerebral cortex of patients with Alzheimer's disease, elicit an inflammatory response, which is related to the progressive accumulation of Aβ [83].

A growing body of experimental evidence points to the prefibrillar, soluble oligomers, which constitute the initial stage of aggregation and are transiently present during the process of amyloid formation, as the most important causative agents of toxicity [84–92b]. According to this hypothesis, mature amyloid fibrillary deposits are inactive proteinaceous reservoirs that are in equilibrium with smaller toxic assemblies.

This aspect has been studied in detail in the case of transthyretin in ATTR amyloidosis [91] and in case of the Aβ protein [92a, 93], in which soluble precursors have been shown to be the specific mediators of damage, through generation of oxidative stress, activation of the apoptotic pathway and interference with synaptic function and neurotransmission. In ATTR, the presence of non-fibrillar TTR aggregates was demonstrated in sciatic nerves of asymptomatic individuals, which also presented increased caspase-3 activation [94]. Soluble oligomers, or even the amyloidogenic light chains, have also been shown to exert cytotoxicity and contribute to organ dysfunction in AL amyloidosis. This observation derives from direct clinical evidence: it was observed, in fact, that the reduction of the amyloidogenic free light chain concentration caused by chemotherapy translates into a simultaneous reduction of the serum concentration of the amino terminal fragment of pro-brain natriuretic peptide (NT-proBNP), a marker of cardiac dysfunction, and a concomitant echocardiographic improvement in heart function, associated with clinical amelioration, despite unaltered amyloid deposits in the myocardium as assessed by echocardiography [90, 95].

Possibly, tissue damage requires the presence of both components: amyloid fibrils and prefibrillar aggregates. There is no sign of disease in the absence of deposits, whereas the elimination of the soluble fibrillar precursor may allow the clearance of signs and symptoms of disease, despite the persistence of unmodified amyloid deposits. A proposed unifying hypothesis is the existence of a synergic effect between amyloid fibrils and their precursor. An equilibrium between associating and dissociating molecules has in fact been observed at the growing surface of the fibril [96], creating a high concentration gradient of precursor monomers and oligomers, which can exert their influence on cells situated in proximity of amyloid deposits.

The precise way of interaction between amyloidogenic precursors and cells is another issue still open for debate. Internalization of amyloidogenic light chains by a fluid-phase endocytosis has been documented in live cardiac fibroblasts, in which the protein is subsequently directed to lysosomes and then re-secreted into the extracellular medium [97]. A pore-like activity of annular oligomers, with insertion into the outer cellular membrane and consequent alteration of the ion and metabolite permeability, is an additional mechanism proposed to explain cellular toxicity [98–100]. Once interacting with the cell, different mechanisms of damage may intervene. It has been demonstrated that, in isolated cardiomyocytes, amyloidogenic light chains specifically alter the cellular redox state, causing an increase in intracellular reactive oxygen species and upregulation of the redox-sensitive protein, heme oxygenase-1, with consequent direct impairment of cardiomyocyte contractility and relaxation, associated with alterations in intracellular calcium handling [101a]. Recently, the activation of p38alpha MAPK pathway has been shown to be involved in the contractile dysfunction and apoptosis caused by amyloidogenic light chains [101b]. Other mechanisms, such as activation of nuclear factor kappaB, pro-inflammatory cytokines and pro-apoptotic caspase-3 [82, 94, 102], have been demonstrated in vivo in clinical samples and in cell culture systems. In ATTR amyloidosis, activation of the unfolded protein response pathways has been detected in tissues not specialized in TTR synthesis but presenting extracellular TTR aggregate and fibril deposition [103], and subsequent studied on tissues, cultured cells and animal models confirmed the role of TTR, as well as of other amyloidogenic proteins deposition as an external stimulus to an intracellular unfolded protein response [104, 105].

Finally, important clues on the molecular mechanisms behind amyloid toxicity come from the global analysis of changes in the proteome of tissue and cells. Modifications in the expression of proteins involved in cell survival and energetics have been described both in cerebral and in systemic forms [30, 106]. In subcutaneous fat tissue of patients with AL and ATTR amyloidoses, proteins such as αB-crystallin, a small intracellular chaperone with antiapoptotic activity, aldo-keto reductase I and peroxiredoxin 6, a thiol peroxidase regulated at the transcriptional level by oxidative stress, were found to be underexpressed, in comparison to controls. AlphaB-crystallin, in particular, is able to inhibit the in vivo amyloid fibril formation, specifically the formation of fibrils from the Aβ protein, b2-m and α-synuclein [107–109b]. Considering that adipocytes are not involved in the synthesis of the amyloidogenic precursors, the significance of this finding in the setting of systemic amyloidoses is still unclear, but it does suggest that the extracellular amyloid deposits can influence, or can be influenced by, the expression of intracellular proteins involved in protein folding and cell survival.

Conclusions

The impressive advancement in the understanding of the molecular mechanisms of systemic amyloidoses, witnessed in the last decade, has translated in better care of these severe diseases. The unveiling of the cytotoxicity of amyloid proteins in various aggregated forms, in the prefibrillar state, has led to the development of new paradigms in the treatment of systemic amyloidosis. For instance, in AL amyloidosis a strong relationship between the concentration of the circulating amyloid precursor, the monoclonal light chains, and the sensitive serum biomarkers of heart dysfunction [95, 110] has been observed [90] and formed the basis for a more stringent and effective monitoring of the efficacy of chemotherapy [111].

Several new drugs and novel therapeutic approaches have been developed thanks to the elucidation of the molecular mechanisms of amyloidoses. Molecules capable of interfering with the promoting/protective role played by common constituents of amyloid deposits, such as glycosaminoglycans and SAP, have been designed. Drugs capable of inhibiting the interaction between glycosaminoglycans and amyloid proteins have been mentioned above. Small, palindromic molecules capable of clearing SAP from the circulation and thus displacing SAP from amyloid deposits have been developed and are being tested in patients [112]. In ATTR amyloidosis, drugs binding to the central channel of transthyretin tetramer, such as diflunisal and Fx-1006A®, have proved effective in preventing the tetramer dissociation into monomers, which is considered the prerequisite first step in the amyloidogenic cascade [113, 114]. These drugs are currently tested in clinical trials.

There are grounds for optimism that present progress in understanding the molecular mechanisms of amyloid diseases will lead, in the not too distant future, to effective therapies.

References

1. Merlini G, Bellotti V. Molecular mechanisms of amyloidosis. N Engl J Med. 2003;349:583–96.
2. Westermark P, Benson MD, Buxbaum JN, et al. A primer of amyloid nomenclature. Amyloid 2007;14:179–83.
3. Dobson CM. Protein folding and misfolding. Nature 2003;426:884–90.
4. Relini A, Rolandi R, Bolognesi M, et al. Ultrastructural organization of ex vivo amyloid fibrils formed by the apolipoprotein A-I Leu174Ser variant: an atomic force microscopy study. Biochim Biophys Acta 2004;1690:33–41.
5. Serpell LC, Sunde M, Benson MD, Tennent GA, Pepys MB, Fraser PE. The protofilament substructure of amyloid fibrils. J Mol Biol. 2000;300:1033–9.
6. Chiti F, Webster P, Taddei N, et al. Designing conditions for in vitro formation of amyloid protofilaments and fibrils. Proc Natl Acad Sci USA. 1999;96:3590–4.
7. Ventura S, Zurdo J, Narayanan S, et al. Short amino acid stretches can mediate amyloid formation in globular proteins: the Src homology 3 (SH3) case. Proc Natl Acad Sci USA. 2004;101:7258–63.
8. Trovato A, Chiti F, Maritan A, Seno F. Insight into the structure of amyloid fibrils from the analysis of globular proteins. PLoS Comput Biol. 2006;2:e170.
9. Monsellier E, Chiti F. Prevention of amyloid-like aggregation as a driving force of protein evolution. EMBO Rep. 2007;8:737–42.
10. Chiti F, Dobson CM. Amyloid formation by globular proteins under native conditions. Nat Chem Biol. 2009;5:15–22.
11. Merlini G, Bellotti V. Lysozyme: a paradigmatic molecule for the investigation of protein structure, function and misfolding. Clin Chim Acta 2005;357:168–72.
12. Wetzel R. Domain stability in immunoglobulin light chain deposition disorders. Adv Protein Chem. 1997;50:183–242.
13. Davis DP, Gallo G, Vogen SM, et al. Both the environment and somatic mutations govern the aggregation pathway of pathogenic immunoglobulin light chain. J Mol Biol. 2001;313:1021–34.
14. Bellotti V, Mangione P, Merlini G. Review: immunoglobulin light chain amyloidosis–the archetype of structural and pathogenic variability. J Struct Biol. 2000;130:280–9.
15. Perfetti V, Casarini S, Palladini G, et al. Analysis of V(lambda)-J(lambda) expression in plasma cells from primary (AL) amyloidosis and normal bone marrow identifies 3r (lambdaIII) as a new amyloid-associated germline gene segment. Blood 2002;100:948–53.
16. Comenzo RL, Zhang Y, Martinez C, Osman K, Herrera GA. The tropism of organ involvement in primary systemic amyloidosis: contributions of Ig V(L) germ line gene use and clonal plasma cell burden. Blood 2001;98:714–20.
17. Abraham RS, Geyer SM, Price-Troska TL, et al. Immunoglobulin light chain variable (V) region genes influence clinical presentation and outcome in light chain-associated amyloidosis (AL). Blood 2003;101:3801–8.
18. Abraham RS, Geyer SM, Ramirez-Alvarado M, Price-Troska TL, Gertz MA, Fonseca R. Analysis of somatic hypermutation and antigenic selection in the clonal B cell in immunoglobulin light chain amyloidosis (AL). J Clin Immunol. 2004;24:340–53.
19. Solomon A, Frangione B, Franklin EC. Bence Jones proteins and light chains of immunoglobulins. Preferential association of the V lambda VI subgroup of human light chains with amyloidosis AL (lambda). J Clin Invest. 1982;70:453–60.
20. Perfetti V, Ubbiali P, Vignarelli MC, et al. Evidence that amyloidogenic light chains undergo antigen-driven selection. Blood 1998;91:2948–54.

21. Benson MD, Kincaid JC. The molecular biology and clinical features of amyloid neuropathy. Muscle Nerve 2007;36:411–23.

22. Ando Y, Ueda M. Novel methods for detecting amyloidogenic proteins in transthyretin related amyloidosis. Front Biosci. 2008;13:5548–58.

23. Connors LH, Lim A, Prokaeva T, Roskens VA, Costello CE. Tabulation of human transthyretin (TTR) variants, 2003. Amyloid 2003;10:160–84.

24. Bellotti V, Chiti F. Amyloidogenesis in its biological environment: challenging a fundamental issue in protein misfolding diseases. Curr Opin Struct Biol. 2008;18:771–9.

25. Sitia R, Braakman I. Quality control in the endoplasmic reticulum protein factory. Nature 2003;426:891–4.

26. Sato T, Susuki S, Suico MA, et al. Endoplasmic reticulum quality control regulates the fate of transthyretin variants in the cell. EMBO J. 2007;26:2501–12.

27. Sorgjerd K, Ghafouri B, Jonsson BH, Kelly JW, Blond SY, Hammarstrom P. Retention of misfolded mutant transthyretin by the chaperone BiP/GRP78 mitigates amyloidogenesis. J Mol Biol. 2006;356:469–82.

28. Sekijima Y, Wiseman RL, Matteson J, et al. The biological and chemical basis for tissue-selective amyloid disease. Cell 2005;121:73–85.

29. Bergstrom J, Gustavsson A, Hellman U, et al. Amyloid deposits in transthyretin-derived amyloidosis: cleaved transthyretin is associated with distinct amyloid morphology. J Pathol. 2005;206:224–32.

30. Lavatelli F, Perlman DH, Spencer B, et al. Amyloidogenic and associated proteins in systemic amyloidosis proteome of adipose tissue. Mol Cell Proteomics 2008;7:1570–83.

31. Olsen KE, Sletten K, Westermark P. Extended analysis of AL-amyloid protein from abdominal wall subcutaneous fat biopsy: kappa IV immunoglobulin light chain. Biochem Biophys Res Commun. 1998;245:713–6.

32. Picken MM, Gallo GR, Pruzanski W, Frangione B. Biochemical characterization of amyloid derived from the variable region of the kappa light chain subgroup III. Arthritis Rheum. 1990;33:880–4.

33. Westermark P, Westermark GT. Purification of transthyretin and transthyretin fragments from amyloid-rich human tissues. Methods Mol Biol. 2005;299:255–60.

34. Gustavsson A, Jahr H, Tobiassen R, Jacobson DR, Sletten K, Westermark P. Amyloid fibril composition and transthyretin gene structure in senile systemic amyloidosis. Lab Invest. 1995;73:703–8.

35. Ihse E, Stangou AJ, Heaton ND, et al. Proportion between wild-type and mutant protein in truncated compared to full-length ATTR: an analysis on transplanted transthyretin T60A amyloidosis patients. Biochem Biophys Res Commun. 2009;379:846–50.

36. Ihse E, Ybo A, Suhr O, Lindqvist P, Backman C, Westermark P. Amyloid fibril composition is related to the phenotype of hereditary transthyretin V30M amyloidosis. J Pathol. 2008;216:253–61.

37. Kingsbury JS, Theberge R, Karbassi JA, Lim A, Costello CE, Connors LH. Detailed structural analysis of amyloidogenic wild-type transthyretin using a novel purification strategy and mass spectrometry. Anal Chem. 2007;79:1990–8.

38. Westermark P, Bergstrom J, Solomon A, Murphy C, Sletten K. Transthyretin-derived senile systemic amyloidosis: clinicopathologic and structural considerations. Amyloid 2003;10 Suppl 1:48–54.

39. Lim A, Prokaeva T, Connor LH, Falk RH, Skinner M, Costello CE. Identification of a novel transthyretin Thr59Lys/Arg104His. A case of compound heterozygosity in a Chinese patient diagnosed with familial transthyretin amyloidosis. Amyloid 2002;9:134–40.

40. Stoppini M, Mangione P, Monti M, et al. Proteomics of beta2-microglobulin amyloid fibrils. Biochim Biophys Acta 2005;1753:23–33.

41. Giorgetti S, Stoppini M, Tennent GA, et al. Lysine 58-cleaved beta2-microglobulin is not detectable by 2D electrophoresis in ex vivo amyloid fibrils of two patients affected by dialysis-related amyloidosis. Protein Sci. 2007;16:343–9.

42. Obici L, Franceschini G, Calabresi L, et al. Structure, function and amyloidogenic propensity of apolipoprotein A-I. Amyloid 2006;13:191–205.

43. Connors LH, Jiang Y, Budnik M, et al. Heterogeneity in primary structure, post-translational modifications, and germline gene usage of nine full-length amyloidogenic kappa1 immunoglobulin light chains. Biochemistry 2007;46:14259–71.

44. Merlini G, Mastanduno M, Moy PW, Hauschka PV, Osserman EF. Molecular hetero-geneity and gamma-carboxyglutamic acid content of Bence-Jones proteins: possible relevance to amyloidogenicity. In: Glenner GG, Osserman EF, Benditt EP, Calkins E, Cohen AS, Zucker-Franklin D, editors. Amyloidosis. New York: Plenum; 1986, pp. 25–34.

45. Haass C, De Strooper B. The presenilins in Alzheimer's disease–proteolysis holds the key. Science 1999;286:916–9.

46. Miller DL, Papayannopoulos IA, Styles J, et al. Peptide compositions of the cerebrovas-cular and senile plaque core amyloid deposits of Alzheimer's disease. Arch Biochem Biophys. 1993;301:41–52.

47. Lim A, Prokaeva T, McComb ME, Connors LH, Skinner M, Costello CE. Identi-fication of S-sulfonation and S-thiolation of a novel transthyretin Phe33Cys variant from a patient diagnosed with familial transthyretin amyloidosis. Protein Sci. 2003;12: 1775–85.

48. Kingsbury JS, Klimtchuk ES, Theberge R, Costello CE, Connors LH. Expression, purification, and in vitro cysteine-10 modification of native sequence recombinant human transthyretin. Protein Expr Purif. 2007;53:370–7.

49. Morante S. The role of metals in beta-amyloid peptide aggregation: X-Ray spec-troscopy and numerical simulations. Curr Alzheimer Res. 2008;5:508–24.

50. Drago D, Bolognin S, Zatta P. Role of metal ions in the abeta oligomerization in Alzheimer's disease and in other neurological disorders. Curr Alzheimer Res. 2008;5:500–7.

51. Zatta P, Drago D, Zambenedetti P, et al. Accumulation of copper and other metal ions, and metallothionein I/II expression in the bovine brain as a function of aging. J Chem Neuroanat. 2008;36:1–5.

52. Hamazaki H. Ca(2+)-dependent binding of human serum amyloid P component to Alzheimer's beta-amyloid peptide. J Biol Chem. 1995;270:10392–4.

53. Tennent GA, Lovat LB, Pepys MB. Serum amyloid P component prevents proteolysis of the amyloid fibrils of Alzheimer disease and systemic amyloidosis. Proc Natl Acad Sci USA. 1995;92:4299–303.

54. Pepys MB. Pathogenesis, diagnosis and treatment of systemic amyloidosis. Philos Trans R Soc Lond B Biol Sci. 2001;356:203–10; discussion 10–1.

55. Gallo G, Wisniewski T, Choi-Miura NH, Ghiso J, Frangione B. Potential role of apolipoprotein-E in fibrillogenesis. Am J Pathol. 1994;145:526–30.

56. Kisilevsky R. The relation of proteoglycans, serum amyloid P and apo E to amyloidosis current status, 2000. Amyloid 2000;7:23–5.

57. Ohashi K, Kawai R, Hara M, Okada Y, Tachibana S, Ogura Y. Increased matrix metalloproteinases as possible cause of osseoarticular tissue destruction in long-term haemodialysis and beta 2-microglobulin amyloidosis. Virchows Arch. 1996;428:37–46.

58. Ancsin JB. Amyloidogenesis: historical and modern observations point to heparan sul-fate proteoglycans as a major culprit. Amyloid 2003;10:67–79.

59a. Kisilevsky R. Review: amyloidogenesis-unquestioned answers and unanswered ques-tions. J Struct Biol. 2000;130:99–108.

59b. Elimova E, Kisilevsky R, Ancsin JB. Heparan sulfate promotes the aggregation of HDL-associated serum amyloid A: evidence for a proamyloidogenic histidine molecu-lar switch. FASEB J. 2009;23:3436–48.

60. McCubbin WD, Kay CM, Narindrasorasak S, Kisilevsky R. Circular-dichroism studies on two murine serum amyloid A proteins. Biochem J. 1988;256:775–83.

61. Fraser PE, Nguyen JT, Chin DT, Kirschner DA. Effects of sulfate ions on Alzheimer beta/A4 peptide assemblies: implications for amyloid fibril-proteoglycan interactions. J Neurochem. 1992;59:1531–40.

62. McLaurin J, Franklin T, Zhang X, Deng J, Fraser PE. Interactions of Alzheimer amyloid-beta peptides with glycosaminoglycans effects on fibril nucleation and growth. Eur J Biochem. 1999;266:1101–10.

63. Castillo GM, Cummings JA, Yang W, et al. Sulfate content and specific glycosaminoglycan backbone of perlecan are critical for perlecan's enhancement of islet amyloid polypeptide (amylin) fibril formation. Diabetes 1998;47:612–20.

64. Yamamoto S, Yamaguchi I, Hasegawa K, et al. Glycosaminoglycans enhance the trifluoroethanol-induced extension of beta 2-microglobulin-related amyloid fibrils at a neutral pH. J Am Soc Nephrol. 2004;15:126–33.

65. Suk JY, Zhang F, Balch WE, Linhardt RJ, Kelly JW. Heparin accelerates gelsolin amyloidogenesis. Biochemistry 2006;45:2234–42.

66. McLaughlin RW, De Stigter JK, Sikkink LA, Baden EM, Ramirez-Alvarado M. The effects of sodium sulfate, glycosaminoglycans, and Congo red on the structure, stability, and amyloid formation of an immunoglobulin light-chain protein. Protein Sci. 2006;15:1710–22.

67a. Calamai M, Kumita JR, Mifsud J, et al. Nature and significance of the interactions between amyloid fibrils and biological polyelectrolytes. Biochemistry 2006;45: 12806–15.

67b. Motamedi-Shad N, Monsellier E, Torrassa S, Relini A, Chiti F. Kinetic analysis of amyloid formation in the presence of heparan sulfate: faster unfolding and change of pathway. J Biol Chem. 2009;284:29921–34.

68. Inoue S, Kuroiwa M, Saraiva MJ, Guimaraes A, Kisilevsky R. Ultrastructure of familial amyloid polyneuropathy amyloid fibrils: examination with high-resolution electron microscopy. J Struct Biol. 1998;124:1–12.

69. Elimova E, Kisilevsky R, Szarek WA, Ancsin JB. Amyloidogenesis recapitulated in cell culture: a peptide inhibitor provides direct evidence for the role of heparan sulfate and suggests a new treatment strategy. FASEB J. 2004;18:1749–51.

70. Li JP, Galvis ML, Gong F, et al. In vivo fragmentation of heparan sulfate by heparanase overexpression renders mice resistant to amyloid protein A amyloidosis. Proc Natl Acad Sci USA. 2005;102:6473–7.

71. Kisilevsky R, Lemieux LJ, Fraser PE, Kong X, Hultin PG, Szarek WA. Arresting amyloidosis in vivo using small-molecule anionic sulphonates or sulphates: implications for Alzheimer's disease. Nat Med. 1995;1:143–8.

72. Ancsin JB, Kisilevsky R. The heparin/heparan sulfate-binding site on apo-serum amyloid A. Implications for the therapeutic intervention of amyloidosis. J Biol Chem. 1999;274:7172–81.

73. Dember LM, Hawkins PN, Hazenberg BP, et al. Eprodisate for the treatment of renal disease in AA amyloidosis. N Engl J Med. 2007;356:2349–60.

74. Goldsbury C, Kistler J, Aebi U, Arvinte T, Cooper GJ. Watching amyloid fibrils grow by time-lapse atomic force microscopy. J Mol Biol. 1999;285:33–9.

75. Zhu M, Souillac PO, Ionescu-Zanetti C, Carter SA, Fink AL. Surface-catalyzed amyloid fibril formation. J Biol Chem. 2002;277:50914–22.

76. Linse S, Cabaleiro-Lago C, Xue WF, et al. Nucleation of protein fibrillation by nanoparticles. Proc Natl Acad Sci USA. 2007;104:8691–6.

77. Relini A, Canale C, De Stefano S, et al. Collagen plays an active role in the aggregation of beta2-microglobulin under physiopathological conditions of dialysis-related amyloidosis. J Biol Chem. 2006;281:16521–9.

78. Harris DL, King E, Ramsland PA, Edmundson AB. Binding of nascent collagen by amyloidogenic light chains and amyloid fibrillogenesis in monolayers of human fibrocytes. J Mol Recognit. 2000;13:198–212.

79. Meng X, Fink AL, Uversky VN. The effect of membranes on the in vitro fibrillation of an amyloidogenic light-chain variable-domain SMA. J Mol Biol. 2008;381:989–99.

80. Pepys MB. Amyloidosis. Annu Rev Med. 2006;57:223–41.

81. Yan SD, Zhu H, Zhu A, et al. Receptor-dependent cell stress and amyloid accumulation in systemic amyloidosis. Nat Med. 2000;6:643–51.

82. Sousa MM, Du Yan S, Fernandes R, Guimaraes A, Stern D, Saraiva MJ. Familial amyloid polyneuropathy: receptor for advanced glycation end products-dependent triggering of neuronal inflammatory and apoptotic pathways. J Neurosci. 2001;21:7576–86.

83. Rogers J, Webster S, Lue LF, et al. Inflammation and Alzheimer's disease pathogenesis. Neurobiol Aging 1996;17:681–6.

84. Cecchi C, Pensalfini A, Baglioni S, et al. Differing molecular mechanisms appear to underlie early toxicity of prefibrillar HypF-N aggregates to different cell types. Febs J. 2006;273:2206–22.

85. Haass C, Selkoe DJ. Soluble protein oligomers in neurodegeneration: lessons from the Alzheimer's amyloid beta-peptide. Nat Rev Mol Cell Biol. 2007;8:101–12.

86. Townsend M, Shankar GM, Mehta T, Walsh DM, Selkoe DJ. Effects of secreted oligomers of amyloid beta-protein on hippocampal synaptic plasticity: a potent role for trimers. J Physiol. 2006;572:477–92.

87. Klyubin I, Walsh DM, Lemere CA, et al. Amyloid beta protein immunotherapy neutralizes Abeta oligomers that disrupt synaptic plasticity in vivo. Nat Med. 2005;11:556–61.

88. Cleary JP, Walsh DM, Hofmeister JJ, et al. Natural oligomers of the amyloid-beta protein specifically disrupt cognitive function. Nat Neurosci. 2005;8:79–84.

89. Walsh DM, Selkoe DJ. Oligomers on the brain: the emerging role of soluble protein aggregates in neurodegeneration. Protein Pept Lett. 2004;11:213–28.

90. Palladini G, Lavatelli F, Russo P, et al. Circulating amyloidogenic free light chains and serum N-terminal natriuretic peptide type B decrease simultaneously in association with improvement of survival in AL. Blood 2006;107:3854–8.

91. Andersson K, Olofsson A, Nielsen EH, Svehag SE, Lundgren E. Only amyloidogenic intermediates of transthyretin induce apoptosis. Biochem Biophys Res Commun. 2002;294:309–14.

92a. Lambert MP, Barlow AK, Chromy BA, et al. Diffusible, nonfibrillar ligands derived from Abeta1-42 are potent central nervous system neurotoxins. Proc Natl Acad Sci USA. 1998;95:6448–53.

92b. Sakono M, Zako T. Amyloid oligomers: formation and toxicity of Abeta oligomers. FEBS J. 2010;277:1348–58.

93. Hartley DM, Walsh DM, Ye CP, et al. Protofibrillar intermediates of amyloid beta-protein induce acute electrophysiological changes and progressive neurotoxicity in cortical neurons. J Neurosci. 1999;19:8876–84.

94. Sousa MM, Cardoso I, Fernandes R, Guimaraes A, Saraiva MJ. Deposition of transthyretin in early stages of familial amyloidotic polyneuropathy: evidence for toxicity of nonfibrillar aggregates. Am J Pathol. 2001;159:1993–2000.

95. Palladini G, Campana C, Klersy C, et al. Serum N-terminal pro-brain natriuretic peptide is a sensitive marker of myocardial dysfunction in AL amyloidosis. Circulation 2003;107:2440–5.

96. Carulla N, Caddy GL, Hall DR, et al. Molecular recycling within amyloid fibrils. Nature 2005;436:554–8.

97. Monis GF, Schultz C, Ren R, et al. Role of endocytic inhibitory drugs on internalization of amyloidogenic light chains by cardiac fibroblasts. Am J Pathol. 2006;169:1939–52.

98. Caughey B, Lansbury PT. Protofibrils, pores, fibrils, and neurodegeneration: separating the responsible protein aggregates from the innocent bystanders. Annu Rev Neurosci. 2003;26:267–98.

99. Lashuel HA, Hartley D, Petre BM, Walz T, Lansbury PT, Jr. Neurodegenerative disease: amyloid pores from pathogenic mutations. Nature 2002;418:291.

100. Lashuel HA, Lansbury PT, Jr. Are amyloid diseases caused by protein aggregates that mimic bacterial pore-forming toxins? Q Rev Biophys. 2006;39:167–201.

101a. Brenner DA, Jain M, Pimentel DR, et al. Human amyloidogenic light chains directly impair cardiomyocyte function through an increase in cellular oxidant stress. Circ Res. 2004;94:1008–10.

101b. Shi J, Guan J, Jiang B, Brenner DA, Del Monte F, Ward JE, Connors LH, Sawyer DB, Semigran MJ, Macgillivray TE, Seldin DC, Falk R, Liao R. Amyloidogenic light chains induce cardiomyocyte contractile dysfunction and apoptosis via a non-canonical p38alpha MAPK pathway. Proc Natl Acad Sci USA. 2010;107:4188–93.

102. Sousa MM, do Amaral JB, Guimaraes A, Saraiva MJ. Up-regulation of the extracellular matrix remodeling genes, biglycan, neutrophil gelatinase-associated lipocalin, and matrix metalloproteinase-9 in familial amyloid polyneuropathy. FASEB J. 2005;19:124–6.

103. Teixeira PF, Cerca F, Santos SD, Saraiva MJ. Endoplasmic reticulum stress associated with extracellular aggregates. Evidence from transthyretin deposition in familial amyloid polyneuropathy. J Biol Chem. 2006;281:21998–2003.

104. Santos SD, Cardoso I, Magalhaes J, Saraiva MJ. Impairment of the ubiquitin-proteasome system associated with extracellular transthyretin aggregates in familial amyloidotic polyneuropathy. J Pathol. 2007;213:200–9.

105. Casas S, Gomis R, Gribble FM, Altirriba J, Knuutila S, Novials A. Impairment of the ubiquitin-proteasome pathway is a downstream endoplasmic reticulum stress response induced by extracellular human islet amyloid polypeptide and contributes to pancreatic beta-cell apoptosis. Diabetes 2007;56:2284–94.

106. Zabel C, Sagi D, Kaindl AM, et al. Comparative proteomics in neurodegenerative and non-neurodegenerative diseases suggest nodal point proteins in regulatory networking. J Proteome Res. 2006;5:1948–58.

107. Rekas A, Adda CG, Andrew Aquilina J, et al. Interaction of the molecular chaperone alphaB-crystallin with alpha-synuclein: effects on amyloid fibril formation and chaperone activity. J Mol Biol. 2004;340:1167–83.

108. Raman B, Ban T, Sakai M, et al. AlphaB-crystallin, a small heat-shock protein, prevents the amyloid fibril growth of an amyloid beta-peptide and beta2-microglobulin. Biochem J. 2005;392:573–81.

109a. Lee S, Carson K, Rice-Ficht A, Good T. Small heat shock proteins differentially affect Abeta aggregation and toxicity. Biochem Biophys Res Commun. 2006;347:527–33.

109b. Waudby CA, Knowles TP, Devlin GL, Skepper JN, Ecroyd H, Carver JA, Welland ME, Christodoulou J, Dobson CM, Meehan S. The interaction of alphaB-crystallin with mature alpha-synuclein amyloid fibrils inhibits their elongation. Biophys J. 2010;98:843–51.

110. Dispenzieri A, Kyle RA, Gertz MA, et al. Survival in patients with primary systemic amyloidosis and raised serum cardiac troponins. Lancet 2003;361:1787–9.

111. Wechalekar A, Merlini G, Gillmore JD, et al. Role of NT-ProBNP to assess the adequacy of treatment response in AL amyloidosis. Blood 2008;112:596–7.

112. Pepys MB, Herbert J, Hutchinson WL, et al. Targeted pharmacological depletion of serum amyloid P component for treatment of human amyloidosis. Nature 2002;417:254–9.

113. Tojo K, Sekijima Y, Kelly JW, Ikeda S. Diflunisal stabilizes familial amyloid polyneuropathy-associated transthyretin variant tetramers in serum against dissociation required for amyloidogenesis. Neurosci Res. 2006;56:441–9.

114. Sekijima Y, Kelly JW, Ikeda S. Pathogenesis of and therapeutic strategies to ameliorate the transthyretin amyloidoses. Curr Pharm Design. 2008;14:3219–30.

Chapter 5

Supportive Care for Amyloidosis

Martha Q. Lacy and Nelson Leung

Abstract Supportive measures for the care of amyloid patients are reviewed here. Cardiac issues include medical management of congestive heart failure and arrhythmias including the use of defibrillators and the use of pleural catheters for diuretic-refractory effusions. The indications for solid organ transplant are reviewed including heart transplant for AL and non-AL amyloid, liver transplant for ATTR and non-ATTR familial amyloid, and kidney transplant for AL, AA, and AFib. Medical management of renal issues including agents to reduce proteinuria and the use of eprodisate to slow progression of AA amyloid is discussed.

Keywords Amyloidosis, Heart transplant, Liver transplant, Kidney transplant, Implantable defibrillator

Introduction

The major focus of care for the patient with amyloidosis remains pursuing curative strategies. However, there are significant interventions that can impact the care of the patient with amyloidosis. This chapter focuses on this aspect of care. We will discuss both medical and surgical interventions that are currently in use for supportive care of patients with amyloidosis.

Cardiac Issues

Use of Cardiovascular Drugs

Considerable caution has to be exercised in the use of certain cardiac amyloid medications. Amyloid fibrils bind to both digitalis [1] and nifedipine [2]. Care must be taken because these drugs may be associated with excessive toxicity in amyloid patients, including increased susceptibility to digitalis toxicity and to hemodynamic deterioration after calcium channel blockers [3, 4]. Angiotensin-converting enzyme (ACE) inhibitors have been used to improve symptoms of congestive heart failure but may provoke profound hypotension in AL amyloidosis. Caution must also be taken when using beta blockers. These drugs are often useful in the management of tachyarrhythmias but one study has shown that the use of beta blockers in patients with cardiac amyloid is associated with a higher mortality rate [5].

From: *Amyloidosis*, Contemporary Hematology,
Edited by: M.A. Gertz and S.V. Rajkumar, DOI 10.1007/978-1-60761-631-3_5,
© Springer Science+Business Media, LLC 2010

Management of Pleural Effusions

Management of patients with systemic amyloidosis (AL) who present with diuretic-refractory pleural effusions is challenging and is associated with a poor prognosis. Aggressive diuresis is often complicated by hypotension and intravascular volume depletion. Other options include repeated large-volume thoracentesis, chest tube placement, pleurodesis by tube thoracostomy, and video-assisted thoracoscopy with talc insufflation. Serial thoracenteses are often unsatisfactory to patients due to recurrence and the need to perform the procedure repeatedly which increase the risk of complications. Pleural catheters (PleurX), small-bore chest tubes designed to remain in place for prolonged periods, have been reported to be useful in the management of recurrent pleural effusions [6] but are associated with risk of infection including empyema.

Recent reports have suggested a role for bevacizumab in the management of pleural effusions in AL amyloid [7, 8]. Vascular endothelial growth factor (VEGF) has been implicated to play a role in both malignant and non-malignant pleural effusions through its ability to regulate vascular permeability. Moreover, VEGF levels are high in patients with plasma cell disorders including AL amyloidosis [9–11]. Bevacizumab is an antibody directed against vascular endothelial growth factor. However, caution must be used because the safety of utilizing bevacizumab in patients with preexisting nephrotic syndrome and renal failure has not been determined.

Implantable Cardioverter Defibrillator

Cardiac involvement occurs in approximately 60% of patients with AL amyloidosis and is associated with a poor prognosis [12]. Approximately two-thirds of patients with cardiac amyloidosis die of "sudden" types of death, presumably due to heart arrhythmias [13]. Prophylactic implantable cardioverter defibrillators (ICDs) have been suggested as an option to reduce this risk. In one study, 19 cardiac AL amyloidosis patients with history of syncope or high-grade ventricular arrhythmias received an ICD. Two patients with sustained ventricular tachyarrhythmias were successfully treated with the ICD. Two subsequently underwent cardiac transplant and one died of an unrelated disease. There were six cardiac deaths, all sudden despite the ICD and all due to electromechanical dissociation. Thus, the limited available clinical data do not support widespread use of ICDs.

Heart Transplant for Amyloidosis

Heart transplant for amyloid was first described in 1988 [14]. In recent years it has been increasingly accepted as a treatment modality for patients with amyloid cardiomyopathy. Initially amyloid heart disease was considered a contraindication for cardiac transplant based on the hypothesis that amyloid deposition would recur in the cardiac allograft. Early reports generated from a survey of heart transplant centers in the United States, Canada, and Europe showed results inferior to what is seen in heart transplant for primary cardiomyopathy [15, 16]. Survival at 4 years was 39% and systemic progression was seen in the majority of patients. However, it is difficult to draw conclusions based on their experience because patients were seen at a number of different centers and were not screened to exclude those with extensive systemic involvement or treated with chemotherapy following the heart transplant. In addition many of the early reports did not distinguish outcomes in patients with AL versus non-AL amyloidosis. Heart transplantation for amyloid cardiomyopathy continues to generate controversy because of the donor shortage and concerns about recurrence either in the transplanted heart or other vital organs.

Heart Transplant for AL Amyloidosis

Dubrey and colleagues [17] reported 5-year survival rates following heart transplant of 38% among amyloidosis patients and 67% among patients without amyloidosis. In that series 8 of 10 patients had AL amyloid and only 1 of the 8 had chemotherapy following heart transplant. That patient had significant regression of amyloid deposits in extracardiac organs documented by radiolabeled SAP scanning. A follow-up study from the same group [18] described results in 24 patients with amyloid heart disease who had heart transplants. The group of AL patients who received chemotherapy after heart transplant had improved survival compared to the group who received no chemotherapy, but survival was still inferior to what has been reported with heart transplant for primary cardiomyopathy. UNOS data [19] including 69 heart transplants performed in 24 different centers in the United States also suggest inferior outcomes for heart transplant in patients with amyloidosis compared to those undergoing heart transplants for other reasons. One-and five-year actuarial survival rates are 75 and 54% among amyloidosis patients and 82 and 64% among others, respectively. However, in that series, no distinction was made between patients having transplant for AL versus non-AL amyloidosis. In addition there was no information regarding whether systemic chemotherapy or SCT was given to patients with AL amyloidosis.

In recent years there have been a number of reports of sequential heart transplant followed by SCT for patients with AL amyloid cardiomyopathy [20–23] The largest series was from Mayo Clinic and reported 11 patients who underwent sequential orthotopic heart transplant followed by autologous peripheral blood stem cell transplant [24]. The 1- and 5-year survival from heart transplant was 82 and 65%, respectively. The median survival was 76 months from heart transplant and 57 months from SCT (Fig. 5-1). Similar results have been reported in patients who underwent heart transplant and were treated with oral melphalan and dexamethasone [25, 26]. These data suggest that careful screening to include only those patients without significant other organ involvement followed by effective treatment of the underlying monoclonal plasma cell dyscrasia may improve outcomes of heart transplant in AL patients.

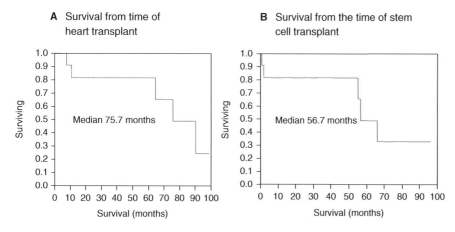

Fig. 5-1. (**a**) Survival after orthotopic heart transplantation. (**b**) Survival from the time of high-dose therapy and stem cell transplantation according to the Kaplan–Meier method. Reprinted from Lacy et al. [46].

Heart Transplant for ATTR Amyloidosis

Using the same rationale, some centers have advocated combined heart/liver transplant (CHLT) for ATTR amyloid cardiomyopathy. More than 99% of transthyretin is synthesized in the liver and secreted into circulation. Orthotopic liver transplantation removes the source for the pathologic protein. Multiple reports [21, 27] suggest that CHLT is a feasible treatment option for ATTR amyloid. Between 1987 and 2006, 47 cases of combined heart–liver and heart–liver–kidney were reported to the United Network for Sharing (UNOS). The most common reason for CHLT was amyloidosis (30%). Patient, heart, and liver graft survival rates were 75.6, 75.6, and 73.5% at 5 years respectively, rates comparable to outcomes in patients with single organ transplants.

Others have suggested that isolated heart transplant is more appropriate. Patients with ATTR amyloid mutations typically do not get symptomatic cardiac involvement until their 5th or 6th decade, suggesting that the patient is unlikely to immediately develop amyloid in the transplanted heart. CHLT presents more logistical obstacles as well as potential morbidity. A caution to those advocating this approach is the finding that the heart involvement in ATTR amyloidosis can progress even after liver transplant [28, 29]. The hypothesis is that once there is a nidus of amyloid, wild type TTR can deposit onto it and extend the amyloid matrix [29].

Liver Transplantation for ATTR Amyloid

Orthotopic liver transplant (OLT) was first performed as treatment for ATTR amyloid in 1990 by investigators at the Karolinska Institute in Stockholm, Sweden [30]. In 1995 the Familial Amyloidotic Polyneuropathy World Transplant Registry (FAP-WTR) was started. In the 10 years since the creation of the registry, 539 patients underwent 579 OLTs [31]. Four hundred and fifty (83%) of the patients carried the Val30Met mutation. Other mutations represented 12% of the patients and 5% had missing or unknown mutations. The overall 5-year survival was 77% and was significantly better on the patients with the Val30Met mutation compared to the non-Val30Met mutations (79 versus 56%, $p < 0.001$).

It takes an average of 5–6 decades for patients with an amyloidogenic TTR mutation to develop clinically significant amyloidosis and the liver in such patients is usually not compromised. In many carriers, the genetic disorder never manifests during lifetime and only a proportion of patients with FAP develop disease symptoms. Based on this, centers have been willing to do the so-called domino or sequential liver transplantation procedure. This procedure means that the removed FAP liver is reused for transplantation in another patient in need of a liver. Reports from Domino Liver Transplantation Registry (DLTR) indicate that patient survival is excellent and comparable to the survival with OLT performed for other chronic liver disorders [32, 33]. Domino liver transplantation is a tool that makes it possible to increase the number of liver grafts available for transplantation for patients with ATTR.

Organ Transplantation for Hereditary Non-ATTR Amyloidosis

Hereditary non-ATTR systemic amyloidosis is a rare autosomal dominant condition in which progressive amyloid deposition in the viscera, especially the kidneys, frequently leads to organ failure. Mutations in the genes encoding apolipoprotein

AI (apoAI), apolipoprotein AII (apoAII), fibrinogen Aα-chain, and lysozyme have been identified as the cause of the disease in different kindreds. Apolipoprotein AI is secreted by liver and intestine, catabolized in the liver and kidneys and is the main protein in high-density lipoprotein. At least 16 different mutations in apoAI have been reported as causes of hereditary amyloidosis [34]. Six variants (Gly26Arg, Trp50Arg, Leu60Arg, Del70-72, Leu75Pro, and Leu64Pro) have been reported to cause an amyloid phenotype characterized by renal manifestations in association with extensive visceral amyloid deposits and hepatosplenomegaly. Gillmore initially reported combined hepatorenal transplant in a patient with ApoAI amyloidosis in 2001 [35]. Since then there have been 10 other patients reported [36, 37] who underwent either renal transplant or dual organ transplant (liver/kidney, heart/kidney) with good results reported in eight. Two patients died from complications of the transplant. It is estimated that approximately 50% of plasma ApoAI is secreted from liver. Regression after liver transplant suggests that amyloid deposition is a dynamic equilibrium. Reducing the supply of the amyloidogenic variant alters the balance between accumulation and regression of amyloid in favor of regression.

Renal Involvement with Amyloid

Renal involvement is common in AL and AA. In a study of 474 patients with AL, 73% of the patients presented with proteinuria with half in the nephrotic range [12]. Fifty percent of the patients also presented with abnormal serum creatinine. In patients with AA, 97% were found to have renal involvement as defined by >500 mg/day of proteinuria or serum creatinine of >1.5 mg/dL [38]. In this study, 23% of those with glomerular filtration rate >20 mL/min at baseline progressed to end-stage renal disease (ESRD). This is compared to a rate of 47% from a 15-year study of 78 Italian patients with AA [39].The rate of ESRD for patients with AL ranges between 26 and 39% [39, 40]. Median survival of these patients after initiation of dialysis is 11 months with 20% of the mortality occurring within the first month. The median survival of AA patients after starting dialysis was 17 months but was not statistically different from the patients with AL [39].

Medical Strategies to Reduce Proteinuria

Proteinuria may cause worsening of accompanying renal disease. Reduction of proteinuria that is toxic to glomeruli and the tubules is one of the main objectives of the therapy. Many drugs have been tried for this purpose. Angiotensin-converting enzyme inhibitors (ACEI) show promise for their antiproteinuric and renoprotective effects [41]. Losartan, an angiotensin receptor blocker (AT1ra), has also been shown to reduce proteinuria in AA amyloidosis [42, 43]. Non-steroidal anti-inflammatory drugs (NSAIDs) have been studied but have not shown any benefit [42]. Cytokine-directed therapies including infliximab [44] and etanercept [45] have also been successfully used, but reports are largely anecdotal and large trials have not been done.

Eprodisate is a member of a new class of compounds designed to interfere with interactions between amyloidogenic proteins and glycosaminoglycans and thereby inhibit polymerization of amyloid fibrils and deposition of the fibrils in tissues. A randomized trial established that eprodisate given orally slows the decline of renal function in AA amyloidosis [46] (Fig. 5-2). Further studies are planned to confirm this finding.

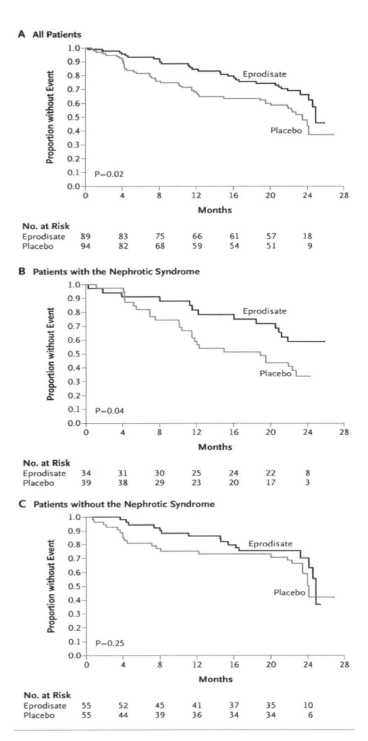

Fig. 5-2. Kaplan–Meier estimates of event-free survival (**Panel A**) show survival for all patients. Survival for patients with (**Panel B**) and for those without (**Panel C**) the nephrotic syndrome is also shown. An event is any component of the composite end point of worsened disease. The number of patients at risk for the end point drops markedly between 20 and 24 months because many patients completed their final study visit just before 24 months. Only patients who completed their final study visit at 24 months or later are included in the at-risk population at 24 months. Dember et al. [46]. Copyright © 2007 Massachusetts Medical Society. All rights reserved.

Kidney Transplant for Amyloid

Kidney transplantation is an option and has been successfully performed in selected patients with amyloidosis. Disease progression and recurrence are two major obstacles that prevent the wider use of kidney transplantation in this population. Early death is particularly problematic in AL where patients can succumb rapidly to their disease [47]. Even in less aggressive forms of amyloidosis (AA), patient survival can be inferior to the non-amyloidosis patients [48]. Deaths were most commonly the result of cardiovascular and infectious complications followed by progression of amyloidosis.

Recurrence of amyloidosis is a major obstacle to kidney transplantation. Recurrence can result in graft loss and has been reported in multiple types of amyloidosis including AL, AA particularly secondary to familial Mediterranean fever (FMF), fibrinogen Aα-chain (AFib), and apolipoprotein AI (AApoAI) [36, 49–51]. The usual time for recurrence is 2–5 years.

Several strategies have been employed to prevent recurrence and disease progression after kidney transplantation. In AL where the source of the amyloid is a plasma cell dyscrasia, the goal of hematologic complete response should be achieved. This has been done successfully with high-dose therapy followed by autologous stem cell transplantation either before or after kidney transplantation [51, 52]. In AA secondary FMF, colchicine at doses of 1–2 mg/day successfully reduced recurrence down to less than 10% from 40% [53, 54]. Lower doses (0.5–1.0 mg/day) may also be effective although may be less reliable [55]. Anakinra, an interleukin 1 receptor antagonist, has been reported to be beneficial in preventing AA from recurring after kidney transplant in a patient with AA due to FMF [56].

For hereditary amyloidosis (i.e., AFib) where the amyloid precursor is synthesized by the liver, combined liver kidney transplantation has been found to be effective at preventing recurrence [49]. Delayed progression has been observed in patients with AFib who received a liver transplantation [36]. Similar strategy has also been used in AApoAI but since the liver accounts for only a portion of the synthesis, long-term effectiveness is unknown [36].

Organ Transplant for Hereditary Fibrinogen Amyloidosis

Kidney transplantation has been used in patients with hereditary fibrinogen amyloidosis (AFib) who typically progress to end-stage renal disease (ESRD) but rarely have significant extra-renal disease. Typically the time from onset of proteinuria to ESRD is approximately 5 years and the survival is approximately 15 years from onset of symptoms. In a series of 71 patients with AFib, kidney transplant was described in 10 patients, two of whom received two grafts [49]. Three grafts failed for technical reasons and never worked. At the time of publication, five of the nine grafts were still functioning with a median graft survival of 5.9 years. Three of the grafts failed because of recurrent amyloidosis. Seven patients underwent combined hepatorenal transplantation. One died of perioperative complications; the remaining six did well with no evidence of recurrence at 2 years. Similar results were reported with AApoAI. Five of the eight patients who received kidney transplantation without liver allograft recurred versus no recurrence in two patients who received combined liver kidney transplantation [36]. Combined hepatorenal transplant removes the source of the circulating amyloidogenic fibrinogen variant and prevents recurrence of the amyloid in the transplanted kidney but is associated with increased perioperative risks. Given the benefit of isolated renal transplant, combined hepatorenal transplant is recommended only in younger, healthier patients.

Conclusions

While the primary goal of treatment for all forms of amyloidosis remains cure, important gains have been made in supportive care for these patients. Optimal medical management can improve cardiac symptoms, proteinuria, and management of volume status. Devices such as the PleurX catheter can improve the management of refractory effusions. Careful and judicious use of organ transplantation, including heart, lung, and kidneys, can improve both survival and quality of life in patients with amyloidosis. Studies need to be designed to further refine which patients are appropriate to consider for these options.

References

1. Rubinow A, Skinner M, Cohen AS. Digoxin sensitivity in amyloid cardiomyopathy. Circulation 1981;63:1285–8.
2. Gertz MA, Skinner M, Connors LH, Falk RH, Cohen AS, Kyle RA. Selective binding of nifedipine to amyloid fibrils. Am J Cardiol. 1985;55:1646.
3. Pollak A, Falk RH. Left ventricular systolic dysfunction precipitated by verapamil in cardiac amyloidosis. Chest 1993;104:618–20.
4. Gertz MA, Falk RH, Skinner M, Cohen AS, Kyle RA. Worsening of congestive heart failure in amyloid heart disease treated by calcium channel-blocking agents. Am J Cardiol. 1985;55:1645.
5. Austin BA, Duffy B, Tan C, Rodriguez ER, Starling RC, Desai MY. Comparison of functional status, electrocardiographic, and echocardiographic parameters to mortality in endomyocardial-biopsy proven cardiac amyloidosis. Am J Cardiol. 2009;103:1429–33.
6. Herlihy JP, Loyalka P, Gnananandh J, Gregoric ID, Dahlberg CG, Kar B, Delgado RM 3rd. PleurX catheter for the management of refractory pleural effusions in congestive heart failure. Tex Heart Inst J. 2009;36:38–43.
7. Hoyer RJ, Leung N, Witzig TE, Lacy MQ. Treatment of diuretic refractory pleural effusions with bevacizumab in four patients with primary systemic amyloidosis. Am J Hematol. 2007;82:409–13.
8. Pichelmayer O, Zielinski C, Raderer M. Response of a nonmalignant pleural effusion to bevacizumab. N Engl J Med. 2005;353:740–1.
9. Kimlinger T, Kline M, Kumar S, Lust J, Witzig T, Rajkumar SV. Differential expression of vascular endothelial growth factors and their receptors in multiple myeloma. Haematologica 2006;91:1033–40.
10. Rajkumar SV, Kyle RA. Angiogenesis in multiple myeloma. Semin Oncol. 2001;28:560–4.
11. Shulman K, Rosen S, Tognazzi K, Manseau EJ, Brown LF. Expression of vascular permeability factor (VPF/VEGF) is altered in many glomerular diseases. J Am Soc Nephrol. 1996;7:661–6.
12. Kyle RA, Gertz MA. Primary systemic amyloidosis: clinical and laboratory features in 474 cases. Semin Hematol. 1995;32:45–59.
13. Dubrey SW, Cha K, Skinner M, LaValley M, Falk RH. Familial and primary (AL) cardiac amyloidosis: echocardiographically similar diseases with distinctly different clinical outcomes. Heart 1997;78:74–82.
14. Conner R, Hosenpud JD, Norman DJ, Pantely GA, Cobanoglu A, Starr A. Heart transplantation for cardiac amyloidosis: successful one-year outcome despite recurrence of the disease. J Heart Transplant. 1988;7:165–7.
15. Hosenpud JD, DeMarco T, Frazier OH, Griffith BP, Uretsky BF, Menkis AH, O'Connell JB, Olivari MT, Valantine HA. Progression of systemic disease and reduced long-term survival in patients with cardiac amyloidosis undergoing heart transplantation. Follow-up results of a multicenter survey. Circulation 1991;84:III338–43.

16. Hosenpud JD, Uretsky BF, Griffith BP, O'Connell JB, Olivari MT, Valantine HA. Successful intermediate-term outcome for patients with cardiac amyloidosis undergoing heart transplantation: results of a multicenter survey. J Heart Transplant. 1990;9:346–50.

17. Dubrey SW, Burke MM, Khaghani A, Hawkins PN, Yacoub MH, Banner NR. Long term results of heart transplantation in patients with amyloid heart disease 10.1136/heart.85.2.202. Heart 2001;85:202–7.

18. Dubrey SW, Burke MM, Hawkins PN, Banner NR. Cardiac transplantation for amyloid heart disease: the United Kingdom experience. J Heart Lung Transplant. 2004;23:1142–53.

19. Kpodonu J, Massad MG, Caines A, Geha AS. Outcome of heart transplantation in patients with amyloid cardiomyopathy. J Heart Lung Transplant. 2005;24:1763–5.

20. Gillmore JD, Goodman HJ, Lachmann HJ, Offer M, Wechalekar AD, Joshi J, Pepys MB, Hawkins PN. Sequential heart and autologous stem cell transplantation for systemic AL amyloidosis. Blood 2006;107:1227–9.

21. Sack FU, Kristen A, Goldschmidt H, Schnabel PA, Dengler T, Koch A, Karck M. Treatment options for severe cardiac amyloidosis: heart transplantation combined with chemotherapy and stem cell transplantation for patients with AL-amyloidosis and heart and liver transplantation for patients with ATTR-amyloidosis. Eur J Cardiothorac Surg. 2008;33:257–62.

22. Perz JB, Kristen AV, Rahemtulla A, Parameshwar J, Sack FU, Apperley JF, Goldschmidt H, Katus HA, Dengler TJ. Long-term survival in a patient with AL amyloidosis after cardiac transplantation followed by autologous stem cell transplantation. Clin Res Cardiol. 2006;95:671–4.

23. Maurer MS, Raina A, Hesdorffer C, Bijou R, Colombo P, Deng M, Drusin R, Haythe J, Horn E, Lee SH, Marboe C, Naka Y, Schulman L, Scully B, Shapiro P, Prager K, Radhakrishnan J, Restaino S, Mancini D. Cardiac transplantation using extended-donor criteria organs for systemic amyloidosis complicated by heart failure. Transplantation 2007;83:539–45.

24. Lacy MQ, Dispenzieri A, Hayman SR, Kumar S, Kyle RA, Rajkumar SV, Edwards BS, Rodeheffer RJ, Frantz RP, Kushwaha SS, Clavell AL, Dearani JA, Sundt TM, Daly RC, McGregor CG, Gastineau DA, Litzow MR, Gertz MA. Autologous stem cell transplant after heart transplant for light chain (Al) amyloid cardiomyopathy. J Heart Lung Transplant. 2008;27:823–9.

25. Mignot A, Varnous S, Redonnet M, Jaccard A, Epailly E, Vermes E, Boissonnat P, Gandjbakhch I, Herpin D, Touchard G, Bridoux F. Heart transplantation in systemic (AL) amyloidosis: a retrospective study of eight French patients. Arch Cardiovasc Dis. 2008;101:523–32.

26. Mignot A, Bridoux F, Thierry A, Varnous S, Pujo M, Delcourt A, Gombert JM, Goujon JM, Favreau F, Touchard G, Herpin D, Jaccard A. Successful heart transplantation following melphalan plus dexamethasone therapy in systemic AL amyloidosis. Haematologica 2008;93:e32–5.

27. Grazi GL, Cescon M, Salvi F, Ercolani G, Ravaioli M, Arpesella G, Magelli C, Grigioni F, Cavallari A. Combined heart and liver transplantation for familial amyloidotic neuropathy: considerations from the hepatic point of view. Liver Transpl. 2003;9:986–92.

28. Dubrey SW, Davidoff R, Skinner M, Bergethon P, Lewis D, Falk RH. Progression of ventricular wall thickening after liver transplantation for familial amyloidosis. Transplantation 1997;64:74–80.

29. Yazaki M, Mitsuhashi S, Tokuda T, Kametani F, Takei YI, Koyama J, Kawamorita A, Kanno H, Ikeda SI. Progressive wild-type transthyretin deposition after liver transplantation preferentially occurs onto myocardium in FAP patients. Am J Transplant. 2007;7:235–42.

30. Holmgren G, Steen L, Ekstedt J, Groth CG, Ericzon BG, Eriksson S, Andersen O, Karlberg I, Norden G, Nakazato M, et al. Biochemical effect of liver transplantation in two Swedish patients with familial amyloidotic polyneuropathy (FAP-met30). Clin Genet. 1991;40:242–6.

31. Herlenius G, Wilczek HE, Larsson M, Ericzon BG. Ten years of international experience with liver transplantation for familial amyloidotic polyneuropathy: results from the Familial Amyloidotic Polyneuropathy World Transplant Registry. Transplantation 2004;77: 64–71.

32. Ericzon BG, Larsson M, Wilczek HE. Domino liver transplantation: risks and benefits. Transplant Proc. 2008;40:1130–1.

33. Ericzon BG, Larsson M, Herlenius G, Wilczek HE. Report from the Familial Amyloidotic Polyneuropathy World Transplant Registry (FAPWTR) and the Domino Liver Transplant Registry (DLTR). Amyloid 2003;10 Suppl 1:67–76.

34. Eriksson M, Schonland S, Yumlu S, Hegenbart U, von Hutten H, Gioeva Z, Lohse P, Buttner J, Schmidt H, Rocken C. Hereditary apolipoprotein AI-associated amyloidosis in surgical pathology specimens. Identification of three novel mutations in the APOA1 gene. J Mol Diagn. 2009;11(3):257–62.

35. Gillmore JD, Stangou AJ, Tennent GA, Booth DR, O'Grady J, Rela M, Heaton ND, Wall CA, Keogh JA, Hawkins PN. Clinical and biochemical outcome of hepatorenal transplantation for hereditary systemic amyloidosis associated with apolipoprotein AI Gly26Arg. Transplantation 2001;71:986–92.

36. Gillmore JD, Stangou AJ, Lachmann HJ, Goodman HJ, Wechalekar AD, Acheson J, Tennent GA, Bybee A, Gilbertson J, Rowczenio D, O'Grady J, Heaton ND, Pepys MB, Hawkins PN. Organ transplantation in hereditary apolipoprotein AI amyloidosis. Am J Transplant. 2006;6:2342–7.

37. Testro AG, Brennan SO, Macdonell RA, Hawkins PN, Angus PW. Hereditary amyloidosis with progressive peripheral neuropathy associated with apolipoprotein AI Gly26Arg: outcome of hepatorenal transplantation. Liver Transpl. 2007;13:1028–31.

38. Lachmann HJ, Goodman HJ, Gilbertson JA, Gallimore JR, Sabin CA, Gillmore JD, Hawkins PN. Natural history and outcome in systemic AA amyloidosis. N Engl J Med. 2007;356:2361–71.

39. Bergesio F, Ciciani AM, Manganaro M, Palladini G, Santostefano M, Brugnano R, Di Palma AM, Gallo M, Rosati A, Tosi PL, Salvadori M. Renal involvement in systemic amyloidosis: an Italian collaborative study on survival and renal outcome. Nephrol Dial Transplant. 2008;23:941–51.

40. Gertz MA, Leung N, Lacy MQ, Dispenzieri A, Zeldenrust SR, Hayman SR, Buadi FK, Dingli D, Greipp PR, Kumar SK, Lust JA, Rajkumar SV, Russell SJ, Witzig TE. Clinical outcome of immunoglobulin light chain amyloidosis affecting the kidney. Nephrol Dial Transplant. 2009 Oct;24(10):3132–7. Epub 2009 Apr 29.

41. Ruggenenti P, Perna A, Gherardi G, Gaspari F, Benini R, Remuzzi G. Renal function and requirement for dialysis in chronic nephropathy patients on long-term ramipril: REIN follow-up trial. Gruppo Italiano di Studi Epidemiologici in Nefrologia (GISEN). Ramipril efficacy in nephropathy. Lancet 1998;352:1252–6.

42. Kahvecioglu S, Dilek K, Akdag I, Gullulu M, Demircan C, Ersoy A, Yurtkuran M. Effect of indomethacin and selective cyclooxygenase-2 inhibitors on proteinuria and renal function in patients with AA type renal amyloidosis. Nephrology (Carlton) 2006;11:232–7.

43. Odabas AR, Cetinkaya R, Selcuk Y, Bilen H. Effect of losartan treatment on the proteinuria in normotensive patients having proteinuria due to secondary amyloidosis. Ups J Med Sci. 2001;106:183–8.

44. Elkayam O, Hawkins PN, Lachmann H, Yaron M, Caspi D. Rapid and complete resolution of proteinuria due to renal amyloidosis in a patient with rheumatoid arthritis treated with infliximab. Arthritis Rheum. 2002;46:2571–3.

45. Serratrice J, Granel B, Disdier P, Weiller PJ, Dussol B. Resolution with etanercept of nephrotic syndrome due to renal AA amyloidosis in adult Still's disease. Am J Med. 2003;115:589–90.

46. Dember LM, Hawkins PN, Hazenberg BP, Gorevic PD, Merlini G, Butrimiene I, Livneh A, Lesnyak O, Puechal X, Lachmann HJ, Obici L, Balshaw R, Garceau D, Hauck W, Skinner M. Eprodisate for the treatment of renal disease in AA amyloidosis. N Engl J Med. 2007;356:2349–60.

47. Brown JH, Maxwell AP, Bruce I, Murphy BG, Doherty CC. Renal replacement therapy in multiple myeloma and systemic amyloidosis. Ir J Med Sci. 1993;162:213–7.
48. Pasternack A, Ahonen J, Kuhlback B. Renal transplantation in 45 patients with amyloidosis. Transplantation. 1986;42:598–601.
49. Gillmore JD, Lachmann HJ, Rowczenio D, Gilbertson JA, Zeng CH, Liu ZH, Li LS, Wechalekar A, Hawkins PN. Diagnosis, pathogenesis, treatment, and prognosis of hereditary fibrinogen A alpha-chain amyloidosis. J Am Soc Nephrol. 2009;20:444–51.
50. Helin H, Pasternack A, Falck H, Kuhlback B. Recurrence of renal amyloid and de novo membranous glomerulonephritis after transplantation. Transplantation 1981;32:6–9.
51. Leung N, Griffin MD, Dispenzieri A, Haugen EN, Gloor JM, Schwab TR, Textor SC, Lacy MQ, Litzow MR, Cosio FG, Larson TS, Gertz MA, Stegall MD. Living donor kidney and autologous stem cell transplantation for primary systemic amyloidosis (AL) with predominant renal involvement. Am J Transplant. 2005;5:1660–70.
52. Casserly LF, Fadia A, Sanchorawala V, Seldin DC, Wright DG, Skinner M, Dember LM. High-dose intravenous melphalan with autologous stem cell transplantation in AL amyloidosis-associated end-stage renal disease. Kidney Int. 2003;63:1051–7.
53. Livneh A, Zemer D, Siegal B, Laor A, Sohar E, Pras M. Colchicine prevents kidney transplant amyloidosis in familial Mediterranean fever. Nephron 1992;60:418–22.
54. Sherif AM, Refaie AF, Sheashaa HA, El-Tantawy AE, Sobh MA. Long-term evaluation of neuromyopathy in live donor FMF amyloidotic kidney transplant recipients. Am J Nephrol. 2004;24:582–6.
55. Celik A, Saglam F, Dolek D, Sifil A, Soylu A, Cavdar C, Temizkan A, Bora S, Gulay H, Camsari T. Outcome of kidney transplantation for renal amyloidosis: a single-center experience. Transplant Proc. 2006;38:435–9.
56. Moser C, Pohl G, Haslinger I, Knapp S, Rowczenio D, Russel T, Lachmann HJ, Lang U, Kovarik J. Successful treatment of familial Mediterranean fever with Anakinra and outcome after renal transplantation. Nephrol Dial Transplant. 2009;24:676–8.

Chapter 6

Assessing Response and Prognosis in AL Amyloidosis

Angela Dispenzieri

Abstract Advances in assessing response and assigning risk to patients with AL amyloidosis have been made in the past several decades. Historically the most important predictor of overall survival has been the presence and extent of cardiac involvement. Most recently there have been advances for better stratifying cardiac risk; other risk factors have also been identified. Methods for assessing clinical response criteria have also improved with readily available means to measure changes of the serum immunoglobulin free light chain. These developments have been integral for improving outcomes for these patients.

Keywords Amyloidosis, Prognosis, Response, Cardiac, Free light chain, Biomarkers

Introduction

Immunoglobulin light chain amyloidosis (AL) is a low tumor burden plasma cell disorder characterized by deposition of insoluble fibrils composed of immunoglobulin light chains. Without treatment, it has an inexorable progressive course due to uncontrolled tissue damage [1]. Patients have been observed to survive from days to decades, but historically the most important predictor of overall survival has been the presence and extent of cardiac involvement [2]. As early as 1991, it was evident that those patients treated with and responding to chemotherapy survived longest [3–5]. Response criteria have evolved over time, first with an eye toward symptomatic organ improvement [6], but later to hematologic responses using conventional myeloma-type response criteria [7, 8] and later to an emphasis on changes of the serum immunoglobulin free light chain concentrations (FLCs) [9]. In addition, there has been progress in predicting prognosis based on other baseline characteristics, which will be the focus of this chapter.

Assessing Response

Quantifying "response" in patients with AL is a major challenge. Since most patients have "low tumor burden," with bone marrows and serum and urine M-proteins more akin to monoclonal gammopathy of undetermined significance (MGUS) than myeloma [10], meaningful typical hematologic response assessment had not been feasible in the majority of patients. Moreover, since these patients do not die due

From: *Amyloidosis*, Contemporary Hematology,
Edited by: M.A. Gertz and S.V. Rajkumar, DOI 10.1007/978-1-60761-631-3_6,
© Springer Science+Business Media, LLC 2010

to bone marrow crowding from high "tumor burden," the major focus for response was improvement in organ function rather than hematologic response. There are several challenges associated with assessing organ response. First, since amyloid proteins are insoluble proteins with variable rates of dissolution, organ response is often delayed with objective improvement occurring after discontinuation of effective chemotherapy. Second, there are no standardized measures of improvement for many of the amyloidosis-related abnormalities (e.g., macroglossia, purpura, and pulmonary involvement).

There have been several major breakthroughs in response assessment in the past two decades. The first was realization that hematologic response was a valuable endpoint [7, 8]. The second was introduction of the serum immunoglobulin free light chain, which made patients heretofore unevaluable for hematologic response evaluable for hematologic response [11–13]. The third advance was the publication of an international consensus for measurement of amyloid response [9]. Finally, the recognition of the soluble cardiac biomarker, N-terminal-pro B-type natriuretic peptide (NT-proBNP), as a helpful gauge of cardiac response is an important [14], but yet to be validated, advancement in measuring response. Table 6-1 summarizes the first iteration of the internationally accepted amyloid response criteria. More than likely, these response criteria will be revised to incorporate more modern parameters and to address deficiencies in the ensuing decade.

Hematologic Response

It is now recognized that hematologic response not only is important for "real-time" assessment of the efficacy of therapy, but is one of the most important prognostic determinants for both organ response and overall survival [15, 16]. When bone marrow biopsy, electrophoresis, and immunofixation electrophoresis of the serum and urine were the only tools available for measurement of hematologic response, fewer than 50% had "measurable" disease as defined by the multiple myeloma response criteria (i.e., serum M-protein greater than or equal to 1 g/dL or urine M-protein greater than 200 mg/24 h). Moreover, urine M-protein measurement is not very reliable in a patient with nephrotic syndrome due to contamination with background non-specific proteinuria. Many patients were destined to have their hematologic "measurement" limited to a binary determination of positive or negative immunofixation studies. However, with introduction of the serum FLC measurement, nearly 75% of patients now had truly measurable disease [11–13].

Organ Response

Improvement of organ function is clearly the most important response for patients in terms of both quality of life and overall survival. The internationally accepted organ response criteria for patients with AL amyloidosis are shown in Table 6-1 [9]. Median time to organ response is 6–12 months, depending on the treatment [4, 15]. The organ response criteria focus on renal, cardiac, and liver responses. Hematologic response typically precedes organ response (Fig. 6-1). Of those patients who achieve a complete hematologic response—be it through high-dose chemotherapy with autologous peripheral blood stem cell transplantation or through a simpler oral regimen like melphalan and dexamethasone—approximately 66–87% will achieve an organ response [15, 16]. Of those who achieve a partial hematologic response, 30–56% will achieve an organ response. It is rare to have an organ response in the absence of a hematologic response. The fact that the odds of achieving organ response are lower in

Table 6-1. Defining amyloid organ involvement and response to therapy.

Organ system	Involvement[a]	Improvement	Worsening
Kidney	24-h urine protein >0.5 g/day, predominantly albumin	50% reduction in 24-h urine protein excretion (at least 0.5 g/day) without worsening of creatinine or creatinine clearance by 25% over baseline	50% increase in urinary protein loss (at least 1 g/24 h) or 25% worsening of creatinine or creatinine clearance
Heart	Echo: mean wall thickness >12 mm, no other cardiac cause	≥2 mm reduction in the interventricular septal (IVS) thickness by echocardiogram, or Improvement of ejection fraction by ≥20%, or Improvement by two New York Heart Association classes without an increase in diuretic use or in wall thickness	Increase in cardiac wall thickness by ≥2 mm (2D ECHO), or Increase in New York Heart Association class by 1 grade with a decreasing ejection fraction of ≥10%
Liver	Total liver span >15 cm in the absence of heart failure or alkaline phosphatase >1.5 times institutional upper limit of normal	≥50% decrease in an initially elevated alkaline phosphatase level, or Decrease in liver size by at least 2 cm (radiographic determination)	≥50% increase of alkaline phosphatase above lowest level
Nerve, peripheral	Clinical symmetric lower extremity sensorimotor peripheral neuropathy	Improvement in electromyogram nerve conduction velocity (rare)	Not defined
Nerve, autonomic	Gastric-emptying disorder, pseudo-obstruction, voiding dysfunction not related to direct organ infiltration	Not defined	Not defined
Gastrointestinal tract	Direct biopsy verification with symptoms	Not defined	Not defined
Lung	Direct biopsy verification with symptoms Interstitial radiographic pattern	Not defined	Not defined

(continued)

Table 6-1. (continued)

Organ system	Involvement[a]	Improvement	Worsening
Soft tissue	Tongue enlargement, clinical Arthropathy Claudication, presumed vascular amyloid Skin Myopathy by biopsy or pseudohypertrophy Lymph node (may be localized) Carpal tunnel	Not defined	Not defined
Hematologic		Complete response (CR): Serum and urine negative for monoclonal protein by immunofixation Free light chain ratio normal Marrow < 5% plasma cells Partial response (PR): If serum M component > 05. g/dL, a 50% reduction If urine light chain in urine with a visible peak and >100 mg/day and 50% reduction If free light chain >10 mg/dL and 50% reduction	Progression from CR: any detectable monoclonal protein or abnormal free light chain ratio (light chain must double) Progression from PR or stable disease, 50% increase in serum M-protein to >0.5 g/dL or 50% increase in urine M-protein to >200 mg/day, or free light chain increase of 50% to >10 mg/dL

[a]Biopsy of affected organ or biopsy at an alternate site with clinical involvement
Summarized from Gertz et al. [9]

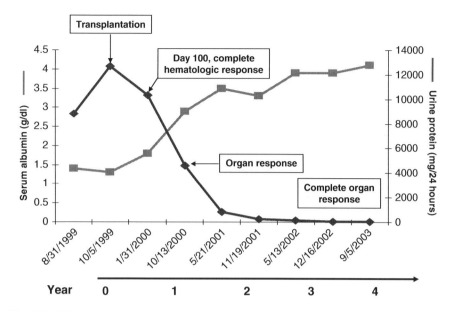

Fig. 6-1. Time lag between hematologic response and organ response.

partial hematologic response cohort makes decision making difficult in this group of patients. Does one give additional treatment to convert partial hematologic responses to complete hematologic responses? Some authors have taken this approach [17], but toxicity must be taken into consideration in these very fragile patients.

Aside from the lack of inclusion of criteria for nervous system, soft tissue, and pulmonary response, the current criteria are limited by the precision and interoperator variability of measuring liver size and of estimating cardiac interventricular septum and left ventricular septum by echocardiography. Palladini and colleagues have attempted to address part of the challenge in measuring cardiac response by evaluating serial measurements of serum N-terminal-pro B-type natriuretic peptide (NT-proBNP) [14], a marker of cardiac dysfunction in light chain amyloidosis (AL) and a powerful prognostic determinant [18–20]. The authors measured serum NT-proBNP and circulating FLCs at enrollment and after three cycles of chemotherapy in 51 patients with cardiac AL. In patients in whom FLCs decreased by more than 50% (partial hematologic response), NT-proBNP concentration decreased by a median of 48%, whereas in the remaining patients it increased by 47% ($P = 0.01$). The reduction of NT-proBNP was greater in patients ($n = 9$) in whom amyloidogenic FLCs disappeared at immunofixation (median 53%) than in the remaining responding patients (median 31%, $P = 0.04$). Cardiac function in AL appeared to rapidly improve due to a reduction of the circulating amyloidogenic precursor, despite the amount of cardiac amyloid deposits remaining apparently unaltered, as measured by echocardiography. Once these data are validated by others, they should be accepted by the amyloidosis community as an additional cardiac response criterion.

Prognosis

Prognostic factors can be separated into those existing at diagnosis and those that occur after or during therapy. Hematologic and organ responses are examples of the latter and will be discussed first.

Hematologic and Organ Responses as Prognostic Factors

Achieving organ response is the most important prognostic factor in patients with AL amyloidosis. Gertz and colleagues first reported in a series of 151 patients treated with alkylator-based therapy that those 27 patients (18%) with an organ response had significantly better overall survivals than did those without organ response (Fig. 6-2) [4]. The median time to achieve organ response was 11.7 months. For the responders, the median overall survival was 89.4 months with 21 of 27 (78%) surviving 5 years. This was in stark contrast to a median overall survival of 14.7 months seen in the 126 patients who showed no response to alkylator-based therapy.

Because of the frequent time lag in organ response, hematologic response has become an important prognostic measure [7, 8]. Not only does hematologic response using serum and urine M-proteins predict for organ response, it also predicts for overall survival (Fig. 6-3) [21–23]. Those patients achieving the deepest responses have longest overall survival. There is debate as to whether the means by which one arrives at partial or complete hematologic response matter [21]. This is most notable

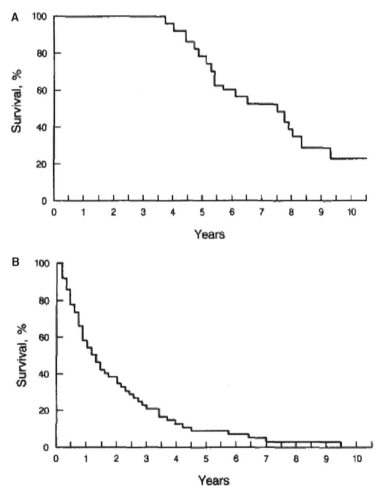

Fig. 6-2. Organ response predicts for overall survival. (**a**) Survival from time of diagnosis of 27 patients with AL with organ response. (**b**) Survival from time of diagnosis of 126 patients with AL treated with melphalan who failed to have organ response. Modified from Gertz et al. [4].

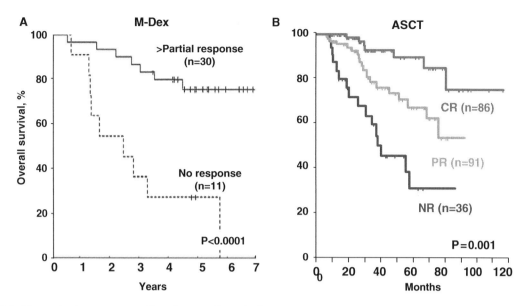

Fig. 6-3. Hematologic response predicts for overall survival. (**a**) Response achieved with M-Dex (melphalan and dexamethasone). Modified from Palladini et al. [23]. (**b**) Effect of hematologic response on outcome of patients undergoing transplantation for primary amyloidosis (Landmark analysis). Modified from Gertz et al. [22].

in the context of high-dose chemotherapy with autologous stem cell transplant versus standard-dose melphalan and dexamethasone. For patients achieving hematologic CR, the 5-year overall survival is about 70% regardless of the treatment modality used to arrive at hematologic CR [22–24]. For patients undergoing ASCT and achieving CR, 10-year survival rates approach 60% [24].

Because of the apparent importance of achieving complete hematologic response, investigators at Memorial Sloan Kettering have looked at treating those patients who did not achieve a complete hematological response at 3 months after their ASCT with adjuvant thalidomide and dexamethasone. Thirty-one patients began adjuvant therapy, with 16 (52%) completing 9 months of treatment and 13 (42%) achieving an improvement in hematological response. By intention to treat, overall hematological response rate was 71% (36% complete response), with 44% having organ responses. With a median follow-up of 31 months, 2-year survival was 84% (95% confidence interval: 73, 94) [17].

Until recently, standard multiple myeloma response criteria were used to assess hematologic response but were limited in that the majority of AL patients did not have adequate tumor burden to be considered to have measurable disease. Fortunately, the serum immunoglobulin FLC is measurable in the majority of patients and a 50% reduction of it predicted for eventual organ response and better overall survival [11–13]. Those patients with the deepest free light chain responses, i.e., normalization of their involved FLC and/or their FLC ratio, had the best overall survival, especially after high-dose chemotherapy with peripheral blood stem cell transplantation [12, 17]. Even using a cutoff of less than or equal to 10 mg/dL at day 100 was prognostic (Fig. 6-4). Although the current response criteria rely primarily on the M-spike and secondarily on the serum FLC, there are data that changes in the FLC outperform changes in the intact immunoglobulin [12]. This, however, will have to be validated in larger series.

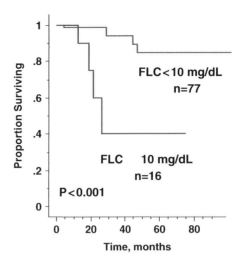

Fig. 6-4. Overall survival based on actual serum free light chain concentration at day 100 post-autologous stem cell transplantation.

Baseline Characteristics as Prognostic Factors

A list of baseline prognostic factors is shown in Table 6-2. An interesting observation made in the 1980s is that the baseline risk factors predicting for overall survival

Table 6-2. Prognostic factors in AL.

Category	Factor
Referral bias	Surviving long enough to attend a tertiary center selects for healthier patients [26]
Cardiac	Congestive heart failure (4 months) [26, 49]
	Exertional syncope [57]
	LV hypertrophy [32, 58]
	LV diastolic dysfunction [33]
	Reduced systolic function [32, 58]
	Troponins [19]
	N-terminal (brain) B-type natriuretic peptide [18–20] or brain natriuretic peptide [59]
	LV outflow obstruction [34]
	RV dysfunction [35, 36]
	RV dilatation [37]
	Atrial dysfunction [38]
Clone	Co-existent multiple myeloma [27]
	Bone marrow plasma cells [12, 47, 48]
	Plasma cell labeling index [47]
	Circulating peripheral blood plasma cells [48]
	Urine monoclonal light chain in urine [49, 50]
	Immunoglobulin free light chain [12]
	Presence of t(11;14) translocation [51]
Number of organs involved	Number of organs involved [4, 8]
Other	Weight loss [49]
	Male gender [10]
	Howell–Jolly bodies [60]
	β_2-microglobulin [48, 54]
	123-I-labeled serum amyloid P component extravascular retention [55, 56]
	Uric acid [61]

during the first year and after the first year differed [25]. In this multivariate analysis of 168 individuals with AL amyloidosis, the risk factors for early death included the presence of congestive heart failure, urine light chains, hepatomegaly, and multiple myeloma. In contrast, serum creatinine, multiple myeloma, orthostatic hypotension, and monoclonal serum protein were the most important variables adversely affecting survival for patients surviving 1 year. Additional prognostic factors have been identified, which are categorized into five major categories: (1) referral bias; (2) cardiac factors; (3) factors directly related to the clone; (4) number of organs involved; and (5) other factors.

Referral Bias

Referral bias exists at large amyloid treatment centers. To be seen at a distant center, a priori, a patient must be physically able to travel. When we evaluated overall survival of the 474 AL amyloidosis patients seen at the Mayo Clinic from 1981 to 1992, the median survival was 2 years; however, the median survival of those patients seen at the Mayo Clinic within 30 days of diagnosis was only 13 months [26].

Cardiac Factors

In the first published clinical trials, median survival for patients with AL was approximately 15–18 months [27–29]. Patients presenting with CHF or syncope had median survivals of 4–6 months. It was clear that patients with significant cardiac disease did worse since they were at the highest risk for sudden cardiac death [30, 31]. Attempts to better dissect patients' risk based on the extent of cardiac disease remain a work in progress, but echocardiography and Doppler studies were the first objective tools used to define cardiac amyloidosis and predict outcomes. By using echocardiographic studies (2D and Doppler), 40% of AL patients have cardiac involvement, but only 17% have symptoms of heart failure [30].

As described in Chapter 8, a variety of cardiac abnormalities may be seen in these patients including left ventricular (LV) hypertrophy [32], LV diastolic dysfunction [33], LV outflow obstruction [34], right ventricular (RV) dysfunction [35, 36], RV dilatation [37], atrial dysfunction [38], abnormal strain imaging and strain rate imaging [39–41], reduced ejection time [42], late gadolinium enhancement and abnormal gadolinium kinetics on cardiac magnetic imaging [43, 44], and rhythm and conduction abnormalities [45].

The most commonly used echocardiographic features are the measurements of the interventricular septal thickness and left ventricular ejection fraction [32]. Cueto-Garcia studied 132 patients with biopsy-proven systemic amyloidosis and subgrouped them by left ventricular wall thickness: group I, mean wall thickness 12 mm or less; group II, mean wall thickness greater than 12 mm but less than 15 mm; group III, mean wall thickness 15 mm or greater; and group IV, atypical features such as wall motion abnormalities or left ventricular dilatation. Survival was negatively influenced both by greater wall thickness and by reduced systolic function.

Doppler-derived left ventricular diastolic filling variables are also important predictors of survival in cardiac amyloidosis [33]. Klein and colleagues performed pulsed-wave Doppler studies of the left ventricular inflow and obtained clinical follow-up data in 63 consecutive patients with biopsy-proven systemic amyloidosis. The patients were subdivided into two groups according to deceleration time: group 1 (33 patients) had a deceleration time of 150 ms or less, indicative of restrictive physiology, and group 2 (30 patients) had a deceleration time of more than 150 ms. Of the 25 cardiac deaths, 19 (76%) were from group 1. The 1-year probability of survival in group 1 was significantly less than that in group 2 (49 versus 92%, $P < 0.001$). Bivariate analysis revealed that the combination of the Doppler variables of shortened deceleration time and increased early diastolic filling velocity to atrial filling velocity ratio were stronger predictors of cardiac death than were the 2D echocardiographic variables of mean left ventricular wall thickness and fractional shortening.

Major limitations of echocardiography and Doppler measurements are that they do not detect early involvement and that there are issues with inter-observer variability. More recently, Doppler myocardial imaging including strain imaging and strain rate imaging have been used to detect early regional left ventricular systolic dysfunction in cardiac amyloidosis at a time when fractional shortening remains normal [39–41]. These abnormalities precede the onset of congestive heart failure and can be detected by strain and strain rate but are not apparent by tissue velocity imaging. Longitudinal systolic strain most accurately detects longitudinal systolic dysfunction in AL amyloidosis [41]. Interrogation of six middle segments was sufficient in identifying patients with advanced amyloid cardiomyopathy [40, 41].

Cardiovascular magnetic resonance (CMR) is also proving to be of use in diagnosing and predicting prognosis in patients with AL amyloidosis, but it is an early science. Two small studies have evaluated the prognostic value of CMR and found that gadolinium kinetics [43], but not late gadolinium enhancement [43, 44], predict for overall survival [43]. The 2-min post-gadolinium intramyocardial T1 difference between subepicardium and subendocardium predicts mortality with 85% accuracy at a threshold value of 23 ms (the lower the difference the worse the prognosis) [43]. LGE volume was positively correlated with serum level of B-type natriuretic peptide (BNP; $R = 0.64$, $P \leq 0.001$), and in multivariate analysis, LGE volume proved the strongest independent predictor of BNP [44].

In addition to structural abnormalities, rhythm and conduction abnormalities play a significant role in these patients in that they are typically the terminal event [45]. Palladini and colleagues studied the spectrum of Holter abnormalities found in AL amyloidosis and assessed their prognostic significance. Fifty-one patients were included and 55% had echographic signs of heart involvement and 23% had heart failure. Complex ventricular arrhythmias were found in 57% of patients, couplets in 29%, and non-sustained ventricular tachycardia in 18%. Overall median survival was 23.4 months. The multivariate analysis demonstrated that interventricular septum thickness and couplets were independent predictors of survival.

More recently, soluble cardiac biomarkers [troponin T, troponin I, NT-proBNP, and brain naturietic factor (BNP)] have been shown to be excellent predictors of prognosis [18–20, 46]. The system was tested both in a transplant cohort and in a non-transplant cohort. The former group included 242 patients with newly diagnosed AL who were seen at the Mayo Clinic between April 1979 and November 2000 and who had echocardiograms and stored serum samples at presentation. Two prognostic models were designed using threshold values of NT-proBNP and either cTnT or cTnI (NT-proBNP < 332 ng/L, cTnT < 0.035 mcg/L, and cTnI < 0.1 mcg/L). Depending on whether NT-proBNP and troponin levels were both low, were high for only one test, or were both high, patients were classified as stage I, II, or III, respectively. Using the cTnT+NT-proBNP model 33, 30, and 37% of patients were stages I, II, and III, respectively, with median survivals of 26.4, 10.5, and 3.5 months, respectively. The alternate cTnI+NT-proBNP model predicted median survivals of 27.2, 11.1, and 4.1 months, respectively [19]. In the transplanted cohort of 98 patients, 49, 38, and 13% of patients were in stage I, stage II, and stage III, respectively [20]. Their updated

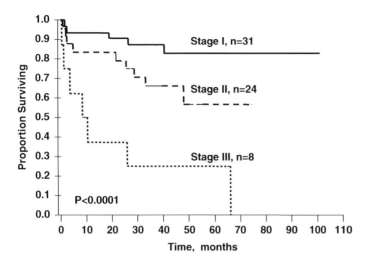

Fig. 6-5. Predicting outcome post-autologous peripheral blood stem cell transplant based on cardiac biomarker staging system. *Stage 1*, both below biomarkers below cutoff; *stage 2*, one of the two biomarkers below cutoff; and *stage 3*, both biomarkers above cutoffs. Cutoffs troponin $T < 0.035$ mcg/L and NT-proBNP < 332 ng/L (39 pmol/L). Results updated from original publication published in Blood 2004;104:1881–7. Median follow-up of surviving patients is 35.5 months. Modified from Dispenzieri et al. [20]. Median follow-up of surviving patients is 35.5 months.

survival with a median follow-up of 35 months is shown in Fig. 6-5. The 3-year overall survival rates are 87, 66, and 24%, respectively. These routine laboratory tests are reproducible and relatively inexpensive and will play a major role in assessing prognosis in patients with AL amyloidosis.

Prognosis as It Relates to the Plasma Cell Clone

The observation made in 1975 that the size of the underlying plasma cell clone was prognostic was tied into the observation that patients with coexisting multiple myeloma, which was largely defined based on bone marrow plasmacytosis, had inferior overall survivals. The respective median survival rates with and without coexisting multiple myeloma were at 1 year, 26 and 54%; and at 5 years, 3 and 17% [27]. This observation has withstood the test of time [30, 31]. Bone marrow plasmacytosis, the proliferative rate of the bone marrow plasma cells, and the presence of circulating plasma cells are all adverse prognostic markers for overall survival [47].

Circulating peripheral blood plasma cells (PBPCs) detected by a sensitive slide-based immunofluorescence technique were found in 16% (24 of 147) patients with AL amyloidosis. Overall survival for patients with high PBPC% (>1%) was poor (median survival, 10 versus 29 months; $P = 0.002$). Multivariate analysis revealed that circulating PBPCs and extent of bone marrow plasmacytosis were independent prognostic factors for survival. Patients with PBPC% of 2% or higher were significantly more likely to have a coexisting clinical diagnosis of multiple myeloma (50 versus 12%, $P = 0.008$) [48].

The plasma cells of patients with AL amyloidosis tend to have a very low proliferative rate. The plasma cell labeling index is a slide-based immunofluorescent test capable of assessing the proliferative potential of the bone marrow plasma cells in patients with AL. In one study of 125 patients, 37% had a proliferative index over 0.

These individuals had a median survival of 15 months in contrast to those with a labeling index of 0, who had a median survival of 30 months [47].

The presence of light chains in the urine was also noted to be an adverse prognostic factor for patients with AL [49, 50]. Whether this is a function of "tumor burden" or renal damage is not clear. The absolute level of serum immunoglobulin free light chains has also been reported to be prognostic [12]. Finally, the presence of translocation 11;14 appears to be an adverse prognostic factor in one small series [51]. If validated this is an important observation since the translocation 11;14 is found in 40–50% of patients with AL amyloidosis [51, 52].

Number of Organs Involved

It has long been recognized that the more organs involved, the worse the prognosis for the patient regardless of the treatment [4, 8]. Figure 6-6 illustrates the impact that the number of organs involved by amyloidosis based on clinical parameters has on overall survival in 270 patients undergoing ASCT. Whereas median survival had not been reached at 6 years in those patients with one affected organ, the respective median survival rates for patients with two and three affected organs, respectively, were 55 and 25.5 months [53]. In a proportional hazards model, overall survival is associated with the number of organs involved and the free immunoglobulin light chain protein level before treatment [12].

The hope is that more objective criteria delineating the *extent* of organ involvement rather than merely the presence or absence or organ involvement will supplant the current system of counting organs. The cardiac biomarker system may offer a viable alternative since elevations of them reflect not only cardiac dysfunction, but also renal dysfunction [18–20]. Another motivation for migrating away from merely counting the number of organs involved is that outcomes vary not only due to extent of involvement, but also based on organ type [26, 49]. In a cohort of 474 patients with AL seen at the Mayo Clinic between 1981 and 1992 within 30 days of diagnosis, the respective median overall survival for patients with congestive heart failure, orthostatic hypotension, nephrotic syndrome, and peripheral neuropathy was 4, 12, 16, and 28 months, while the median survival of the entire group was 13.1 months and the 5-year survival was 7% (Fig. 6-7).

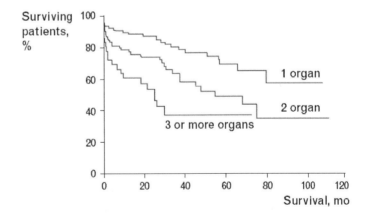

Fig. 6-6. The number of affected organs predicts for outcome in 270 patients undergoing autologous stem cell transplant. Modified from Gertz et al. [53].

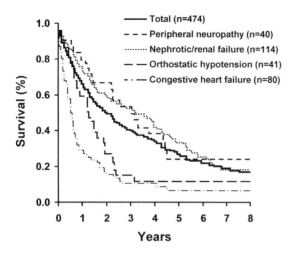

Fig. 6-7. Probability of survival depends on organ involvement at presentation: 474 patients seen between 1981 and 1992. Modified from Kyle and Gertz [26].

Other Prognostic Factors

Several other important prognostic factors are listed in Table 6-2. Among them, β_2-microglobulin and serum amyloid protein scan retention are among the most interesting and are discussed below.

Patients with normal levels of serum β_2-microglobulin have better outcomes than those with elevated values (median overall survival of 33 and 11 months, respectively) [54]. The value of β_2-microglobulin was independent of the presence of renal failure or heart failure in assessing prognosis. The median survival of patients who have normal renal function and an elevated β_2-microglobulin value was 9 months compared with 39 months for those patients with a normal β_2-microglobulin value.

Serum amyloid P (SAP) component binds to amyloid. SAP scintigraphy is used to evaluate the extent and distribution of amyloid. Two studies demonstrate the prognostic utility of the extravascular retention of 123-I-SAP after 24 h in patients with AL [55, 56]. Hachulla and colleagues studied 24 patients with AL amyloidosis and found that 24-h tissue retention was elevated in all patients. In addition, the mean survival in patients with tissue retention greater than 50% was 11.3 versus 24.5 months in patients with levels less than or equal to 50% [56]. Similarly, Hazenberg and colleagues studied the extravascular retention of 123-I-SAP at 24 h in 80 patients with AL amyloidosis [55]. They found that the extravascular retention of 123-I-SAP after 24 h was strongly associated with the number of organs involved. On multivariate analysis, both cardiac involvement (hazard ratio, 3.9; 95% CI, 2.0–7.8) and extravascular retention of 123-I-SAP after 24 h of greater than 50% (hazard ratio, 2.0; 95% CI, 1.1–3.9) were independent predictors of survival. The authors concluded that although this measurement is prognostic, its sensitivity is only 61%.

Concluding Remarks

Considerable advancements in assessing response and assigning risk to patients with AL amyloidosis have been made in the past several decades. This progress has been integral for improving outcomes for these patients. Figure 6-8 demonstrates

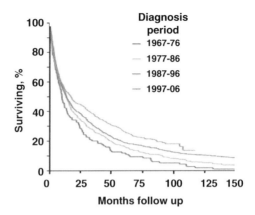

Fig. 6-8. Improved overall survival over time. Overall survival for newly diagnosed patients with AL amyloidosis seen at the Mayo Clinic between 1967 and 2006 in 9-year increments [62].

the doubling in the 4-year overall survival enjoyed by patients diagnosed in the past decade as compared to those diagnosed 40 years earlier.

Acknowledgments This work was supported in part by the Hematologic Malignancies Fund.

Financial support: AD is supported in part by grants CA125614, CA062242, CA111345, and CA107476 from the National Cancer Institute.

References

1. Kyle RA, Greipp PR. Primary systemic amyloidosis: comparison of melphalan and prednisone versus placebo. Blood 1978;52:818–27.
2. Gertz MA, Lacy MQ, Dispenzieri A, Hayman SR. Amyloidosis. Best Pract Res Clin Haematol. 2005;18:709–27.
3. Benson MD. Treatment of AL amyloidosis with melphalan, prednisone, and colchicine. Arthritis rheum. 1986;29:683–7.
4. Gertz MA, Kyle RA, Greipp PR. Response rates and survival in primary systemic amyloidosis. Blood 1991;77:257–62.
5. Kyle RA, Gertz MA, Greipp PR, et al. Long-term survival (10 years or more) in 30 patients with primary amyloidosis. Blood 1999;93:1062–6.
6. Kyle RA, Gertz MA, Greipp PR, et al. A trial of three regimens for primary amyloidosis: colchicine alone, melphalan and prednisone, and melphalan, prednisone, and colchicine. N Engl J Med. 1997;336:1202–7.
7. Comenzo RL, Vosburgh E, Falk RH, et al. Dose-intensive melphalan with blood stem-cell support for the treatment of AL (amyloid light-chain) amyloidosis: survival and responses in 25 patients. Blood 1998;91:3662–70.
8. Moreau P, Leblond V, Bourquelot P, et al. Prognostic factors for survival and response after high-dose therapy and autologous stem cell transplantation in systemic AL amyloidosis: a report on 21 patients. Br J Haematol. 1998;101:766–9.
9. Gertz MA, Comenzo R, Falk RH, et al. Definition of organ involvement and treatment response in immunoglobulin light chain amyloidosis (AL): a consensus opinion from the 10th International Symposium on Amyloid and Amyloidosis, Tours, France, 18–22 April 2004. Am J Hematol. 2005;79:319–28.
10. Gertz MA, Kyle RA. Primary systemic amyloidosis – a diagnostic primer. Mayo Clin Proc. 1989;64:1505–19.
11. Lachmann HJ, Gallimore R, Gillmore JD, et al. Outcome in systemic AL amyloidosis in relation to changes in concentration of circulating free immunoglobulin light chains following chemotherapy. Br J Haematol. 2003;122:78–84.

12. Dispenzieri A, Lacy MQ, Katzmann JA, et al. Absolute values of immunoglobulin free light chains are prognostic in patients with primary systemic amyloidosis undergoing peripheral blood stem cell transplantation. Blood 2006;107:3378–83.

13. Sanchorawala V, Seldin DC, Magnani B, Skinner M, Wright DG. Serum free light-chain responses after high-dose intravenous melphalan and autologous stem cell transplantation for AL (primary) amyloidosis. Bone Marrow Transplant. 2005;36:597–600.

14. Palladini G, Lavatelli F, Russo P, et al. Circulating amyloidogenic free light chains and serum N-terminal natriuretic peptide type B decrease simultaneously in association with improvement of survival in AL. Blood 2006;107:3854–8.

15. Palladini G, Perfetti V, Obici L, et al. Association of melphalan and high-dose dexamethasone is effective and well tolerated in patients with AL (primary) amyloidosis who are ineligible for stem cell transplantation. Blood 2004;103:2936–8.

16. Skinner M, Sanchorawala V, Seldin DC, et al. High-dose melphalan and autologous stem-cell transplantation in patients with AL amyloidosis: an 8-year study. Ann Intern Med. 2004;140:85–93.

17. Cohen AD, Zhou P, Chou J, et al. Risk-adapted autologous stem cell transplantation with adjuvant dexamethasone +/– thalidomide for systemic light-chain amyloidosis: results of a phase II trial. Br J Haematol. 2007;139:224–33.

18. Palladini G, Campana C, Klersy C, et al. Serum N-terminal pro-brain natriuretic peptide is a sensitive marker of myocardial dysfunction in AL amyloidosis. Circulation 2003;107:2440–5.

19. Dispenzieri A, Gertz MA, Kyle RA, et al. Serum cardiac troponins and N-terminal pro-brain natriuretic peptide: a staging system for primary systemic amyloidosis. J Clin Oncol. 2004;22:3751–7.

20. Dispenzieri A, Gertz MA, Kyle RA, et al. Prognostication of survival using cardiac troponins and N-terminal pro-brain natriuretic peptide in patients with primary systemic amyloidosis undergoing peripheral blood stem cell transplantation. Blood 2004;104:1881–7.

21. Jaccard A, Moreau P, Leblond V, et al. High-dose melphalan versus melphalan plus dexamethasone for AL amyloidosis. N Engl J Med. 2007;357:1083–93.

22. Gertz MA, Lacy MQ, Dispenzieri A, et al. Effect of hematologic response on outcome of patients undergoing transplantation for primary amyloidosis: importance of achieving a complete response. Haematologica 2007;92:1415–8.

23. Palladini G, Russo P, Nuvolone M, et al. Treatment with oral melphalan plus dexamethasone produces long-term remissions in AL amyloidosis. Blood 2007;110:787–8.

24. Sanchorawala V, Skinner M, Quillen K, Finn KT, Doros G, Seldin DC. Long-term outcome of patients with AL amyloidosis treated with high-dose melphalan and stem-cell transplantation. Blood 2007;110:3561–3.

25. Kyle RA, Greipp PR, O'Fallon WM. Primary systemic amyloidosis: multivariate analysis for prognostic factors in 168 cases. Blood 1986;68:220–4.

26. Kyle RA, Gertz MA. Primary systemic amyloidosis: clinical and laboratory features in 474 cases. Semin Hematol. 1995;32:45–59.

27. Kyle RA, Bayrd ED. Amyloidosis: review of 236 cases. Medicine 1975;54:271–99.

28. Kyle RA, Greipp PR, Garton JP, Gertz MA. Primary systemic amyloidosis. Comparison of melphalan/prednisone versus colchicine. Am J Med. 1985;79:708–16.

29. Cohen AS, Rubinow A, Anderson JJ, Skinner M, Mason JH, Libbey C, Kayne H. Survival of patients with primary (AL) amyloidosis. Colchicine-treated cases from 1976 to 1983 compared with cases seen in previous years (1961 to 1973). Am J Med. 1987;82:1182–90.

30. Gertz MA, Kyle RA. Amyloidosis: prognosis and treatment. Semin Arthritis Rheum. 1994;24:124–38.

31. Gertz MA, Lacy MQ, Dispenzieri A. Amyloidosis: recognition, confirmation, prognosis, and therapy. Mayo Clin Proc. 1999;74:490–4.

32. Cueto-Garcia L, Reeder GS, Kyle RA, et al. Echocardiographic findings in systemic amyloidosis: spectrum of cardiac involvement and relation to survival. J Am Coll Cardiol. 1985;6:737–43.

33. Klein AL, Hatle LK, Taliercio CP, et al. Prognostic significance of Doppler measures of diastolic function in cardiac amyloidosis. A Doppler echocardiography study. Circulation 1991;83:808–16.

34. Oh JK, Tajik AJ, Edwards WD, Bresnahan JF, Kyle RA. Dynamic left ventricular outflow tract obstruction in cardiac amyloidosis detected by continuous-wave Doppler echocardiography. Am J Cardiol. 1987;59:1008–10.

35. Klein AL, Hatle LK, Burstow DJ, et al. Comprehensive Doppler assessment of right ventricular diastolic function in cardiac amyloidosis. J Am Coll Cardiol. 1990;15:99–108.

36. Ghio S, Perlini S, Palladini G, et al. Importance of the echocardiographic evaluation of right ventricular function in patients with AL amyloidosis. Eur J Heart Fail. 2007;9: 808–13.

37. Patel AR, Dubrey SW, Mendes LA, et al. Right ventricular dilation in primary amyloidosis: an independent predictor of survival. Am J Cardiol. 1997;80:486–92.

38. Modesto KM, Dispenzieri A, Cauduro SA, et al. Left atrial myopathy in cardiac amyloidosis: implications of novel echocardiographic techniques. Eur Heart J. 2005;26:173–9.

39. Koyama J, Ray-Sequin PA, Falk RH. Longitudinal myocardial function assessed by tissue velocity, strain, and strain rate tissue Doppler echocardiography in patients with AL (primary) cardiac amyloidosis. Circulation 2003;107:2446–52.

40. Bellavia D, Abraham TP, Pellikka PA, et al. Detection of left ventricular systolic dysfunction in cardiac amyloidosis with strain rate echocardiography. J Am Soc Echocardiogr. 2007;20:1194–202.

41. Bellavia D, Pellikka PA, Abraham TP, et al. Evidence of impaired left ventricular systolic function by Doppler myocardial imaging in patients with systemic amyloidosis and no evidence of cardiac involvement by standard two-dimensional and Doppler echocardiography. Am J Cardiol. 2008;101:1039–45.

42. Bellavia D, Pellikka PA, Abraham TP, et al. 'Hypersynchronisation' by tissue velocity imaging in patients with cardiac amyloidosis. Heart 2009;95:234–40.

43. Maceira AM, Prasad SK, Hawkins PN, Roughton M, Pennell DJ. Cardiovascular magnetic resonance and prognosis in cardiac amyloidosis. J Cardiovasc Magn Reson. 2008;10:54.

44. Ruberg FL, Appelbaum E, Davidoff R, et al. Diagnostic and prognostic utility of cardiovascular magnetic resonance imaging in light-chain cardiac amyloidosis. Am J Cardiol. 2009;103:544–9.

45. Palladini G, Malamani G, Co F, et al. Holter monitoring in AL amyloidosis: prognostic implications. Pacing Clin Electrophysiol. 2001;24:1228–33.

46. Dispenzieri A, Kyle RA, Gertz MA, et al. Survival in patients with primary systemic amyloidosis and raised serum cardiac troponins. Lancet 2003;361:1787–9.

47. Gertz MA, Kyle RA, Greipp PR. The plasma cell labeling index: a valuable tool in primary systemic amyloidosis. Blood 1989;74:1108–11.

48. Pardanani A, Witzig TE, Schroeder G, et al. Circulating peripheral blood plasma cells as a prognostic indicator in patients with primary systemic amyloidosis. Blood 2003;101: 827–30.

49. Kyle RA, Greipp PR. Amyloidosis (AL). Clinical and laboratory features in 229 cases. Mayo Clin Proc. 1983;58:665–83.

50. Gertz MA, Kyle RA. Prognostic value of urinary protein in primary systemic amyloidosis (AL). Am J Clin Pathol. 1990;94:313–7.

51. Bryce AH, Ketterling R, Gertz MA, et al. Association of translocation t(11;14) with survival in patients with light chain (AL) amyloidosis [Abstract 8549]. J Clin Oncol. 2008;26.

52. Bochtler T, Hegenbart U, Cremer FW, et al. Evaluation of the cytogenetic aberration pattern in amyloid light chain amyloidosis as compared with monoclonal gammopathy of undetermined significance reveals common pathways of karyotypic instability. Blood 2008;111:4700–5.

53. Gertz MA, Lacy MQ, Dispenzieri A, Hayman SR, Kumar S. Transplantation for amyloidosis. Curr Opin Oncol. 2007;19:136–41.

54. Gertz MA, Kyle RA, Greipp PR, Katzmann JA, O'Fallon WM. Beta 2-microglobulin predicts survival in primary systemic amyloidosis. Am J Med. 1990;89:609–14.

55. Hazenberg BP, van Rijswijk MH, Lub-de Hooge MN, et al. Diagnostic performance and prognostic value of extravascular retention of 123I-labeled serum amyloid P component in systemic amyloidosis. J Nucl Med. 2007;48:865–72.

56. Hachulla E, Maulin L, Deveaux M, et al. Prospective and serial study of primary amyloidosis with serum amyloid P component scintigraphy: from diagnosis to prognosis. Am J Med. 1996;101:77–87.

57. Chamarthi B, Dubrey SW, Cha K, Skinner M, Falk RH. Features and prognosis of exertional syncope in light-chain associated AL cardiac amyloidosis. Am J Cardiol. 1997;80:1242–5.

58. Dubrey SW, Cha K, Anderson J, et al. The clinical features of immunoglobulin light-chain (AL) amyloidosis with heart involvement. QJM. 1998;91:141–57.

59. Lebovic D, Hoffman J, Levine BM, et al. Predictors of survival in patients with systemic light-chain amyloidosis and cardiac involvement initially ineligible for stem cell transplantation and treated with oral melphalan and dexamethasone. Br J Haematol. 2008;143:369–73.

60. Gertz MA, Kyle RA, Greipp PR. Hyposplenism in primary systemic amyloidosis. Ann Intern Med. 1983;98:475–7.

61. Kumar S, Dispenzieri A, Lacy MQ, et al. Serum uric acid: novel prognostic factor in primary systemic amyloidosis. Mayo Clin Proc. 2008;83:297–303.

62. Kumar S, Dispenzieri A, Lacy MQ, et al. Improved survival in light chain amyloidosis. Amyloid 2010;17(Suppl 1):89.

Chapter 7

Localized Amyloidosis

Francis Buadi

Abstract The amyloid workshop group has defined guidelines to help differentiate the various forms of amyloidosis. In localized amyloidosis the amyloidogenic protein is typically deposited at the site of production and not transported in the bloodstream. Localized amyloidosis is usually immunoglobulin light chain associated (AL type), although serum amyloid A protein and transthyretin have been reported as causing localized disease. Localized amyloidosis typically involves the laryngo-tracheobronchial tree, urogenital tract, and skin. However, all tissues may be involved, and other sites described include orbit, gastrointestinal, spine/bone, breast, and soft tissues. The true incidence and prevalence of localized amyloidosis are unknown. Localized amyloidosis is less common than systemic amyloidosis and accounts for about 10–20% of all cases of amyloidosis. The median age at diagnosis seems to be in the 6th or 7th decade and there appears to be a slight male predominance. The etiology of localized amyloidosis is unknown, although multiple pathophysiologic mechanisms have been suggested. Localized and systemic amyloidoses have different clinical presentation, clinical course, prognosis, and treatment. It is therefore vital that all cases of suspected localized amyloid do have an extensive evaluation to rule out system disease, since this will impact on therapy.

Keywords Localized, Amyloidosis, Amyloidoma, Urogenital, Tracheobronchial, Amyloid, Cutaneous, Laryngo-tracheobronchial, Immunoglobulin, Transthyretin

Introduction

Amyloidosis is the extracellular deposition of amyloid which is an eosinophilic amorphous material with a high affinity for Congo red dye. This may be hereditary or acquired, and the deposits may be localized or systemic in distribution. The amyloid workshop group has defined guidelines to help differentiate these two forms of the disease [1]. In systemic amyloidosis the amyloid fibril protein is typically produced at distant sites and carried in the bloodstream with deposition at multiple sites, whereas in localized amyloidosis the protein is typically deposited at the site of production and not transported in the bloodstream. The amyloid deposits are composed of insoluble proteins, with beta-pleated sheet conformation in association with serum amyloid P protein (SAP). SAP is a non-fibrillar serum glycoprotein which binds in a calcium-dependent manner to amyloid fibrils of all types. The amyloid deposits stain positive with Congo red dye and show apple green birefringence when viewed under polarized light. Under electron microscope these are seen as non-branching fibrils 8–10 nm in

From: *Amyloidosis*, Contemporary Hematology,
Edited by: M.A. Gertz and S.V. Rajkumar, DOI 10.1007/978-1-60761-631-3_7,
© Springer Science+Business Media, LLC 2010

width. The origin of the amyloid protein varies. They may be constituted from normal protein such as prealbumin (wild-type transthyretin), beta-2 microglobulin, serum amyloid A protein (SAA) or abnormal protein such as mutated transthyretin (TTR), monoclonal immunoglobulin light chains, lysozyme, and apolipoprotein A1. Amyloidosis is usually classified based on the constituent protein and whether it is localized or systemic. Although the true incidence of amyloidosis is unknown it is estimated to be about 6–14 cases per million [2, 3]. In autopsy series, varying rates range from 0.2%, as reported in the Massachusetts General Hospital and Johns Hopkins Hospital studies, to as high as 50% in a South African study [4]. Localized amyloidosis is less common than systemic amyloidosis and accounts for about 10–20% of all cases of amyloidosis [4, 5]. Ravid reported an incidence of 18.4% in 392 consecutive autopsy cases [6]. The median age at diagnosis seems to be in the 6th or 7th decade [4, 7, 8]. There appears to be a slight male predominance [7, 8].

The constituent of an amyloid deposit can be determined by using immuno-histochemical staining, enzyme-linked immunosorbent assay, or liquid chromatography tandem mass spectrometry testing [9]. Localized amyloidosis is typically immunoglobulin light chain associated (AL type), [10–12], although serum amyloid A protein and transthyretin have been reported as causing localized disease [13–16]. Localized amyloidosis typically involves the laryngo-tracheobronchial tree, urogenital tract, and skin. However, all tissues may be involved, and other sites described include orbit, gastrointestinal, spine/bone, breast, and soft tissues [17–21]. Amyloid deposits have also been seen in association with certain malignancies, such as nasopharyngeal carcinoma, breast carcinoma, transitional cell carcinoma of bladder, and medullary thyroid carcinoma with histopathology showing amyloid deposits at the local sites of the tumor [22–27]. The etiology of localized amyloidosis is unknown, although multiple pathophysiologic mechanisms have been suggested. Histopathologic review of biopsy samples in cases of localized AL amyloid has shown infiltration with clonal and occasionally polyclonal plasma cells or lymphocytes [28–30]. In these cases the suggestion is that these cells do produce the abnormal protein responsible for the amyloid [31]. What initiates the migration of these cells into these areas is not clearly understood. Chronic inflammation and chronic infection may play a role. There is certainly more to this than chronic inflammation since these amyloid deposits tend to recur after initial treatment even in the absence of any chronic infection or inflammation. In the case of TTR-localized amyloid it may be associated with the avidity of such proteins for certain tissues as is seen in amyloid-associated carpal tunnel syndrome. In insulin-associated cutaneous amyloidoma it is clear that this is associated with exogenous insulin injection into the subcutaneous tissue which starts a cascade of events leading to amyloid formation.

Localized and systemic amyloidoses have different clinical presentation, clinical course, prognosis, and treatment [32–35]. It is therefore vital that all cases of suspected localized amyloid do have an extensive evaluation to rule out system disease, since this will impact on therapy. Localized amyloidosis is primarily a localized disease [36] without progression to systemic disease although rare cases of development of systemic disease several years after initial diagnosis have been reported [13].

Laryngo-tracheobronchial Amyloidosis

Laryngo-tracheobronchial amyloidosis is an uncommon localized form of amyloidosis, characterized by amyloid deposits restricted to the larynx, trachea, main bronchi, and segmental bronchi [7, 37, 38]. The actual incidence of localized laryngo-tracheobronchial amyloidosis in the general population is unknown.

Laryngo-tracheobronchial amyloidosis represents about 0.5% of all symptomatic laryngo-tracheobronchial lesions. Most patients usually present with symptoms and signs of upper airway inflammation or obstruction, which are intermittent and slowly progressive. The pathogenesis of localized laryngo-tracheobronchial amyloidosis in the upper airways has not been well defined. Chronic inflammatory conditions such as infection, allergens, and irritants in the upper airways may play a role in the pathogenesis of laryngo-tracheobronchial amyloidosis. Most cases are immunoglobulin light chain associated suggesting the possibility of chronic infection. Detailed histologic evaluation of biopsy specimen in most cases has shown local infiltration with clonal plasma cells most probably involved in the production of the amyloidogenic protein [28]. Cases of SAA laryngo-tracheobronchial amyloidosis support the chronic inflammation theory, but these are in the minority.

Diagnosis and Treatment

Presenting signs and symptoms usually depend on the location of the amyloid deposits. The most common site is the larynx. More than 50% of patients do present with hoarseness of voice [36, 39]. In severe cases complete loss of phonation may occur. Airway obstruction symptoms such as wheezing, stridor, and dyspnea at rest or on exertion are usually seen in these patients and may limit activity [40]. In these patients pulmonary function test may show features of proximal or upper airways obstruction. Dysphagia may occur although uncommon. The amyloid deposits tend to be friable and may bleed causing recurrent hemoptysis. Some patients do present with recurrent respiratory tract infection with persistent coughing [37, 39–42]. Most of these patients will have received various therapeutic interventions for respiratory infection or asthma without improve and may carry a diagnosis of reactive upper airway disease. Amyloidosis should be among the differential diagnosis in such patients during their evaluation.

Chest X-ray may show narrowing of the airway but most often is normal. Computer tomography offers the best radiologic evaluation and may help determine the extent of disease to aid in surgical treatment [43]. In most cases it will show nodules, plaques, or thickening of the airways with calcification. Severe narrowing of the airways with post-obstruction collapse may occur [44–46]. On laryngo-tracheobronchoscopy these may appear as firm, non-ulcerated epithelial nodule, submucosal plaques, tumors, or circumferential wall thickening [7]. Although certain morphologic characteristics may suggest amyloidosis, the definitive diagnosis is made on a histologic evaluation of a biopsy specimen. There appears to be an increased risk of bleeding with biopsy of the amyloid tissue [47], although some studies have shown no increased risk of bleeding [48]; however, care must be taken to reduce this complication. The diagnosis is confirmed by a biopsy specimen staining positive with Congo red dye and showing apple green birefringence when viewed under polarized light. Further subtyping by immunohistochemical staining or liquid chromatography tandem mass spectrometry testing of the amyloid deposits will help determine the origin of the amyloidogenic protein [49, 50]. Almost all localized laryngo-tracheobronchial amyloidosis are of immunoglobulin light chain origin, which is either immunoglobulin kappa or lambda light chain [12]. It is essential to rule out system disease in all patients suspected to have localized amyloidosis. Workup to exclude systemic disease should include evaluation for underlying plasma cell or B-cell lymphoproliferative disorder. Serum and 24-h urine protein electrophoresis with immunofixation must be negative for circulating monoclonal protein. Bone marrow biopsy and aspiration should be negative for involvement with clonal plasma cell or B-cell lymphoproliferative disorder and amyloid deposition. Abdominal sub-cutaneous fat aspirated should be negative for amyloid deposition [51].

There is no standard treatment for laryngo-tracheobronchial amyloidosis. The primary goal of therapy is preservation of organ function such as phonation and maintaining a stable patent airway [52]. Therapeutic intervention should be based on symptoms and extent of disease. Since progression may be slow, some patients can be monitored with routine evaluation using laryngo-tracheobronchoscopy and serial CT scans. In cases where therapeutic intervention is indicated, a multidisciplinary approach to evaluation and treatment is vital. This team must include an otolaryngologist, hematologist, and pulmonary physicians. Direct removal of the amyloid deposits is the most effective therapy currently used for localized laryngo-tracheobronchial amyloidosis. The type and distribution of the amyloid deposits do influence surgical treatment options. Nodular deposits can be easily removed whereas diffuse wall deposits cannot be surgically removed without major airway damage. Endoscopic approach such as micro-direct laryngoscopy with excision of amyloid deposits is usually the preferred method, although occasionally an open field surgical intervention is required [42, 43]. Endoscopy with removal of the amyloid deposits by neodymium:yttrium–aluminum–garnet (Nd:YAG) or carbon dioxide (CO_2) [7, 48, 53–55] is usually very effective in most cases and is able to control disease with improvement in symptoms such as stridor, dyspnea, and hoarseness of voice. In a retrospective review of 32 cases published by Piazza, all but 2 patients were endo-scopically treated with a median of two endoscopic procedures using Nd:YAG laser or CO_2 laser required to control initial disease [7]. In severe cases tracheostomy may be required before surgical removal of the amyloid deposits because of risk of bleeding, inflammation, and edema [28]. In Piazza's series 12.5% of patients required a tracheostomy. Stenting of significantly stenosed airways has been done in patients who are deemed not to be surgical candidates and are at significant risk of airway obstruction. External beam radiation therapy has been successfully used in a limited number of cases with prolonged remissions [56, 57]. The rationale has been the identification of clonal plasma cell in the amyloid deposits and the fact that plasma cells are highly radiosensitive. The typical dose has been 20–24 Gy [58]. In most of these case reports improvements in functional status, pulmonary function, bronchoscopic visualization, and CT-based luminal diameters after moderate-dose radiation therapy were achieved. Systemic therapies with corticosteroids, colchicine, and chemotherapy drugs have not shown any benefit and are not recommended [13]. Adjuvant treatment with drugs that reduce mucus secretion, antibiotic prophylaxis, nebulizers, and occasionally inhaled corticosteroid may provide transient symptom relieve. Laryngo-tracheobronchial amyloidosis is incurable and intermittent treatment may be required in a patient's life time [40, 41]. Although the prognosis of localized amyloidosis is better than systemic amyloidosis, it can still cause significant morbidity and mortality [32].

Localized Urogenital Tract Amyloidosis

Localized urogenital tract amyloidosis is a rare disease of the urogenital tract. The bladder appears to be the most common site, although it may involve all parts of the urinary tract such as the renal pelvis, ureter, and urethra [8, 59–61]. Ureteral involvement may be unilateral or bilateral [62, 63]. Amyloid deposition in the seminal vesicles and ejaculatory system has been noted in prostate biopsy specimen, although the clinical significance of this is unknown [64, 65]. The amyloid deposits are predominantly located in the lamina propria and muscularis propria although vessel wall involvement is not unusual. Almost all localized urogenital tract amyloidoses are of immunoglobulin light chain origin, which is either immunoglobulin kappa (25%) or lambda (50%) light chain [11, 61]. A few cases associated with SAA and TTR have been reported [61, 66–68]. The etiology of localized urogenital amyloidosis is unknown. It has been postulated that this may be due to chronic inflammation either from recurrent infection or other bladder irritants. It is essential to exclude systemic amyloidosis since systemic amyloidosis may involve all organs of the body including the urogenital tract. Workup to exclude systemic disease should include evaluation for underlying plasma cell or B-cell lymphoproliferative disorder. Serum and 24-h urine protein electrophoresis with immunofixation must be negative for circulating monoclonal protein. Bone marrow biopsy and aspiration should be negative for involvement with clonal plasma cell or B-cell lymphoproliferative disorder and subcutaneous fat aspirate should be negative for amyloid.

Diagnosis and Treatment

Most patients usually present with gross painless hematuria (62.5%) [8]. Obstructive and irritative urologic symptoms such as pain, anuria, recurrent infections, hydronephrosis, and rarely acute renal failure may occur [69]. Those with ureteral involvement may present with significant ureter obstruction and hydronephrosis resulting in flank pain and occasionally renal failure [62, 63, 70]. In a retrospective study of 31 patients seen at the Mayo Clinic, 24 (77%) had gross painless hematuria. In six of these patients, the hematuria was associated with irritative symptoms of the lower urinary tract such as dysuria, frequency, and nocturia. The remaining seven patients had only irritative lower urinary tract symptoms [61]. Most of these patients are usually suspected to have renal stones or malignancy. Urinalysis, urine culture, and cytology should be obtained as part of initial evaluation. Urinary cytology is an essential part of the evaluation and is usually negative for malignant cells. Evaluation with computer tomography scan, intravenous pyelography, and cytoscopy with biopsy will usually confirm the diagnosis. CT-urography is non-specific and tends to suggest a neoplasm or inflammation. Depending on the site of disease it may show ureteral obstruction, ureteral wall thickening, diffuse bladder wall thickening, filling defects, and focal masses [44]. Scattered calcification of these lesions is not uncommon. Under diagnostic flexible cystoscopy, amyloidosis of the urogenital tract may be seen as nodular masses with ulceration and occasionally active bleeding. It is not always possible to visually differentiate urothelial malignancy from amyloidosis and both have been simultaneously reported in patients [71, 72]. Multiple adequate biopsies are essential in order not to miss an underlying urogenital malignancy. Histologically the biopsies show amorphous eosinophilic material which stains positive with Congo red dye and show apple green birefringence when viewed under polarized light. Immunohistochemical stain typically shows the amyloid to be of immunoglobulin light chain origin consistent with AL amyloid with rare cases of AA and TTR types reported. There is a high predominance of lambda light chain [8, 11, 61, 69].

Transurethral resection followed in certain cases with dimethyl sulfoxide instillation into the bladder is the initial preferred treatment. For small localized lesions, fulguration or laser therapy may be adequate treatment. Transurethral resection alone is usually successful in controlling the disease in a significant number of cases [61, 73]. Extensive bladder surgery is usually not required, although in cases of uncontrollable massive hematuria, partial or total cystectomy has been performed.

The use of intravesical dimethyl sulfoxide therapy (DMSO) administration as an adjuvant may help prevent extensive surgery [74]. DMSO is believed to increase the solubility of amyloid fibrils and may reduce reaccumulation of amyloid protein. Diffuse or locally extensive bladder involvement usually fails to respond to conventional transurethral destructive surgical procedures. Intravesical DMSO can be a bladder saving measure and may help resolve ureterovesical obstruction in some patients [75, 76]. In a Mayo Clinic publication, six patients who continued to have symptomatic disease despite conventional transurethral destructive therapy were treated every 2 weeks with 30-min instillations of 50 mL 50% DMSO intravesically. Four patients had disease stabilization for 2–6 years [77]. Renal autotransplant has been performed in ureter amyloidosis with significant obstruction to help preserve kidney function [63, 70]. Regular follow-up is required because of a recurrence rate of 54% [61]. This should include urinalysis and cystoscopy. Urogenital localized amyloidosis is a localized disease with good prognosis. Systemic progression does not occur and therefore repeated evaluation for systemic disease without new symptoms suggestive of systemic disease is unnecessary and should be avoided [61, 78].

Cutaneous Amyloidosis

Cutaneous deposition of amyloid may represent localized disease or a manifestation of systemic amyloidosis. In primary localized cutaneous amyloidosis there is no visceral involvement and the disease is confined to the skin. Deposition of amyloid in the skin and the subcutaneous tissue can result in a variety of different skin lesions in patients with localized cutaneous amyloidosis. Primary localized cutaneous amyloidosis can be divided into three forms: macular, papula (lichenoid), and nodular forms. Cases having simultaneous features of macular, maculopapular, and lichenoid lesion are not uncommon. Majority of patients usually have the macular or lichenoid form of cutaneous amyloidosis [79–81]. The origin of the amyloid proteins in the macular and lichenoid forms of cutaneous amyloidosis is unknown [82]. It has, however, been postulated that these may arise from epidermal damage and filamentous degradation of keratinocytes with subsequent formation of amyloidogenic proteins. In the nodular form, the amyloid is of immunoglobulin light chain origin. There is, however, no demonstrable monoclonal protein in the serum and the immunoglobulin light chains are produced by clonal plasma cells located in the amyloid deposits [79, 83]. Patients presenting with the nodular form of amyloidosis should have a complete evaluation to exclude the possibility of systemic amyloidosis, including a serum and urine protein electrophoresis with immunofixation, a bone marrow biopsy, and an abdominal fat pad biopsy. In contrast to the lichenoid and macular forms, in the nodular variant the skin is more extensively involved with amyloid, with involvement of the dermal vessels. In lichenoid and macular amyloidosis the amyloid deposits are typically confined to the papillary dermis and do not involve adnexal structures. Macular and lichenoid amyloidosis may present as pruritic skin eruption [83, 84]. In macular amyloidosis, pigmented macules are seen on the back, chest, buttocks, and limbs [84]. These lesions may remain unchanged for several years. On the other hand lichenoid amyloidosis first presents as hyperkeratotic papules or plaques on the extensor surfaces of the limbs, and occasionally the abdominal and chest walls. Nodular localized cutaneous amyloidosis may be more extensive involving the extremities, trunk, genitals, or face [85]. Regional and racial differences in incidence have also been reported, with lichenoid amyloidosis common in the Chinese and macular in Middle Easterners, Central, and South Americans [81, 84, 86].

Diagnosis and Management

Although the history and clinical features of these skin lesions may suggest cutaneous amyloidosis, these are non-specific and a tissue biopsy showing the characteristic histologic features is required. More than one biopsy may be required to arrive at the diagnosis. The amyloid deposits stain positive with Congo red dye and show the characteristic apple green birefringence under polarized light. Other stains such as thioflavin T, periodic acid Schiff (PAS), triphenyl methane dye, and Van Gieson may be used. The fibrillar non-branching ultrastructure of the amyloid deposits can be confirmed by electron microscopy [87]. Lichenoid and macular amyloid may react with anti-keratin antibody, whereas primary systemic amyloid, secondary systemic amyloid, and familial amyloid usually stain negative [88]. This may be helpful in the evaluation of patients and confirmation of localized cutaneous amyloidosis.

Most patients with localized cutaneous amyloidosis can be monitored for several years without the need for therapy. Treatment may be recommended for patients with severe pruritus or for cosmetic reasons. The type of therapy will depend on the form of amyloidosis. Deposits of nodular primary cutaneous amyloidosis can be excised surgically or treated with carbon dioxide laser [89]. These lesions, however, tend to recur locally. For macular and lichenoid amyloid, therapeutic modalities such as antihistamines, intralesional corticosteroids, etretinate, and dermabrasion have been employed with variable success. Topical dimethyl sulfoxide (DMSO) 50% solution in water may offer some benefit. Ozkaya-Bayazit reported marked clinical improvement with rapid improvement of itching and flattening of papules in 9 out of 10 patients after 11 weeks of treatment [90]. However, relapses were seen in the follow-up period. Both PUVA and UVB phototherapy has also shown some promise in the management of this condition [91, 92].

Macular and lichenoid amyloidoses are primarily diseases of the cutaneous tissue and do not progress to systemic amyloidosis [81, 85], although there have been reported cases of progression several years after diagnosis. On the other hand risk of progression appears to be high in patients with the nodular variant of cutaneous amyloidosis. The relationship between this localized form of light chain deposition and primary systemic amyloidosis has been debated. Studies have shown almost no risk to nearly a fifth of these patients going on to develop systemic amyloidosis [85, 93, 94]. Patients with nodular amyloidosis who test negative for systemic involvement should be followed carefully in order to detect any evolution into a systemic disease by monitoring serum and urine with immunofixation annually.

Others Rare Forms of Localized Amyloidosis

Localized cutaneous amyloid deposits have been seen at sites of insulin injection [95, 96]. These are thought to be a reaction to the insulin and immunohistochemical staining with anti-insulin antibody is usually positive. These patients may present with insulin resistance and evaluation of the insulin injection sites usually will show subcutaneous nodules [83]. Changing the type of insulin formulation and rotating the sites of injection may reduce the amyloid deposits and also resolve the insulin resistance.

Localized orbit and adnexal amyloidoses do occur [97, 98]. Most are immunoglobulin light chain associated, but SAA cases have been reported. It should be emphasized for the clinician that localized amyloidosis of the conjunctiva and orbit is a benign disease without systemic implications. Limited surgical intervention for cosmetic reasons maybe indicated [99]. There have been cases of orbital amyloid deposition in association with localized MALT lymphoma. External beam radiotherapy following surgical debulking is an effective treatment [100].

Rarely isolated bone amyloidosis is seen in clinical practice [101]. In purely localized amyloid tumor of the bone there should be no evidence of plasmacytoma or multiple myeloma. The spine seems to be a common site. Depending on its location, emergency resection may be required such as when it involves the spine with cord compression [102–104]. The prognosis of this type of amyloidoma is excellent, and cure can be expected after local resection [103].

References

1. Westermark P, et al. A primer of amyloid nomenclature. Amyloid 2007;14(3):179–83.
2. Magy-Bertrand N, et al. Incidence of amyloidosis over 3 years: the AMYPRO study. Clin Exp Rheumatol. 2008;26(6):1074–8.
3. Kyle RA, et al. Incidence and natural history of primary systemic amyloidosis in Olmsted County, Minnesota, 1950 through 1989. Blood 1992;79(7):1817–22.
4. Mody G, Bowen R, Meyers OL. Amyloidosis at Groote Schuur Hospital, Cape Town. S Afr Med J. 1984;66(2):47–9.
5. Kyle RA, Bayrd ED. Amyloidosis: review of 236 cases. Medicine (Baltimore) 1975;54(4):271–99.
6. Ravid M, et al. Incidence and origin of non-systemic microdeposits of amyloid. J Clin Pathol. 1967;20(1):15–20.
7. Piazza C, et al. Endoscopic management of laryngo-tracheobronchial amyloidosis: a series of 32 patients. Eur Arch Otorhinolaryngol. 2003;260(7):349–54.
8. Merrimen JL, Alkhudair WK, Gupta R. Localized amyloidosis of the urinary tract: case series of nine patients. Urology 2006;67(5):904–9.
9. Olsen KE, Sletten K, Westermark P. The use of subcutaneous fat tissue for amyloid typing by enzyme-linked immunosorbent assay. Am J Clin Pathol. 1999;111(3):355–62.
10. Page DL, et al. Immunoglobulin origin of localized nodular pulmonary amyloidosis. Res Exp Med (Berlin). 1972;159(2):75–86.
11. Fujihara S, Glenner GG. Primary localized amyloidosis of the genitourinary tract: immunohistochemical study on eleven cases. Lab Invest 1981;44(1):55–60.
12. Berg AM, et al. Localized amyloidosis of the larynx: evidence for light chain composition. Ann Otol Rhinol Laryngol. 1993;102(11):884–9.
13. Paccalin M, et al. Localized amyloidosis: a survey of 35 French cases. Amyloid 2005;12(4):239–45.
14. Lew W, Seymour AE. Primary amyloid tumor of the breast. Case report and literature review. Acta Cytol. 1985;29(1):7–11.
15. Hill JC, Maske R, Bowen RM. Secondary localized amyloidosis of the cornea associated with tertiary syphilis. Cornea 1990;9(2):98–101.
16. Kyle RA, Gertz MA, Linke RP. Amyloid localized to tenosynovium at carpal tunnel release. Immunohistochemical identification of amyloid type. Am J Clin Pathol. 1992;97(2):250–53.
17. Lin PY, et al. Localized amyloidosis of the cornea secondary to trichiasis: clinical course and pathogenesis. Cornea 2003;22(5):491–94.
18. Krishnan J, et al. Tumoral presentation of amyloidosis (amyloidomas) in soft tissues. A report of 14 cases. Am J Clin Pathol. 1993;100(2):135–44.
19. Bisceglia M, et al. Primary amyloid tumor of the breast. Case report and review of the literature. Pathologica 1995;87(2):162–7.
20. Pasternak S, Wright BA, Walsh N. Soft tissue amyloidoma of the extremities: report of a case and review of the literature. Am J Dermatopathol. 2007;29(2):152–55.
21. Dutt S, et al. Secondary localized amyloidosis in interstitial keratitis. Clinicopathologic findings. Ophthalmology 1992;99(5):817–23.

22. Looi LM. The pattern of amyloidosis in Malaysia. Malays J Pathol. 1994;16(1):11–13.

23. Melato M, Manconi R, Falconieri G. Amyloidosis and lung cancer. A morphological and histochemical study. Morphol Embryol (Bucur). 1981;27(2):137–42.

24. Lynch LA, Moriarty AT. Localized primary amyloid tumor associated with osseous metaplasia presenting as bilateral breast masses: cytologic and radiologic features. Diagn Cytopathol. 1993;9(5):570–5.

25. Munichor M, et al. Localized amyloidosis in nasopharyngeal carcinoma diagnosed by fine needle aspiration and electron microscopy. A case report. Acta Cytol. 2000;44(4):673–8.

26. Prathap K, Looi LM, Prasad U. Localized amyloidosis in nasopharyngeal carcinoma. Histopathology 1984;8(1):27–34.

27. Sabate JM, et al. Localized amyloidosis of the breast associated with invasive lobular carcinoma. Br J Radiol. 2008;81(970):e252–4.

28. da Costa P, Corrin B. Amyloidosis localized to the lower respiratory tract: probable immunoamyloid nature of the tracheobronchial and nodular pulmonary forms. Histopathology 1985;9(7):703–10.

29. Setoguchi M, et al. Analysis of plasma cell clonality in localized AL amyloidosis. Amyloid 2000;7(1):41–5.

30. Hui AN, et al. Amyloidosis presenting in the lower respiratory tract. Clinicopathologic, radiologic, immunohistochemical, and histochemical studies on 48 cases. Arch Pathol Lab Med. 1986;110(3):212–8.

31. Hamidi Asl K, et al. Organ-specific (localized) synthesis of Ig light chain amyloid. J Immunol. 1999;162(9):5556–60.

32. Kerner MM, et al. Amyloidosis of the head and neck. A clinicopathologic study of the UCLA experience, 1955–1991. Arch Otolaryngol Head Neck Surg. 1995;121(7): 778–82.

33. Kyle RA, et al. Long-term survival (10 years or more) in 30 patients with primary amyloidosis. Blood 1999;93(3):1062–6.

34. Zhong YP, Wu YJ, Zhuang JL. A clinical analysis of 71 cases of amyloidosis. Zhonghua Nei Ke Za Zhi 2003;42(5):303–5.

35. Cazalets C, et al. Epidemiologic description of amyloidosis diagnosed at the University Hospital of Rennes from 1995 to 1999. La Revue de Medecine Interne. 2003;24(7): 424–30.

36. Ma L, et al. Primary localized laryngeal amyloidosis: report of 3 cases with long-term follow-up and review of the literature. Arch Pathol Lab Med. 2005;129(2):215–8.

37. Godbersen GS, et al. Organ-limited laryngeal amyloid deposits: clinical, morphological, and immunohistochemical results of five cases. Ann Otol Rhinol Laryngol. 1992;101(9):770–5.

38. Xu L, et al. Respiratory manifestations in amyloidosis. Chin Med J (Engl). 2005;118(24):2027–33.

39. Pribitkin E, et al. Amyloidosis of the upper aerodigestive tract. Laryngoscope 2003;113(12):2095–101.

40. Lewis JE, et al. Laryngeal amyloidosis: a clinicopathologic and immunohistochemical review. Otolaryngol Head Neck Surg. 1992;106(4):372–7.

41. Bartels H, et al. Laryngeal amyloidosis: localized versus systemic disease and update on diagnosis and therapy. Ann Otol Rhinol Laryngol. 2004;113(9):741–8.

42. Mitrani M, Biller HF. Laryngeal amyloidosis. Laryngoscope 1985;95(11):1346–7.

43. Kennedy TL, Patel NM. Surgical management of localized amyloidosis. Laryngoscope 2000;110(6):918–23.

44. Urban BA, et al. CT evaluation of amyloidosis: spectrum of disease. Radiographics 1993;13(6):1295–308.

45. Kim HY, et al. Localized amyloidosis of the respiratory system: CT features. J Comput Assist Tomogr. 1999;23(4):627–31.

46. Pickford HA, Swensen SJ, Utz JP. Thoracic cross-sectional imaging of amyloidosis. AJR Am J Roentgenol. 1997;168(2):351–5.

47. Yood RA, et al. Bleeding manifestations in 100 patients with amyloidosis. JAMA 1983;249(10):1322–4.
48. Utz JP, Swensen SJ, Gertz MA. Pulmonary amyloidosis. The Mayo Clinic experience from 1980 to 1993. Ann Intern Med. 1996;124(4):407–13.
49. Kebbel A, Rocken C. Immunohistochemical classification of amyloid in surgical pathology revisited. Am J Surg Pathol. 2006;30(6):673–83.
50. Kaplan B, et al. Biochemical subtyping of amyloid in formalin-fixed tissue samples confirms and supplements immunohistologic data. Am J Clin Pathol. 2004;121(6):794–800.
51. Duston MA, et al. Diagnosis of amyloidosis by abdominal fat aspiration. Analysis of four years' experience. Am J Med. 1987;82(3):412–4.
52. Heinritz H, Kraus T, Iro H. Localized amyloidosis in the area of the head-neck. A retrospective study. HNO. 1994;42(12):744–9.
53. Motta G, et al. CO(2)-laser treatment of laryngeal amyloidosis. J Laryngol Otol. 2003;117(8):647–50.
54. Madden BP, Lee M, Paruchuru P. Successful treatment of endobronchial amyloidosis using Nd:YAG laser therapy as an alternative to lobectomy. Monaldi Arch Chest Dis. 2001;56(1):27–9.
55. Capizzi SA, Betancourt E, Prakash UB. Tracheobronchial amyloidosis. Mayo Clin Proc. 2000;75(11):1148–52.
56. Kurrus JA, et al. Radiation therapy for tracheobronchial amyloidosis. Chest 1998;114(5):1489–92.
57. Monroe AT, et al. Tracheobronchial amyloidosis: a case report of successful treatment with external beam radiation therapy. Chest 2004;125(2):784–9.
58. Kalra S, et al. External-beam radiation therapy in the treatment of diffuse tracheobronchial amyloidosis. Mayo Clin Proc. 2001;76(8):853–6.
59. Stillwell TJ, Segura JW, Farrow GM. Amyloidosis of the urethra. J Urol. 1989;141(1):52–3.
60. Esslimani M, et al. Urogenital amyloidosis: clinico-pathological study of 8 cases. Ann Pathol. 1999;19(6):487–91.
61. Tirzaman O, et al. Primary localized amyloidosis of the urinary bladder: a case series of 31 patients. Mayo Clin Proc. 2000;75(12):1264–8.
62. Callaghan P, Asklin B. Ureteral obstruction due to primary localized amyloidosis. Scand J Urol Nephrol. 1993;27(4):535–6.
63. Yazaki T, et al. Renal autotransplantation for localized amyloidosis of the ureter. J Urol. 1982;128(1):119–21.
64. Kee KH, et al. Amyloidosis of seminal vesicles and ejaculatory ducts: a histologic analysis of 21 cases among 447 prostatectomy specimens. Ann Diagn Pathol. 2008;12(4):235–8.
65. Pitkanen P, et al. Amyloid of the seminal vesicles. A distinctive and common localized form of senile amyloidosis. Am J Pathol. 1983;110(1):64–9.
66. Farina Perez LA, Ortiz Rey JA. Secondary bladder amyloidosis with severe recurrent hematuria: transurethral Mikuliz procedure as hemostatic option. Arch Esp Urol. 2005;58(7):665–8.
67. Akram CM, et al. Primary localized AA type amyloidosis of urinary bladder: case report of rare cause of episodic painless hematuria. Urology 2006;68(6):1343 e15–7.
68. Boorjian S, et al. A rare case of painless gross hematuria: primary localized AA-type amyloidosis of the urinary bladder. Urology 2002;59(1):137.
69. Khan SM, et al. Localized amyloidosis of the lower genitourinary tract: a clinicopathological and immunohistochemical study of nine cases. Histopathology 1992;21(2):143–7.
70. Usami T, et al. A case of localized amyloidosis of the ureter treated by renal autotransplantation. Nippon Hinyokika Gakkai Zasshi. 1988;79(12):2031–6.
71. Shiramizu M, et al. Primary localized amyloidosis of the renal pelvis coexisting with transitional cell carcinoma: a case report. Hinyokika Kiyo 1992;38(6):699–702.
72. Johnston PW, Ewen SW. Localized amyloidosis and transitional cell carcinoma of the same ureter. Histopathology 1990;17(6):579–82.

73. Zaman W, et al. Localized primary amyloidosis of the genitourinary tract: does conservatism help? Urol Int. 2004;73(3):280–2.

74. Tokunaka S, et al. Experience with dimethyl sulfoxide treatment for primary localized amyloidosis of the bladder. J Urol. 1986;135(3):580–2.

75. Kato Y, et al. Localized amyloidosis of the ureter and bladder treated effectively by occlusive dressing technique therapy using dimethyl sulfoxide: a case report. Hinyokika Kiyo 2000;46(6):421–4.

76. Takeda T, Kozakai N, Ikeuchi K. Localized amyloidosis of the bladder treated effectively by occlusive dressing technique therapy using dimethyl sulfoxide (DMSO): two case reports. Nippon Hinyokika Gakkai Zasshi 2005;96(7):705–8.

77. Malek RS, et al. Primary localized amyloidosis of the bladder: experience with dimethyl sulfoxide therapy. J Urol. 2002;168(3):1018–20.

78. Duffau P, et al. Primary localized amyloidosis of the urinary tract. A case series of five patients. La Revue de Medecine Interne. 2005;26(4):288–93.

79. MacDonald DM, Black MM, Ramnarain N. Immunofluorescence studies in primary localized cutaneous amyloidosis. Br J Dermatol. 1977;96(6):635–41.

80. Kibbi AG, et al. Primary localized cutaneous amyloidosis. Int J Dermatol. 1992;31(2):95–8.

81. al-Ratrout JT, Satti MB. Primary localized cutaneous amyloidosis: a clinicopathologic study from Saudi Arabia. Int J Dermatol. 1997;36(6):428–34.

82. Eswaramoorthy V, et al. Macular amyloidosis: etiological factors. Tokyo J Dermatol. 1999;26(5):305–10.

83. Salim T, et al. Lichen amyloidosus: a study of clinical, histopathologic and immunofluorescence findings in 30 cases. Indian J Dermatol Venereol Leprol. 2005;71(3):166–9.

84. Rasi A, Khatami A, Javaheri SM. Macular amyloidosis: an assessment of prevalence, sex, and age. Int J Dermatol. 2004;43(12):898–9.

85. Brownstein MH, Helwig EB. The cutaneous amyloidoses. I. Localized forms. Arch Dermatol. 1970;102(1):8–19.

86. Wang WJ, et al. Clinical and histopathological characteristics of primary cutaneous amyloidosis in 794 Chinese patients. Zhonghua Yi Xue Za Zhi (Taipei). 2001;64(2):101–7.

87. Lin CS, Wong CK. Electron microscopy of primary and secondary cutaneous amyloidoses and systemic amyloidosis. Clin Dermatol. 1990;8(2):36–45.

88. Yoneda K, et al. Immunohistochemical staining properties of amyloids with anti-keratin antibodies using formalin-fixed, paraffin-embedded sections. J Cutan Pathol. 1989;16(3):133–6.

89. Alster TS, Manaloto RM. Nodular amyloidosis treated with a pulsed dye laser. Dermatol Surg. 1999;25(2):133–5.

90. Ozkaya-Bayazit E, Bayazit H, Ozarmagan G. Topical provocation in 27 cases of cotrimoxazole-induced fixed drug eruption. Contact Derm. 1999;41(4):185–9.

91. Jin AG, et al. Comparative study of phototherapy (UVB) vs. photochemotherapy (PUVA) vs. topical steroids in the treatment of primary cutaneous lichen amyloidosis. Photodermatol Photoimmunol Photomed. 2001;17(1):42–3.

92. Grimmer J, et al. Successful treatment of lichen amyloidosis with combined bath PUVA photochemotherapy and oral acitretin. Clin Exp Dermatol. 2007;32(1):39–42.

93. Woollons A, Black MM. Nodular localized primary cutaneous amyloidosis: a long-term follow-up study. Br J Dermatol. 2001;145(1):105–9.

94. Moon AO, Calamia KT, Walsh JS. Nodular amyloidosis: review and long-term follow-up of 16 cases. Arch Dermatol. 2003;139(9):1157–9.

95. Storkel S, et al. Iatrogenic, insulin-dependent, local amyloidosis. Lab Invest. 1983;48(1):108–11.

96. Swift B. Examination of insulin injection sites: an unexpected finding of localized amyloidosis. Diabet Med. 2002;19(10):881–2.

97. Hayasaka S, Setogawa T, Ohmura M. Secondary localized amyloidosis of the cornea caused by trichiasis. Ophthalmologica 1987;194(2–3):77–81.

98. Knowles DM II, et al. Amyloidosis of the orbit and adnexae. Surv Ophthalmol. 1975;19(6):367–84.

99. Di Bari R, et al. Primary localized orbital amyloidosis: a case report. Eur J Ophthalmol. 2006;16(6):895–7.

100. Khaira M, et al. The use of radiotherapy for the treatment of localized orbital amyloidosis. Orbit 2008;27(6):432–7.

101. Porchet F, Sonntag VK, Vrodos N. Cervical amyloidoma of C2. Case report and review of the literature. Spine 1998;23(1):133–8.

102. Mulleman D, et al. Primary amyloidoma of the axis and acute spinal cord compression: a case report. Eur Spine J. 2004;13(3):244–8.

103. Mizuno J, et al. Primary amyloidoma of the thoracic spine presenting with acute paraplegia. Surg Neurol. 2001;55(6):378–82.

104. Haridas A, et al. Primary isolated amyloidoma of the lumbar spine causing neurological compromise: case report and literature review. Neurosurgery 2005;57(1):E196 (discussion E196).

Chapter 8

Amyloid Heart Disease

Rodney H. Falk and Simon W. Dubrey

Abstract Cardiac involvement in patients with amyloidosis is common. It produces significant clinical symptoms in about 40% of patients with AL amyloidosis. A significant proportion of patients with familial amyloidosis have clinical involvement of the heart, and heart failure is almost always the presenting feature of senile systemic amyloidosis. The severity of the cardiac symptoms and the response to treatment vary depending upon the type of amyloid deposition. In this chapter, the different types of cardiac amyloidosis are reviewed and the diagnostic workup and appropriate therapies are addressed.

Keywords Amyloidosis, Congestive heart failure, Cardiomyopathy

Amyloid Heart Disease: General Overview

The heart is commonly involved in systemic amyloidosis and, when a diagnosis of amyloidosis in other organs has already been made, symptoms arising from the heart are readily attributable to its involvement by the disease. Unfortunately, when cardiac amyloidosis is an isolated disorder, or even when the cardiac manifestations of undiagnosed multi-organ amyloidosis predominate, the diagnosis is often not entertained and may be considerably delayed. Cardiac involvement varies both in severity and in prevalence among the various subtypes of amyloidosis. AL amyloidosis is associated with clinical cardiac involvement in about half the cases, although subclinical involvement may be detected in almost every case at autopsy or on endomyocardial biopsy. Transthyretin amyloidosis due to a mutant transthyretin is frequently associated with amyloid cardiomyopathy, although the prevalence of clinically significant cardiac disease varies depending upon the specific mutation. Several less common forms of amyloidosis are also associated with cardiac disease. Senile systemic amyloidosis is universally associated with cardiac disease which, other than carpal tunnel syndrome, is virtually the exclusive manifestation of the disease.

Common to all types of cardiac amyloidosis is a cardiomyopathy characterized by ventricular wall thickening in the absence of left ventricular dilation (Fig. 8-1). This thickening is due to amyloid infiltration of the myocardium and the greater the left ventricular mass, the greater the amyloid burden. As echocardiography is almost universally available and is usually one of the earliest tests employed in the investigation of suspected heart disease, the disease can be suspected by its echocardiographic appearance (Fig. 8-2). Unfortunately, even advanced cases of cardiac amyloidosis are sometimes misdiagnosed by cardiologists who are not attuned to these echocardiographic findings, and early stages of the disease are often

From: *Amyloidosis*, Contemporary Hematology,
Edited by: M.A. Gertz and S.V. Rajkumar, DOI 10.1007/978-1-60761-631-3_8,
© Springer Science+Business Media, LLC 2010

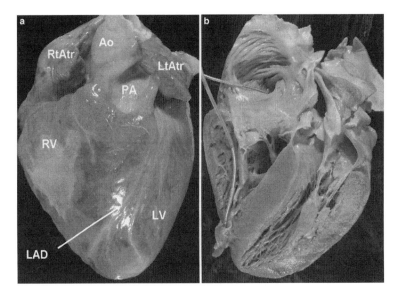

Fig. 8-1. (**a**) View of the heart in a patient with severe amyloid cardiomyopathy. The atria (*top* portion of the specimen) are firm and have not collapsed post-mortem, due to stiffening from amyloid infiltration. (**b**) Cut section of the same heart. ICD/pacing wires are seen in the right atrium (*upper* portion of figure) and right ventricular apex. Note the small right and left ventricular cavities with markedly thickened septum and LV free wall typical of amyloidosis.

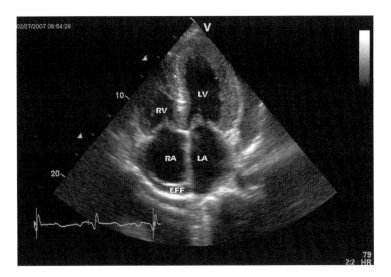

Fig. 8-2. Apical four chamber view of a 2D echocardiogram in a patient with advanced AL cardiomyopathy. The left ventricle (LV) and right ventricle (RV) have a normal cavity size with thick walls, whereas there is enlargement of both the right atrium (RA) and the left atrium (LA). A small pericardial effusion (PE) is present.

unrecognized despite a fairly typical appearance. This is most commonly because the wall thickening seen on echocardiography is mistakenly attributed to left ventricular hypertrophy, which is by far the commonest cause of thickened left ventricular walls. In true left ventricular hypertrophy, the electrocardiogram will show normal or increased QRS voltage, whereas the infiltrative nature of amyloidosis frequently results in low voltage [1, 2], which may on occasion be extreme (Fig. 8-3). Additional

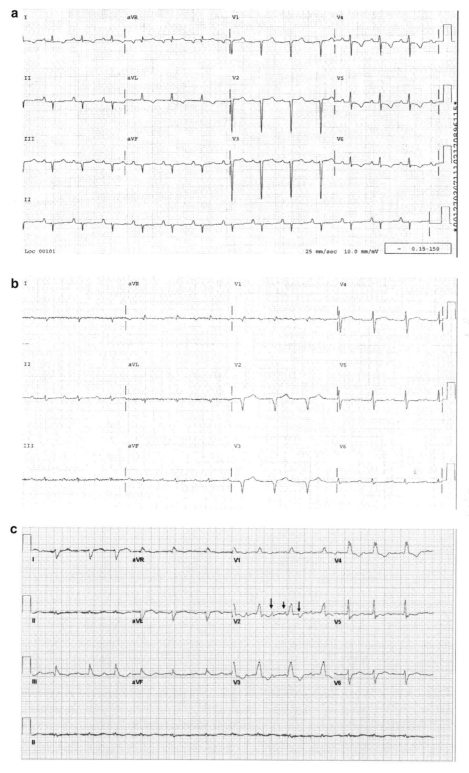

Fig. 8-3. Typical ECG appearances in cardiac amyloidosis. (**a**) Q waves in leads 2, 3 and aVf and in V1-3, suggestive of an old infarction. The patient had normal epicardial coronary arteries and AL amyloid cardiomyopathy. (**b**) Extreme low voltage in a patient with AL amyloidosis. (**c**) Low normal voltage with a marked right axis deviation and right bundle branch block pattern in a patient with senile cardiac amyloidosis. The rhythm is a slow atrial flutter, typical of senile amyloidosis and associated, in this patient, with a clinical deterioration despite a relatively well-controlled ventricular rate.

clues to an infiltrative cardiomyopathy on echocardiography include right ventricular free wall thickening (something that is rarely seen in hypertensive or valvular disease), prominent biatrial dilation, and diffuse valvular thickening. Tissue Doppler echocardiography, a technique that measures velocities within the myocardium (as opposed to standard Doppler echocardiography which evaluates velocity of blood flow within the cardiac chambers), is impaired both in true left ventricular hypertrophy and in amyloid heart disease. However, the impairment is much greater in amyloidosis than in other forms of heart disease.

Magnetic resonance imaging (MRI) is becoming a useful tool in assessing suspected or documented cardiac amyloidosis. In addition to the much greater accuracy of MRI compared to echocardiography for measuring right and left ventricular wall thickness, a distinctive pattern has been described in patients with cardiac amyloidosis (Fig. 8-4). This consists of ventricular wall thickening with a diffuse, predominantly subendocardial, "delayed enhancement" pattern of gadolinium uptake in the myocardium. The myocardial and blood pool kinetics of gadolinium uptake are also unusual in patients with cardiac amyloidosis [3]. Several investigators have attempted to correlate the presence of delayed gadolinium enhancement with prognosis in cardiac amyloidosis, but the small series and inclusion of some patients with minimal echocardiographic evidence of cardiac involvement makes interpretation difficult [4, 5]. It appears that the mere presence of delayed enhancement may not be a prognostic indicator when cardiac amyloidosis is present, but analysis of gadolinium kinetics may have prognostic value [6]. Most of the limited literature currently available is in patients with relatively advanced disease and it is unclear whether or not cardiac MR will be helpful in determining early cardiac involvement. The picture is further complicated by recent restrictions on the use of gadolinium in patients with renal impairment due to the potential for causing nephrogenic systemic fibrosis [7]. Despite the need for further work in this area, serial cardiac MR clearly has excellent potential for assessing the progress or regression of amyloidosis in the heart and will likely gain credence as a useful clinical tool.

[123]I-labeled serum amyloid P component has been extensively used in a few centers for imaging amyloid deposits but it does not image amyloid in the heart due to

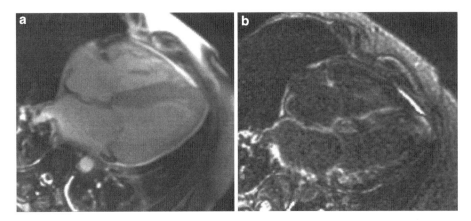

Fig. 8-4. (**a**) Cardiac MRI in advanced amyloid cardiomyopathy showing thickened ventricular and atrial septum. (**b**) Delayed gadolinium enhancement in the same patient—the white areas in the ventricular and atrial walls are abnormal and represent delayed gadolinium uptake in a typical distribution for cardiac amyloidosis.

blood pool uptake [8]. ^{99m}Tc-aprotinin has been quite successful as an isotope for cardiac imaging and may be fairly specific for cardiac amyloidosis [9]. However, experience is limited, and the focus on newer echocardiographic techniques and cardiac MR has steered interest away from radioisotope imaging.

The gross pathologic features of amyloid cardiomyopathy reflect the findings seen on echocardiography. Histologically, the myocardial cells are separated and distorted by amyloid deposition [10] (Fig. 8-5). Intramyocardial vessels are frequently infiltrated by amyloid deposits, resulting in impaired vasodilation, which may result in myocardial ischemia. On very rare occasions, amyloid deposits have been found in epicardial vessels resulting in obstructive coronary artery disease indistinguishable on coronary angiography from cholesterol-laden plaques. Although the predominant manifestation of amyloid heart disease is congestive heart failure due to myocardial infiltration with resultant impairment in left ventricular compliance (diastolic dysfunction), amyloid cardiomyopathy may rarely present with small vessel involvement and minimal or no myocardial infiltration. In such cases, the presenting complaint may be angina pectoris or significant systolic dysfunction (with no or only mild left ventricular dilation) due to chronic myocardial ischemia. Diagnosis of amyloidosis in such cases is extremely difficult unless an endomyocardial biopsy is performed or unless involvement of other organs in the typical fashion suggests the diagnosis. The atria are involved in all types of cardiac amyloidosis, as is the conduction system of the heart [11]. Severe atrial infiltration may lead to atrial standstill in the presence of electrical sinus rhythm [12]. In such cases, the prevalence of atrial thrombus formation is high (Fig. 8-6), and thromboembolism may be the initial manifestation of the disease [13–15]. Atrial arrhythmias (fibrillation, flutter, or atrial tachycardia) tend to occur late in the disease. Significant ventricular arrhythmias have been described, but are uncommonly seen, possibly because the initial episode of ventricular tachycardia or fibrillation in such a compromised heart may cause instantaneous, nonresuscitatable cardiac arrest.

The left ventricular ejection fraction in cardiac amyloidosis is often normal even in the presence of congestive heart failure. However, this does not necessarily reflect pure diastolic dysfunction. Left ventricular ejection fraction is primarily calculated, or estimated visually, from the contraction of the heart along its short axis. However, the subendocardial myocytes are longitudinally oriented and are particularly susceptible to damage. Tissue Doppler imaging can evaluate longitudinal contraction of

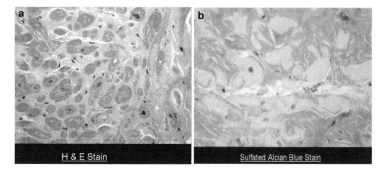

Fig. 8-5. (**a**) H and E stain showing extensive amyloid infiltration of the myocardium (*light pink*) which distorts and separates the myocytes (*darker pink*). (**b**) Staining with sulfated *Alcian blue* (another patient) shows typical amyloid staining with turquoise staining of the amyloid and yellow myocyte staining.

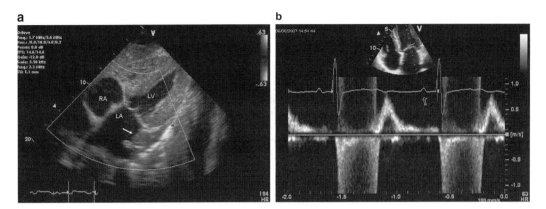

Fig. 8-6. (**a**) Subcostal view of the heart in a patient with sinus rhythm and end-stage amyloid cardiomyopathy. The *arrow* points to a thrombus filling the left atrial appendage. (**b**) Doppler echocardiography and ECG in a patient with cardiac amyloidosis and atrial failure. The *arrow* indicates the P-wave of the ECG confirming sinus rhythm, whereas the Doppler flow across the mitral valve, seen between the two downward systolic "bars" of Doppler flow (representing mitral regurgitation), is notable for the absence of any flow following the P-wave, representing atrial failure.

the heart and demonstrates that longitudinal systolic dysfunction is universal, and disproportionately severe, in amyloid heart disease compared both to other types of heart disease and to the degree of left ventricular ejection fraction impairment [16–19]. In addition to direct infiltration by amyloid deposits, there is probably additional myocardial ischemia caused by compression and infiltration of small vessels; there is some evidence that this may be greater in AL amyloidosis than in other types [20].

Clinical Findings

The common clinical feature among the various forms of cardiac amyloidosis is the presence of congestive heart failure associated with a non-dilated left ventricle with thickened walls and a normal or mildly reduced left ventricular ejection fraction. Because the disease affects all parts of the heart, biventricular heart failure is usually present, although the presenting feature is often that of severe right-sided heart failure. Peripheral edema may be profound and ascites is not uncommon. Careful physical examination is important in order not to miss the cardiac etiology of the presenting symptoms. When cardiac ascites or congestive hepatomegaly is present the jugular venous pressure is always elevated, often to the angle of the jaw. However, if attention is not given to the elevated neck veins, a diagnosis of heart failure may initially be missed, particularly if attention is misdirected by the report of a normal ejection fraction on echocardiogram.

Once the disease is suspected, a histological diagnosis needs to be made. In many cases, amyloid deposition can be found in the fat, and an abdominal fat pad biopsy is a simple procedure with a relatively high yield. A higher yield will be obtained from a cardiac biopsy in suspected cardiac amyloidosis although this carries the usual risks of endomyocardial biopsy. A negative cardiac biopsy in suspected cardiac amyloidosis usually rules out the disease, as infiltration is widespread and is almost always found in a biopsy specimen. Once a positive biopsy has been obtained, it is critical to determine the type of amyloid, as this determines the treatment. The specific types of cardiac amyloidosis are discussed below.

Types of Amyloidosis and Heart Involvement

AL Amyloidosis

AL amyloidosis is probably the most commonly recognized form of amyloid heart disease. While organ dysfunction is predominantly due to infiltration of the heart by amyloid deposits, there is evidence that amyloidogenic light chains may also be inherently cytotoxic. Indirect evidence supporting a toxic component in AL amyloidosis comes from clinical observation. Patients with cardiac AL amyloidosis and evidence of active disease have a far worse prognosis than patients with transthyretin amyloidosis despite similar echocardiographic appearances and, after successful chemotherapy, patients with AL amyloidosis frequently have significant improvement in symptoms of heart failure with associated decrease in B-natriuretic peptide (BNP) and serum troponin despite unchanged echocardiographic appearance [21]. Experimental in vitro data also suggest cardiotoxicity of amyloidogenic light chains, possibly related to oxidative stress [22, 23].

The echocardiogram in AL amyloidosis is indistinguishable from that in other forms of cardiac amyloidosis [24] and, as noted above, is characterized by biventricular thickening, biatrial enlargement, restrictive hemodynamics, and a small cavity with a relatively preserved ejection fraction. Most patients have evidence of extracardiac involvement, most commonly heavy proteinuria. Other organs that are commonly involved include the peripheral and autonomic nervous systems, liver, and skin. Periorbital purpura is relatively common and, in the presence of a positive biopsy for amyloid, is virtually pathognomonic for AL amyloidosis. Confirmatory diagnosis of AL cardiac amyloidosis does not necessarily require endomyocardial biopsy if the echocardiogram is typical and if a positive biopsy for amyloid has been obtained from another site. However, cardiac biopsy may be useful if there is no extracardiac disease or in a patient with a history of hypertension and ventricular wall thickening who has evidence of amyloidosis elsewhere but in whom the cause of wall thickening is uncertain. In skilled hands, endomyocardial biopsy is generally a safe procedure and the generalized nature of myocardial involvement in amyloidosis of any type virtually guarantees a positive biopsy if the disease is present in the heart. While we favor immunofluorescence with a panel of antibodies and performed on a fresh, non-preserved biopsy sample [25], to determine the precise type of amyloid, several other techniques, discussed elsewhere in this book, are equally valuable [26].

In the absence of treatment, the natural history of AL amyloidosis is rapidly progressive, with death occurring within 2 years in about 80% of patients [27]. AL amyloid presenting with heart failure has a very poor prognosis, with a median survival as low as 4 months [28]. Merlini and coworkers were the first to suggest that the circulating level of N-terminal pro-B-natriuretic peptide (NT-proBNP), the terminal fragment of the prohormone proBNP, had a prognostic implication in AL amyloidosis [29]. In a multivariate analysis, NT-proBNP appeared to be more sensitive than conventional echocardiographic parameters in detecting clinical improvement or worsening of amyloid cardiomyopathy during follow-up. Other investigators, using either NT-proBNP or BNP, have reported similar results. It has been suggested that elevation of BNP in amyloidosis is not only a function of the presence of congestive heart failure, but may reflect the hormone production by cardiac myocytes compressed by amyloid deposits [30]. Electron microscopy has revealed higher densities of BNP granules in myocytes abutting amyloid deposits [31], and patients with echocardiographic evidence of cardiac amyloidosis have similar BNP elevations to those with overt heart failure, suggesting that left ventricular filling pressure is not the only determinant of BNP levels [30]. Cardiac troponin T (TnT) and cardiac troponin I (TnI) are regulatory proteins of the myofilament that are exclusively expressed by the heart and that are elevated with myocardial injury. Utilizing high-sensitivity troponin assays, it can be shown that a significant proportion of patients with cardiac amyloidosis have elevation of troponin. A staging system, utilizing serum levels of BNP or NT-proBNP in conjunction with serum TnT, has been developed and may be of value in helping to select patients who have a suitable risk for high-dose chemotherapy and autologous stem cell transplant [32, 33]. In the authors' opinion, these serum biomarkers are a useful adjunct to the clinical history and physical examination combined with echocardiography but certainly do not substitute for either.

There are several unusual presentations of cardiac involvement in AL amyloidosis. An occasional patient is seen in whom electrocardiographic features of left ventricular hypertrophy are present on the electrocardiogram despite the absence of hypertension or valve disease [34]. These patients often have a relatively hyperdynamic left ventricle with significant left ventricular thickening. Heart failure may be mild and, despite the increased thickness of the left ventricle, they may, from a cardiac standpoint, tolerate aggressive therapy relatively well. It is not clear whether this ECG finding represents true hypertrophy of the cardiac myocytes as a reaction to the amyloid infiltration or whether there is another mechanism. Cardiac amyloidosis is associated with a small left ventricular cavity and, if the ejection fraction is relatively well preserved and wall thickening is considerable, left ventricular outflow tract obstruction mimicking hypertrophic cardiomyopathy may occasionally occur [35, 36]. If these patients are mistaken for true hypertrophic cardiomyopathy and are treated with verapamil or diltiazem they may experience worsening of heart failure, and this is a clue to the presence of amyloidosis [37]. Classical angina with minimal epicardial coronary artery disease is a feature of cardiac amyloidosis. It is not uncommon in patients with typical amyloid cardiomyopathy but a very small percentage of patients may have normal or minimally thickened walls [38–40]. Unless there is other organ involvement in such cases, the diagnosis is often not apparent and requires an endomyocardial biopsy. Biopsy in such cases reveals perivascular amyloid, which results in impaired small vessel vasodilation. Small vessel amyloid may also occur in the jaw, leading to jaw claudication on chewing and occasionally in the limb muscles resulting in exertional claudication [41–43]. Even more rare is the development of severe systolic dysfunction with minimal or no left ventricular wall thickening. Unlike classical dilated cardiomyopathy in which the ventricular cavity may be markedly enlarged, patients with amyloidosis who present primarily with systolic dysfunction tend to have a normal or minimally dilated left ventricle. The most likely etiology is small vessel amyloid leading to global myocardial ischemia. Valvular involvement with amyloid deposition is not uncommon in systemic amyloidosis but rarely causes significant valvular dysfunction. It almost invariably occurs in the setting of significant myocardial infiltration. Microscopic amyloid deposits have been found in a high proportion of valves excised at the time of valve replacement in patients without systemic amyloidosis. The biochemical composition of these deposits is unclear, but they do not seem to be of clinical importance [44].

Treatment of AL Cardiac Amyloidosis

The approach to management of AL cardiac amyloidosis is twofold: treatment of the heart failure and treatment of the underlying plasma cell dyscrasia. Patients with AL amyloidosis of the heart tend to respond poorly to conventional heart failure therapies. Careful titration of diuretics and salt restriction remains the mainstay of management. Calcium channel blockers have no role in the management and their use is often associated with significant worsening of heart failure [37]. Despite the presence of severe diastolic dysfunction, there is no evidence of a beneficial effect of beta blockers except in atrial fibrillation, in which they should be used with caution due to their negative inotropic effects. There is no role for digoxin in patients with cardiac amyloidosis who are in sinus rhythm. However, for patients with atrial fibrillation, cautious use of digoxin may aid in heart rate control although the risk of digoxin toxicity may be increased, possibly related to abnormal binding of the drug to amyloid fibrils. Angiotensin-converting enzyme (ACE) inhibitors and angiotensin receptor blockers are rarely tolerated in AL amyloidosis and may provoke profound hypotension if used. This may be because vascular tone in this condition is disproportionately related to angiotensin receptors, because of impaired sympathetic nervous system function.

Hypotension in AL cardiac amyloidosis may be due to low cardiac output, autonomic neuropathy, or impaired vascular tone due to amyloid infiltration. If autonomic neuropathy is present, the alpha-agonist midodrine can be effective, although the effect is usually modest. Orthostatic hypotension may require thigh-high support stockings. Fludrocortisone is generally not tolerated in cardiac amyloidosis due to its sodium-retaining effects. If permanent pacing is needed for atrioventricular block, strong consideration should be given to biventricular pacing, as right ventricular pacing alone may further decrease the already impaired stroke volume. Unless sustained ventricular tachycardia has been documented, there appears to be little role for implantable defibrillators as most cases of sudden death in cardiac amyloidosis are due to electromechanical dissociation [45]. We have generally found that, among patients in whom a defibrillator is implanted, the defibrillation threshold is within acceptable range. However, extensive amyloid infiltration has occasionally been associated with elevated defibrillation threshold and, in such cases, novel lead types may be of value [46].

Treatment of the underlying plasma cell dyscrasia currently requires chemotherapy directed toward the underlying clonal plasma cell disease, with the objective of abolishing, or at least significantly reducing, the production of the amyloidogenic monoclonal light chains. Resolution of light chain production with chemotherapy is associated with a reduction of serum NT-proBNP and improvement in survival [21]. High-dose chemotherapy with melphalan supported by autologous stem cell transplantation has been used increasingly in AL amyloidosis [47, 48]. Response rates in terms of clonal disease remission are encouragingly high, but the procedure is associated with a high incidence of treatment-related mortality, which tends to concentrate among patients with cardiac involvement. Of 312/701 AL patients deemed eligible for high-dose chemotherapy, the median survival was 4.6 years. A complete hematologic response was achieved in 40%, although the mortality rate in the first 100 days was 13% [48]. Survival was poorer among patients with cardiac amyloidosis compared to those who had no evidence of heart involvement. In a comparative study of high-dose chemotherapy with melphalan and associated autologous stem cell transplant compared to a regimen of melphalan plus dexamethasone, no difference in survival was found although there was a trend toward better survival among patients with cardiac involvement who were treated with oral therapy [49]. Although high-dose chemotherapy with stem cell transplant has been successfully used in a significant number of patients with cardiac disease, results tend to be better in experienced centers and the published data argue that, for most physicians outside the few specialized centers treating cardiac amyloidosis, therapy should be initiated with an oral regimen and then assessing response.

Regimens using thalidomide, lenalidomide, and bortezomib with or without associated steroid use are showing promise although have been cases of increased congestive heart failure among patients with severe cardiac involvement treated with bortezomib. A report of 22 consecutive patients with AL amyloidosis and New York Heart Association class IV heart failure highlights the very high mortality in this disease despite treatment by expert physicians [50]. All patients were treated with a combination of daily thalidomide, with 4 days per month of melphalan and reduced-intensity dexamethasone. Three patients were unable to tolerate the dexamethasone due to fluid retention and six died before completing the third cycle. The median survival for the whole group was less than 6 months and only four had a durable survival. The authors noted a delay in diagnosis of over a year from the onset of symptoms in 45% of patients and stressed the importance of the need for a high suspicion of amyloidosis in order to lead to an earlier diagnosis. They also addressed the importance of considering heart transplantation in suitable patients, given the dismal prognosis of severe heart failure in AL amyloidosis.

Heart Transplantation

The decision to consider a patient with AL amyloidosis for heart transplantation is a complex one. The majority of patients have significant amyloid involvement of other organs rendering them unsuitable for cardiac transplantation. Cardiac transplantation alone does not affect the underlying systemic disorder and amyloid deposition will continue unless the plasma cell dyscrasia is addressed. Thus, the pros and cons of treatment of the plasma cell dyscrasia in a patient with severe cardiac amyloidosis have to be weighed against possibility of early transplantation of the heart.

Early attempts at cardiac transplantation in AL amyloidosis did not address the underlying disease, resulting in a short-term improvement followed by death from progressive amyloidosis in the majority of patients [51, 52]. Indeed, in some cases the transplanted heart itself was the site of recurrent amyloidosis [53]. The results of heart transplantation in the UK for patients with amyloidosis were reported for a total of 24 patients, of whom 17 had AL and 7 had non-AL amyloid [54]. These 24 patients represent only 0.44% of the heart transplants performed in the UK between 1984 and 2002. Regardless of the use of adjunctive chemotherapy in some cases, the 5-year survival after heart transplantation for cardiac AL amyloidosis was generally poorer than following heart transplantation for other indications as progression of the systemic disease contributed to the increased mortality. The United States' experience was recently summarized based on a retrospective analysis of the national database of United Network of Organ Sharing (UNOS) [55]. Between 1987 and 2001, 69 patients who had been transplanted for amyloid heart disease were identified, with a mean age of 51 years. There were five intra-operative deaths and the 1-year actuarial survival was 74.6% compared to 81.6% for all other patients undergoing cardiac transplantation during the same period. The 5-year survival was 54% versus 63.3%, respectively, and 9 of the 29 late deaths were said to be of amyloid-related complications. However, the authors did not describe the type of amyloidosis, the concomitant disease, or whether or not adjunctive chemotherapy was given. Similar data have been recently reported from Spain, with a suggestion that AL amyloidosis may fare worse after cardiac transplantation than do other types [56].

Heart transplantation followed by autologous stem cell transplantation has been reported in a limited number of patients. A recent report describes five patients undergoing combined sequential transplants, of whom two died of progressive amyloidosis at 33 and 90 months following heart transplantation. The remaining three patients were well at the time the report was published [57]. Physicians at Columbia

Presbyterian Medical Center in New York have described their experience with cardiac transplantation in 12 patients with cardiac amyloidosis who received a heart transplant with "extended donor criteria" [58]. Extended donor criteria hearts were defined as cardiac allografts "not traditionally considered for cardiac transplantation because of advanced donor age, concomitant non-obstructive coronary artery disease, inability to obtain a cardiac catheterization, mild left ventricular hypertrophy, prolonged ischemic time, or positive donor serologies for hepatitis C." The availability and use of such hearts shortens the waiting list and, although possibly associated with a decreased survival compared to more traditional donor hearts [59]. Twelve patients had AL amyloidosis and two had familial amyloidosis. Eight of the ten with AL amyloidosis also underwent high-dose chemotherapy with autologous stem cell transplantation and the two familial patients underwent liver transplantation in addition to heart transplantation. The 1-year survival of the group was 75% compared to 25% in 13 patients who were evaluated for transplantation but did not receive a heart. At the Mayo Clinic between 1994 and 2005, 11 patients with AL amyloidosis underwent sequential orthoptic heart transplantation followed by autologous stem cell transplantation [60]. Two patients died of complications of stem cell transplant. Three patients subsequently died from progressive amyloidosis at 66, 57, and 55 months after stem cell transplant. The 1- and 5-year heart transplant survival rates were 82 and 65%, respectively, with a median survival of 76 months from heart transplantation and 57 months from stem cell therapy. The authors concluded that aggressive treatment of the underlying plasma cell dyscrasia after heart transplant is feasible and may improve long-term outcome in patients with cardiac amyloidosis. At the Massachusetts General Hospital, 16 of 21 patients with AL cardiac amyloidosis evaluated for cardiac transplantation were listed, nine of whom died while waiting for an organ. All of the remaining seven underwent cardiac transplantation followed by high-dose chemotherapy and autologous stem cell transplantation. There was no treatment-related mortality to the chemotherapy but long-term follow-up is still pending (Semigran, personal communication). Similar experiences have recently been reported from groups in Europe [56, 57, 61, 62] and successful cardiac transplantation has been reported following high-dose chemotherapy and autologous transplant [63]. One patient with AL amyloidosis in whom successful combined heart–kidney transplant was performed without subsequent high-dose chemotherapy has been reported [64].

While it appears possible to perform combined cardiac transplantation and autologous stem cell transplantation in patients with light chain amyloidosis, precise criteria for the optimal candidate for this aggressive therapy have not been formalized. There is, however, a general informal consensus among experts in this field that the disease should be clinically isolated to the heart at the time of cardiac transplantation. There should be no significant proteinuria (less than 500 mg/24 h), no significant neuropathy, and clinically significant hepatic involvement should be excluded. Generally, hepatic involvement in amyloidosis is characterized by an elevated alkaline phosphatase in conjunction with hepatomegaly but, as liver enlargement may be secondary to right heart failure without amyloid infiltration, liver biopsy may be needed in equivocal cases. Chemotherapy and autologous stem cell transplantation are generally performed within 6 months to 1 year of heart transplantation in order to avoid further amyloid deposition. Chemotherapy should be performed by hematologists familiar with stem cell transplantation and in a center that also regularly performs cardiac transplantation so that the patient and his/her immunosuppressive therapy can be monitored carefully. Whether or not the extended donor criteria will prove equivalent to standard donor criteria in these patients remains unclear but, in our opinion, precise attention to selection criteria should be performed regardless of the donor heart status.

Prevention of Sudden Cardiac Death

Sudden cardiac death is common in patients with AL amyloidosis involving the heart. In most other cardiac diseases associated with sudden death, such as coronary artery disease, dilated and hypertrophic cardiomyopathy, ventricular fibrillation is the commonest etiology of sudden death and the implantable cardioverter defibrillator (ICD), used either as a prophylactic or therapy or implanted in a survivor of aborted sudden death, has convincingly been shown to prolong life. Although isolated cases of recurrent ventricular arrhythmia with appropriate ICD function have been documented in cardiac amyloidosis, the majority of deaths appear to be due to pulseless electrical activity, an event not generally amenable to therapy [65]. In a series of 19 patients with either non-sustained ventricular tachycardia or high-grade ventricular arrhythmia treated with a prophylactic ICD, only two received shocks for sustained arrhythmia whereas there were six deaths due to electromechanical dissociation [45].

Hereditary Amyloidosis

Hereditary forms of cardiac amyloidosis are usually associated with mutation in the gene for the plasma protein transthyretin (TTR) and are referred to as ATTR. About 100 different amyloidogenic missense point mutations have been described [66], and the heart is a frequent target for deposition in ATTR amyloidosis. The amyloid deposits are composed of a combination of amyloid derived from mutant TTR and wild-type TTR [67, 68].

Patients with ATTR amyloidosis may present with neuropathy, cardiomyopathy, or a combination of both. Neuropathy most frequently presents as a progressive sensorimotor and/or autonomic neuropathy. In some cases, the cardiomyopathy predominates and the patient presents with heart failure. However, myocardial infiltration can be severe in non-AL amyloid before heart failure develops and, if the predominant clinical manifestation is neuropathy, an associated cardiomyopathy may be overlooked unless echocardiography is performed. Macroglossia is not a feature, although carpal tunnel syndrome may be an early indicator of the disease. The penetrance of hereditary forms of amyloidosis is variable, may vary from kindred to kindred despite the same mutation and some individuals with the genotype may not develop clinical disease. The most common transthyretin mutation is the substitution of isoleucine for valine at position 122 (Val122Ile), which is present in up to 4% of African-Americans [69]. Val122Ile is almost exclusively found in patients of African descent, although a single case has been described in a Caucasian [70]. The predominant feature is a severe cardiomyopathy with minimal or no neuropathy, with the age at presentation usually around 60 years. Because of the high prevalence of hypertension and associated left ventricular hypertrophy in the older African-American population, the echocardiogram may be mistaken for hypertensive heart disease. However, hypertensive heart failure rarely presents with right heart failure, whereas this is the commonest manifestation of amyloid heart disease. The presentation in an African-American patient of left ventricular thickening disproportionate to any history or degree of hypertension, particularly when associated with right ventricular thickening and normal to low voltage on the electrocardiogram, should point strongly to amyloidosis.

Variants of apolipoprotein-AI (Apo-AI) can also cause amyloid heart disease [26, 71]. Wild-type Apo-AI has a tendency to form amyloid fibrils, but this is localized within intravascular atherosclerotic plaques [72]. Apo-AI mutations can cause renal disease, which presents with progressive renal failure in the absence of proteinuria. In a proportion of these patients a progressive cardiomyopathy and heart failure occur. The precursor protein of fibrinogen amyloidosis is expressed in the liver and the disease usually presents with progressive renal disease. Combined liver–kidney transplantation has been successfully performed [73]. Amyloidosis due to fibrinogen mutations almost exclusively affects the kidney [74], although rare cases with cardiac involvement have been described [75]. A rarer form of hereditary amyloidosis includes variant gelsolin type [76]. Cardiac involvement by the gelsolin type is usually restricted to conduction disease [77] and may require a permanent cardiac pacemaker.

Management of Hereditary Forms of Amyloid Heart Disease

Although the echocardiographic features of ATTR and AL amyloidosis are indistinguishable, patients with familial cardiac amyloidosis have a much more indolent course, and congestive heart failure is generally easier to control [24]. In the absence of autonomic neuropathy, ACE inhibitors may be tolerated as may low-dose beta blockers. Renal involvement is not a feature of ATTR amyloidosis although significant azotemia may develop late in the disease as cardiac output falls. At present, the only specific treatment for the transthyretin, fibrinogen [78], and apolipoprotein [73] amyloidoses is organ transplantation. Orthotopic liver transplantation is widely performed for TTR-associated familial amyloid polyneuropathy [79]. Although this has proved very successful in halting and even reversing clinical disease associated with TTR Val30Met, particularly when treated early, paradoxical accelerated progression of cardiac amyloidosis has occurred following liver transplantation in many patients with non-Val30Met TTR variants [80–82]. It is believed that this is due to continued deposition of wild-type transthyretin in the heart, and there is now some evidence that wild-type transthyretin cardiac deposition may preferentially occur after liver transplantation [83–85]. If feasible, combined heart and liver transplantation should be considered for selected patients with hereditary TTR amyloidosis who have significant cardiac amyloidosis at presentation [86, 87].

In fibrinogen-related amyloidosis the precursor protein is expressed in the liver, and liver transplantation has been successfully utilized [88]. Limited experience with hereditary apolipoprotein-AI amyloidosis suggests that amyloid recurs in solid organ transplants remarkably slowly in the absence of any measure to reduce production of the respective amyloidogenic apolipoprotein-AI variant. Combined cardiac and renal transplants have been performed in patients with hereditary apolipoprotein-AI amyloidosis, with excellent long-term results [89]. Successful combined liver and kidney transplantation is also described for apolipoprotein-AI amyloidosis [90]. Overall, the 5-year survival after heart transplantation for non-AL amyloid, combined in some cases with liver or kidney transplantation, is similar to that after heart transplantation in general. The major contraindication to heart transplantation in familial amyloidosis is the presence of severe associated neuropathy. In considering cardiac transplantation in patients with ATTR amyloidosis, strong consideration should be given also to transplanting the liver to prevent further mutant transthyretin production. As the liver otherwise functions normally, the explanted organ can be transplanted into another patient requiring liver transplantation (domino transplantation) [91, 92], and there have even been cases of split domino transplantation in which the liver from the amyloid patients is given to two recipients The development of amyloid deposits several years after receiving such a liver has now been described in a small number of patients [93, 94].

Potential New Therapies

Elucidation of aspects of the molecular pathogenesis of amyloid and amyloidosis is generating a variety of novel approaches to therapy [95–98]. Small molecule ligands that stabilize the native tetrameric structure of TTR and prevent its fibrillogenesis are being actively investigated for prophylaxis and therapy in TTR amyloidosis [99–103]. The non-steroidal anti-inflammatory diflunisal has recently been found to stabilize the tetrameric structure of TTR. This action reduces tetramer dissociation and subsequent monomer misfolding and aggregation into amyloid [104–106]. A trial of its clinical efficacy in ATTR is in progress and several similar, and possibly more potent, agents are in development [106]. A major problem with diflunisal in patients with cardiac dysfunction is aggravation of heart failure. Other strategies, with applications in AL or ATTR amyloidosis, include stabilizing native structures of other amyloidogenic proteins and preventing and reversing fibrillogenesis, as well as disrupting established deposits, using antibodies, synthetic peptides, and small molecule drugs [107, 108].

Senile Systemic Amyloid (SSA)

Wild-type TTR amyloid deposition (SSA) is found at autopsy in about 25% of individuals over the age of 80 [67], although, in most cases, the deposits are generally found in small quantities and there is no clinical significance or abnormality during life. The clinical picture of senile systemic amyloidosis (SSA) occurs only when the amyloid deposits are extensive enough to produce an increase in left ventricular wall thickness. There is some evidence that in SSA the TTR is more likely to be composed of fragments of the TTR molecule than in patients with FAP, in whom the deposits appear to contain intact TTR molecules. This difference in architecture may result in distinct patterns of deposition, and the intact TTR molecular deposits (but not the amyloid that they can produce) may penetrate into the myocytes [109]. Wild-type transthyretin (TTR) is deposited in clinically significant quantities almost exclusively in the heart in SSA, despite the term "systemic" in its nomenclature. Although an occasional patient may be detected in an asymptomatic phase, usually because an echocardiogram is done to elucidate an abnormal electrocardiogram, the usual presenting feature is biventricular congestive heart failure. The only other clinical extracardiac feature is a propensity to a history of carpal tunnel syndrome. The echocardiographic appearance is typical of other forms of amyloidosis, but there is no neuropathy or other major extracardiac involvement. Senile cardiac amyloidosis is almost exclusively a disease of elderly men. In a study of 18 patients (17 males) with amyloid heart involvement due to SSA, the median survival was 60 months. Over the same period, patients with AL amyloid heart disease at the same institution had a median survival of only 5.4 months [110]. A report comparing patients with AL and senile amyloid heart involvement found that patients with SSA had thicker ventricular walls than those with AL [111]. Most patients with SSA had normal voltage electrocardiograms, whereas the majority of those with AL had low voltage. Despite thicker walls (mean septal thickness of 17.8 versus 14.3 mm) and despite an older age, the senile amyloid patients had less severe heart failure and a much longer median survival (75 versus 11 months). These SSA patients were all elderly males with amyloid limited to the heart.

Treatment of SSA is symptomatic, with diuretics remaining the mainstay. Not uncommonly severe right-sided heart failure may be present at the time of presentation. Vigorous treatment often results in significant improvement, with long-term freedom from recurrence of severe heart failure. As with ATTR, patients may tolerate ACE inhibitors or angiotensin receptor blockers. Long-acting nitrates, given for pre-load reduction, may have some effect in relieving symptoms of dyspnea. Given the age of the patients, other, non-amyloid, heart disease may co-exist and should not be overlooked. The disease tends to progress slowly, and a sudden worsening of heart failure often represents the onset of atrial arrhythmia. Atrial fibrillation is common and, if present, warfarin anticoagulation should be used as the thromboembolic risk is very high. Strong consideration should be given to electrical cardioversion if atrial fibrillation or flutter occurs, and amiodarone can be safely used in most patients to help maintain sinus rhythm. Progressive distal conduction system disease with high-degree AV block commonly occurs and, if a permanent pacemaker is needed, consideration should be given to biventricular pacing as right ventricular pacing may aggravate the already decreased cardiac output. Generally, the advanced age of patients with SSA is a contraindication to cardiac transplantation. However, an occasional patient presents in the 7th or even 6th decade, and transplantation has been successfully performed in such patients [54, 112].

Secondary (AA) Amyloidosis

AA amyloidosis, previously termed secondary amyloidosis, is a rare complication of chronic inflammatory disorders. The fibrils are derived from the acute phase reactant serum amyloid A protein (SAA). Although cardiac deposits are often present at histology, echocardiographic abnormalities and clinical symptoms of cardiac AA amyloidosis are extremely rare, occurring in only about 2% of cases. The prognosis is thought to be substantially better than in cases of AL amyloid [113]. Treatment involves suppressing the underlying disease.

Isolated Atrial Amyloid (IAA)

Atrial natriuretic peptide (ANP) is synthesized locally by atrial myocytes [114] and can be deposited locally within the atria as amyloid. IAA is a disease of the elderly, with a female preponderance that contrasts with senile TTR amyloid [111]. The incidence of IAA in elderly hearts is high, with one autopsy study describing IAA in 91 of 100 hearts [115]. IAA first appears in the 4th decade and its prevalence increases by approximately 15–20% per subsequent decade, reaching 95% in those of 81–90 years of age [116]. It may be important in the development of atrial conduction abnormalities and atrial fibrillation, particularly after cardiac surgery [117–120]. ANP plays an established integral role in circulatory hemodynamics, although no relationship has been demonstrated to link IAA and measures of cardiac performance, including ejection fraction. This suggests that conditions that increase ANP production do not necessarily promote atrial amyloidogenesis [121].

Isolated atrial amyloidosis can only be diagnosed by pathologic examination of biopsy or autopsy material, and there are no specific non-invasive features. Management of any associated atrial arrhythmia is the appropriate therapy.

Summary and Conclusion

Early detection of cardiac amyloidosis is the best method to obtain the best possible outcome, as it allows for a broader range of therapeutic options. Clinical awareness of the disease and a high index of clinical suspicion are critical to early diagnosis, but, unfortunately, many cases are diagnosed late in the disease. In AL amyloidosis, severe cardiac involvement precludes high-dose chemotherapy but, in the uncommon cases where infiltration is limited to the heart, combined heart transplantation and chemotherapy offer a hope of long-term survival. Newer chemotherapy regimes, with less treatment-related mortality than high-dose chemotherapy and stem cell transplant, show promise, even when cardiac involvement is severe and when multisystem disease precludes consideration of cardiac transplantation. The identification of a patient with familial amyloidosis should lead to genetic counseling, and possibly genetic screening of offspring, as new therapies, currently in clinical trials, may offer a way to prevent or delay the onset of the disease and early detection in offspring may permit better disease management. Senile systemic amyloid still offers a therapeutic challenge, but drugs to stabilize the amyloidogenic TTR offer a future potential for slowing disease progression. Finally, once a case of amyloidosis is recognized, it is vital to precisely determine the type of amyloid as the prognosis and treatment differ considerably among the types.

References

1. Dubrey SW, Cha K, Anderson J, Chamarthi B, Reisinger J, Skinner M, et al. The clinical features of immunoglobulin light-chain (AL) amyloidosis with heart involvement. QJM. 1998 Feb;91(2):141–57.
2. Carroll JD, Gaasch WH, McAdam KP. Amyloid cardiomyopathy: characterization by a distinctive voltage/mass relation. Am J Cardiol. 1982;49(1):9–13.
3. Maceira AM, Joshi J, Prasad SK, Moon JC, Perugini E, Harding I, et al. Cardiovascular magnetic resonance in cardiac amyloidosis. Circulation 2005 Jan 18;111(2): 186–93.
4. Migrino RQ, Christenson R, Szabo A, Bright M, Truran S, Hari P. Prognostic implication of late gadolinium enhancement on cardiac MRI in light chain (AL) amyloidosis on long term follow up. BMC Med Phys. 2009 May 5;9(1):5.
5. Ruberg FL, Appelbaum E, Davidoff R, Ozonoff A, Kissinger KV, Harrigan C, et al. Diagnostic and prognostic utility of cardiovascular magnetic resonance imaging in light-chain cardiac amyloidosis. Am J Cardiol. 2009 Feb 15;103(4):544–9.
6. Maceira AM, Prasad SK, Hawkins PN, Roughton M, Pennell DJ. Cardiovascular magnetic resonance and prognosis in cardiac amyloidosis. J Cardiovasc Magn Reson. 2008;10(1):54.
7. Kribben A, Witzke O, Hillen U, Barkhausen J, Daul AE, Erbel R. Nephrogenic systemic fibrosis: pathogenesis, diagnosis, and therapy. J Am Coll Cardiol. 2009 May 5;53(18):1621–8.
8. Hazenberg BP, van Rijswijk MH, Piers DA, Lub-de Hooge MN, Vellenga E, Haagsma EB, et al. Diagnostic performance of 123I-labeled serum amyloid P component scintigraphy in patients with amyloidosis. Am J Med. 2006 Apr;119(4):355. e15–24.
9. Glaudemans AW, Slart RH, Zeebregts CJ, Veltman NC, Tio RA, Hazenberg BP, et al. Nuclear imaging in cardiac amyloidosis. Eur J Nucl Med Mol Imaging. 2009 Jan 21;36:702–14.
10. Pellikka PA, Holmes DR Jr., Edwards WD, Nishimura RA, Tajik AJ, Kyle RA. Endomyocardial biopsy in 30 patients with primary amyloidosis and suspected cardiac involvement. Arch Intern Med. 1988;148(3):662–6.
11. Reisinger J, Dubrey SW, Lavalley M, Skinner M, Falk RH. Electrophysiologic abnormalities in AL (primary) amyloidosis with cardiac involvement. J Am Coll Cardiol. 1997;30(4):1046–51.
12. Dubrey S, Pollak A, Skinner M, Falk RH. Atrial thrombi occurring during sinus rhythm in cardiac amyloidosis: evidence for atrial electromechanical dissociation [see comments]. Br Heart J. 1995;74(5):541–4.
13. Feng D, Syed IS, Martinez M, Oh JK, Jaffe AS, Grogan M, et al. Intracardiac thrombosis and anticoagulation therapy in cardiac amyloidosis. Circulation. 2009 May 12;119(18):2490–7.

14. Feng D, Edwards WD, Oh JK, Chandrasekaran K, Grogan M, Martinez MW, et al. Intracardiac thrombosis and embolism in patients with cardiac amyloidosis. Circulation 2007 Nov 20;116(21):2420–6.

15. Zubkov AY, Rabinstein AA, Dispenzieri A, Wijdicks EF. Primary systemic amyloidosis with ischemic stroke as a presenting complication. Neurology 2007 Sep 11;69(11): 1136–41.

16. Koyama J, Davidoff R, Falk RH. Longitudinal myocardial velocity gradient derived from pulsed Doppler tissue imaging in AL amyloidosis: a sensitive indicator of systolic and diastolic dysfunction. J Am Soc Echocardiogr. 2004;17(1):36–44.

17. Koyama J, Ray-Sequin PA, Davidoff R, Falk RH. Usefulness of pulsed tissue Doppler imaging for evaluating systolic and diastolic left ventricular function in patients with AL (primary) amyloidosis. Am J Cardiol. 2002;89(9):1067–71.

18. Koyama J, Ray-Sequin PA, Falk RH. Longitudinal myocardial function assessed by tissue velocity, strain, and strain rate tissue Doppler echocardiography in patients with AL (primary) cardiac amyloidosis. Circulation 2003;107(19):2446–52.

19. Ogiwara F, Koyama J, Ikeda S, Kinoshita O, Falk RH. Comparison of the strain Doppler echocardiographic features of familial amyloid polyneuropathy (FAP) and light-chain amyloidosis. Am J Cardiol. 2005 Feb 15;95(4):538–40.

20. Sharma PP, Payvar S, Litovsky SH. Histomorphometric analysis of intramyocardial vessels in primary and senile amyloidosis: epicardium versus endocardium. Cardiovasc Pathol. 2008 Mar–Apr;17(2):65–71.

21. Palladini G, Lavatelli F, Russo P, Perlini S, Perfetti V, Bosoni T, et al. Circulating amyloidogenic free light chains and serum N-terminal natriuretic peptide type B decrease simultaneously in association with improvement of survival in AL. Blood 2006 May 15;107(10):3854–8.

22. Brenner DA, Jain M, Pimentel DR, Wang B, Connors LH, Skinner M, et al. Human amyloidogenic light chains directly impair cardiomyocyte function through an increase in cellular oxidant stress. Circ Res. 2004;94(8):1008–10.

23. Liao RL, Jain M, Teller P, Connors LH, Ngoy S, Skinner M, et al. Infusion of light chains from patients with cardiac amyloidosis causes diastolic dysfunction in isolated mouse hearts. Circulation 2001;104(14):1594–7.

24. Dubrey SW, Cha K, Skinner M, LaValley M, Falk RH. Familial and primary (AL) cardiac amyloidosis: echocardiographically similar diseases with distinctly different clinical outcomes. Heart 1997;78(1):74–82.

25. Collins AB, Smith RN, Stone JR. Classification of amyloid deposits in diagnostic cardiac specimens by immunofluorescence. Cardiovasc Pathol. 2008 Jul 10;18:205–16.

26. Benson MD, Breall J, Cummings OW, Liepnieks JJ. Biochemical characterisation of amyloid by endomyocardial biopsy. Amyloid 2009 Mar;16(1):9–14.

27. Kyle RA, Gertz MA, Greipp PR, Witzig TE, Lust JA, Lacy MQ, et al. A trial of three regimens for primary amyloidosis: colchicine alone, melphalan and prednisone, and melphalan, prednisone, and colchicine. N Engl J Med. 1997 Apr 24;336(17):1202–7.

28. Kyle RA, Gertz MA. Primary systemic amyloidosis: clinical and laboratory features in 474 cases. Semin Hematol. 1995 Jan;32(1):45–59.

29. Palladini G, Campana C, Klersy C, Balduini A, Vadacca G, Perfetti V, et al. Serum N-terminal pro-brain natriuretic peptide is a sensitive marker of myocardial dysfunction in AL amyloidosis. Circulation 2003;107(19):2440–5.

30. Nordlinger M, Magnani B, Skinner M, Falk RH. Is elevated plasma B-natriuretic peptide in amyloidosis simply a function of the presence of heart failure?. Am J Cardiol. 2005;96(7):982–4.

31. Takemura G, Takatsu Y, Doyama K, Itoh H, Saito Y, Koshiji M, et al. Expression of atrial and brain natriuretic peptides and their genes in hearts of patients with cardiac amyloidosis. J Am Coll Cardiol. 1998;31(4):754–65.

32. Dispenzieri A, Gertz MA, Kyle RA, Lacy MQ, Burritt MF, Therneau TM, et al. Serum cardiac troponins and N-terminal pro-brain natriuretic peptide: a staging system for primary systemic amyloidosis. J Clin Oncol. 2004;22(18):3751–7.

33. Dispenzieri A, Gertz MA, Kyle RA, Lacy MQ, Burritt MF, Therneau TM, et al. Prognostication of survival using cardiac troponins and N-terminal pro-brain natriuretic peptide in patients with primary systemic amyloidosis undergoing peripheral blood stem cell transplantation. Blood 2004;104(6):1881–7.

34. Murtagh B, Hammill SC, Gertz MA, Kyle RA, Tajik AJ, Grogan M. Electrocardiographic findings in primary systemic amyloidosis and biopsy-proven cardiac involvement. Am J Cardiol. 2005;95(4):535–7.

35. Velazquez-Cecena JL, Lubell DL, Nagajothi N, Al-Masri H, Siddiqui M, Khosla S. Syncope from dynamic left ventricular outflow tract obstruction simulating hypertrophic cardiomyopathy in a patient with primary AL-type amyloid heart disease. Tex Heart Inst J. 2009;36(1):50–4.

36. Dinwoodey DL, Skinner M, Maron MS, Davidoff R, Ruberg FL. Light-chain amyloidosis with echocardiographic features of hypertrophic cardiomyopathy. Am J Cardiol. 2008 Mar 1;101(5):674–6.

37. Pollak A, Falk RH. Left ventricular systolic dysfunction precipitated by verapamil in cardiac amyloidosis. Chest 1993;104(2):618–20.

38. Al Suwaidi J, Velianou JL, Gertz MA, Cannon RO, Higano ST, Holmes DR, et al. Systemic amyloidosis presenting with angina pectoris. Ann Intern Med. 1999;131(11): 838–41.

39. Hongo M, Yamamoto H, Kohda T, Takeda M, Kinoshita O, Uchikawa S, et al. Comparison of electrocardiographic findings in patients with AL (primary) amyloidosis and in familial amyloid polyneuropathy and anginal pain and their relation to histopathologic findings. Am J Cardiol. 2000;85(7):849–53.

40. Narang R, Chopra P, Wasir HS. Cardiac amyloidosis presenting as ischemic heart disease. A case report and review of literature. Cardiology 1993;82(4):294–300.

41. Mesquita T, Chorao M, Soares I, Mello e Silva A, Abecasis P. Primary amyloidosis as a cause of microvascular angina and intermittent claudication. Rev Port Cardiol. 2005 Dec;24(12):1521–31.

42. Churchill CH, Abril A, Krishna M, Callman ML, Ginsburg WW. Jaw claudication in primary amyloidosis: unusual presentation of a rare disease. J Rheumatol. 2003;30(10):2283–6.

43. Schneider BF, Normansell D, Ayers CR, Hess CE. Intermittent claudication as the presenting symptom in primary amyloidosis. Acta Haematologica 1993;90(2):106–7.

44. Yokota T, Okabayashi H, Ishihara T, Kawano H, Wakabayashi F, Miyamoto AT, et al. Immunohistochemical and pathological characteristics of dystrophic amyloid in surgically excised cardiac valves. Pathol Int. 1994;44(3):182–5.

45. Kristen AV, Dengler TJ, Hegenbart U, Schonland SO, Goldschmidt H, Sack FU, et al. Prophylactic implantation of cardioverter-defibrillator in patients with severe cardiac amyloidosis and high risk for sudden cardiac death. Heart Rhythm 2008 Feb;5(2): 235–40.

46. Dhoble A, Khasnis A, Olomu A, Thakur R. Cardiac amyloidosis treated with an implantable cardioverter defibrillator and subcutaneous array lead system: report of a case and literature review. Clin Cardiol. 2009 May 19;32:E63–5.

47. Comenzo RL, Vosburgh E, Falk RH, Sanchorawala V, Reisinger J, Dubrey S, et al. Dose-intensive melphalan with blood stem-cell support for the treatment of AL (amyloid light-chain) amyloidosis: survival and responses in 25 patients. Blood 1998 May 15;91(10):3662–70.

48. Skinner M, Sanchorawala V, Seldin DC, Dember LM, Falk RH, Berk JL, et al. High-dose melphalan and autologous stem-cell transplantation in patients with AL amyloidosis: an 8-year study. Ann Intern Med. 2004 Jan 20;140(2):85–93.

49. Jaccard A, Moreau P, Leblond V, Leleu X, Benboubker L, Hermine O, et al. High-dose melphalan versus melphalan plus dexamethasone for AL amyloidosis. N Engl J Med. 2007 Sep 13;357(11):1083–93.

50. Palladini G, Russo P, Lavatelli F, Nuvolone M, Albertini R, Bosoni T, et al. Treatment of patients with advanced cardiac AL amyloidosis with oral melphalan, dexamethasone, and thalidomide. Ann Hematol. 2009 Apr;88(4):347–50.

51. Hosenpud JD, DeMarco T, Frazier OH, Griffith BP, Uretsky BF, Menkis AH, et al. Progression of systemic disease and reduced long-term survival in patients with cardiac amyloidosis undergoing heart transplantation. Follow-up results of a multicenter survey. Circulation 1991;84 Suppl 5:III338–43.

52. Hosenpud JD, Uretsky BF, Griffith BP, O'Connell JB, Olivari MT, Valantine HA. Successful intermediate-term outcome for patients with cardiac amyloidosis undergoing heart transplantation: results of a multicenter survey. J Heart Transplant. 1990;9(4): 346–50.

53. Dubrey S, Simms RW, Skinner M, Falk RH. Recurrence of primary (AL) amyloidosis in a transplanted heart with four-year survival. Am J Cardiol. 1995;76(10):739–41.

54. Dubrey S, Burke M, Hawkins P, Banner N. Cardiac transplantation for amyloid heart disease: the United Kingdom experience. J Heart Lung Transplant. 2004;23(10): 1142–53.

55. Kpodonu J, Massad MG, Caines A, Geha AS. Outcome of heart transplantation in patients with amyloid cardiomyopathy. J Heart Lung Transplant. 2005 Nov;24(11): 1763–5.

56. Roig E, Almenar L, Gonzalez-Vilchez F, Rabago G, Delgado J, Gomez-Bueno M, et al. Outcomes of heart transplantation for cardiac amyloidosis: subanalysis of the Spanish registry for heart transplantation. Am J Transplant. 2009 May 6;9:1414–9.

57. Gillmore JD, Goodman HJ, Lachmann HJ, Offer M, Wechalekar AD, Joshi J, et al. Sequential heart and autologous stem cell transplantation for systemic AL amyloidosis. Blood. 2006 Feb 1;107(3):1227–9.

58. Maurer MS, Raina A, Hesdorffer C, Bijou R, Colombo P, Deng M, et al. Cardiac transplantation using extended-donor criteria organs for systemic amyloidosis complicated by heart failure. Transplantation 2007 Mar 15;83(5):539–45.

59. Chen JM, Russo MJ, Hammond KM, Mancini DM, Kherani AR, Fal JM, et al. Alternate waiting list strategies for heart transplantation maximize donor organ utilization. Ann Thorac Surg. 2005 Jul;80(1):224–8.

60. Lacy MQ, Dispenzieri A, Hayman SR, Kumar S, Kyle RA, Rajkumar SV, et al. Autologous stem cell transplant after heart transplant for light chain (Al) amyloid cardiomyopathy. J Heart Lung Transplant. 2008 Aug;27(8):823–9.

61. Mignot A, Varnous S, Redonnet M, Jaccard A, Epailly E, Vermes E, et al. Heart transplantation in systemic (AL) amyloidosis: a retrospective study of eight French patients. Arch Cardiovasc Dis. 2008 Sep;101(9):523–32.

62. Sack FU, Kristen A, Goldschmidt H, Schnabel PA, Dengler T, Koch A, et al. Treatment options for severe cardiac amyloidosis: heart transplantation combined with chemotherapy and stem cell transplantation for patients with AL-amyloidosis and heart and liver transplantation for patients with ATTR-amyloidosis. Eur J Cardiothorac Surg. 2008 Feb;33(2):257–62.

63. Mignot A, Bridoux F, Thierry A, Varnous S, Pujo M, Delcourt A, et al. Successful heart transplantation following melphalan plus dexamethasone therapy in systemic AL amyloidosis. Haematologica 2008 Mar;93(3):e32–5.

64. Audard V, Matignon M, Weiss L, Remy P, Pardon A, Haioun C, et al. Successful long-term outcome of the first combined heart and kidney transplant in a patient with systemic Al amyloidosis. Am J Transplant. 2009 Jan;9(1):236–40.

65. Hess EP, White RD. Out-of-hospital cardiac arrest in patients with cardiac amyloidosis: presenting rhythms, management and outcomes in four patients. Resuscitation 2004;60(1):105–11.

66. Connors LH, Lim A, Prokaeva T, Roskens VA, Costello CE. Tabulation of human transthyretin (TTR) variants, 2003. Amyloid 2003 Sep;10(3):160–84.

67. Westermark P, Sletten K, Johansson B, Cornwell GG III.. Fibril in senile systemic amyloidosis is derived from normal transthyretin. Proc Natl Acad Sci USA 1990 Apr;87(7):2843–5.

68. Yazaki M, Tokuda T, Nakamura A, Higashikata T, Koyama J, Higuchi K, et al. Cardiac amyloid in patients with familial amyloid polyneuropathy consists of abundant wild-type transthyretin. Biochem Biophys Res Commun. 2000 Aug 11;274(3):702–6.

69. Jacobson DR, Pastore RD, Yaghoubian R, Kane I, Gallo G, Buck FS, et al. Variant-sequence transthyretin (isoleucine 122) in late-onset cardiac amyloidosis in black Americans. New Engl J Med. 1997 Feb 13;336(7):466–73.

70. Gillmore JD, Booth DR, Pepys MB, Hawkins PN. Hereditary cardiac amyloidosis associated with the transthyretin Ile122 mutation in a white man. Heart (Br Card Soc). 1999 Sep;82(3):e2.

71. Eriksson M, Schonland S, Yumlu S, Hegenbart U, von Hutten H, Gioeva Z, et al. Hereditary apolipoprotein AI-associated amyloidosis in surgical pathology specimens: identification of three novel mutations in the APOA1 gene. J Mol Diagn. 2009 May;11(3): 257–62.

72. Westermark P, Mucchiano G, Marthin T, Johnson KH, Sletten K. Apolipoprotein A1-derived amyloid in human aortic atherosclerotic plaques. Am J Pathol. 1995 Nov;147(5):1186–92.

73. Gillmore JD, Stangou AJ, Tennent GA, Booth DR, O'Grady J, Rela M, et al. Clinical and biochemical outcome of hepatorenal transplantation for hereditary systemic amyloidosis associated with apolipoprotein AI Gly26Arg. Transplantation 2001;71(7): 986–92.

74. Gillmore JD, Lachmann HJ, Rowczenio D, Gilbertson JA, Zeng CH, Liu ZH, et al. Diagnosis, pathogenesis, treatment, and prognosis of hereditary fibrinogen A alpha-chain amyloidosis. J Am Soc Nephrol. 2009 Feb;20(2):444–51.

75. Mourad G, Delabre JP, Garrigue V. Cardiac amyloidosis with the E526V mutation of the fibrinogen A alpha-chain. N Engl J Med. 2008 Dec 25;359(26):2847–8.

76. Kiuru S, Matikainen E, Kupari M, Haltia M, Palo J. Autonomic nervous system and cardiac involvement in familial amyloidosis, Finnish type (FAF). J Neurol Sci. 1994 Oct;126(1):40–8.

77. Chastan N, Baert-Desurmont S, Saugier-Veber P, Derumeaux G, Cabot A, Frebourg T, et al. Cardiac conduction alterations in a French family with amyloidosis of the Finnish type with the p.Asp187Tyr mutation in the GSN gene. Muscle Nerve 2006 Jan;33(1):113–9.

78. Zeldenrust S, Gertz M, Uemichi T, Bjornsson J, Wiesner R, Schwab T, et al. Orthotopic liver transplantation for hereditary fibrinogen amyloidosis. Transplantation 2003;75(4):560–1.

79. Holmgren G, Ericzon BG, Groth CG, Steen L, Suhr O, Andersen O, et al. Clinical improvement and amyloid regression after liver transplantation in hereditary transthyretin amyloidosis. Lancet 1993 May 1;341(8853):1113–6.

80. Dubrey SW, Davidoff R, Skinner M, Bergethon P, Lewis D, Falk RH. Progression of ventricular wall thickening after liver transplantation for familial amyloidosis. Transplantation 1997 Jul 15;64(1):74–80.

81. Stangou AJ, Hawkins PN, Heaton ND, Rela M, Monaghan M, Nihoyannopoulos P, et al. Progressive cardiac amyloidosis following liver transplantation for familial amyloid polyneuropathy: implications for amyloid fibrillogenesis. Transplantation 1998 Jul 27;66(2):229–33.

82. Pomfret EA, Lewis WD, Jenkins RL, Bergethon P, Dubrey SW, Reisinger J, et al. Effect of orthotopic liver transplantation on the progression of familial amyloidotic polyneuropathy. Transplantation 1998 Apr 15,65(7):918–25.

83. Yazaki M, Mitsuhashi S, Tokuda T, Kametani F, Takei YI, Koyama J, et al. Progressive wild-type transthyretin deposition after liver transplantation preferentially occurs onto myocardium in FAP patients. Am J Transplant. 2007 Jan;7(1):235–42.

84. Liepnieks JJ, Benson MD. Progression of cardiac amyloid deposition in hereditary transthyretin amyloidosis patients after liver transplantation. Amyloid 2007 Dec;14(4):277–82.

85. Ihse E, Stangou AJ, Heaton ND, O'Grady J, Ybo A, Hellman U, et al. Proportion between wild-type and mutant protein in truncated compared to full-length ATTR: an analysis on transplanted transthyretin T60A amyloidosis patients. Biochem Biophys Res Commun. 2009 Feb 20;379(4):846–50.

86. Arpesella G, Chiappini B, Marinelli G, Mikus PM, Dozza F, Pierangeli A, et al. Combined heart and liver transplantation for familial amyloidotic polyneuropathy. J Thorac Cardiovasc Surg. 2003 May;125(5):1165–6.

87. Grazi GL, Cescon M, Salvi F, Ercolani G, Ravaioli M, Arpesella G, et al. Combined heart and liver transplantation for familial amyloidotic neuropathy: considerations from the hepatic point of view. Liver Transplant. 2003 Sep;9(9):986–92.

88. Zeldenrust S, Gertz M, Uemichi T, Bjornsson J, Wiesner R, Schwab T, et al. Orthotopic liver transplantation for hereditary fibrinogen amyloidosis. Transplantation 2003;75:560–1.

89. Dubrey SW, Burke MM, Hawkins PN, Banner NR. Cardiac transplantation for amyloid heart disease: the United Kingdom experience. J Heart Lung Transplant. 2004 Oct;23(10):1142–53.

90. Gillmore JD, Stangou AJ, Tennent GA, Booth DR, O'Grady J, Rela M, et al. Clinical and biochemical outcome of hepatorenal transplantation for hereditary systemic amyloidosis associated with apolipoprotein AI Gly26Arg. Transplantation 2001 Apr 15;71(7): 986–92.

91. Inomata Y, Zeledon ME, Asonuma K, Okajima H, Takeichi T, Ishiko T, et al. Whole-liver graft without the retrohepatic inferior vena cava for sequential (domino) living donor liver transplantation. Am J Transplant. 2007 Jun;7(6):1629–32.

92. Singer R, Mehrabi A, Schemmer P, Kashfi A, Hegenbart U, Goldschmidt H, et al. Indications for liver transplantation in patients with amyloidosis: a single-center experience with 11 cases. Transplantation 2005 Sep 27;80 Suppl 1:S156–9.

93. Goto T, Yamashita T, Ueda M, Ohshima S, Yoneyama K, Nakamura M, et al. Iatrogenic amyloid neuropathy in a Japanese patient after sequential liver transplantation. Am J Transplant. 2006 Oct;6(10):2512–5.

94. Stangou AJ, Heaton ND, Hawkins PN. Transmission of systemic transthyretin amyloidosis by means of domino liver transplantation. N Engl J Med. 2005 Jun 2;352(22): 2356.

95. Cardoso I, Merlini G, Saraiva MJ. 4'-iodo-4'-deoxydoxorubicin and tetracyclines disrupt transthyretin amyloid fibrils in vitro producing noncytotoxic species: screening for TTR fibril disrupters. FASEB J. 2003 May;17(8):803–9.

96. Palha JA, Ballinari D, Amboldi N, Cardoso I, Fernandes R, Bellotti V, et al.. 4'-Iodo-4'-deoxydoxorubicin disrupts the fibrillar structure of transthyretin amyloid. Am J Pathol. 2000 Jun;156(6):1919–25.

97. Peterson SA, Klabunde T, Lashuel HA, Purkey H, Sacchettini JC, Kelly JW. Inhibiting transthyretin conformational changes that lead to amyloid fibril formation. Proc Natl Acad Sci USA 1998 Oct 27;95(22):12956–60.

98. Saraiva MJ. Transthyretin mutations in hyperthyroxinemia and amyloid diseases. Human Mutation 2001 Jun;17(6):493–503.

99. Oza VB, Smith C, Raman P, Koepf EK, Lashuel HA, Petrassi HM, et al. Synthesis, structure, and activity of diclofenac analogues as transthyretin amyloid fibril formation inhibitors. J Med Chem. 2002 Jan 17;45(2):321–32.

100. Almeida MR, Gales L, Damas AM, Cardoso I, Saraiva MJ. Small transthyretin (TTR) ligands as possible therapeutic agents in TTR amyloidoses. Curr Drug targets. CNS Neurol Disord. 2005 Oct;4(5):587–96.

101. Gillmore JD, Hawkins PN. Drug Insight: emerging therapies for amyloidosis. Nat Clin Pract Nephrol. 2006 May;2(5):263–70.

102. Coelho T, Coelho T, Maia L, da Silva AM, et al. A landmark clinical trial of a novel small molecule transthyretin (TTR) stabilizer, Fx-1006A, in patients with TTR amyloid polyneuropathy: a phase II/III, randomized, double-blind, placebo-controlled study. Neurology 2009;72 Suppl. 3:A205.

103. Coelho T, Waddington-Cruz M, Plante-Bordeneuve V, et al. Correlation of clinical outcomes and disease burden in patients with transthyretin (TTR) amyloid polyneuropathy: study Fx-005, a landmark clinical trail of Fx-1006A, a novel small molecule TTR stabilizer. J Neurol. 2008;255 Suppl 1:78.

104. Sekijima Y, Dendle MA, Kelly JW. Orally administered diflunisal stabilizes transthyretin against dissociation required for amyloidogenesis. Amyloid 2006 Dec;13(4):236–49.

105. Tojo K, Sekijima Y, Kelly JW, Ikeda SI. Diflunisal stabilizes familial amyloid polyneuropathy-associated transthyretin variant tetramers in serum against dissociation required for amyloidogenesis. Neurosci Res. 2006 Oct 5;56:441–9.

106. Mairal T, Nieto J, Pinto M, Almeida MR, Gales L, Ballesteros A, et al. Iodine atoms: a new molecular feature for the design of potent transthyretin fibrillogenesis inhibitors. PLoS ONE 2009;4(1):e4124.

107. Miller SR, Sekijima Y, Kelly JW. Native state stabilization by NSAIDs inhibits transthyretin amyloidogenesis from the most common familial disease variants. Lab Invest. 2004 May;84(5):545–52.

108. Miroy GJ, Lai Z, Lashuel HA, Peterson SA, Strang C, Kelly JW. Inhibiting transthyretin amyloid fibril formation via protein stabilization. Proc Natl Acad Sci USA 1996 Dec 24;93(26):15051–6.

109. Bergstrom J, Gustavsson A, Hellman U, Sletten K, Murphy CL, Weiss DT, et al. Amyloid deposits in transthyretin-derived amyloidosis: cleaved transthyretin is associated with distinct amyloid morphology. J Pathol. 2005 Jun;206(2):224–32.

110. Kyle RA, Spittell PC, Gertz MA, Li CY, Edwards WD, Olson LJ, et al. The premortem recognition of systemic senile amyloidosis with cardiac involvement. Am J Med. 1996 Oct;101(4):395–400.

111. Ng B, Connors LH, Davidoff R, Skinner M, Falk RH. Senile systemic amyloidosis presenting with heart failure: a comparison with light chain-associated amyloidosis. Arch Intern Med. 2005 Jun 27;165(12):1425–9.

112. Fuchs U, Zittermann A, Suhr O, Holmgren G, Tenderich G, Minami K, et al. Heart transplantation in a 68-year-old patient with senile systemic amyloidosis. Am J Transplant. 2005 May;5(5):1159–62.

113. Dubrey SW, Cha K, Simms RW, Skinner M, Falk RH. Electrocardiography and Doppler echocardiography in secondary (AA) amyloidosis. Am J Cardiol. 1996 Feb 1;77(4):313–5.

114. Kaye GC, Butler MG, d'Ardenne AJ, Edmondson SJ, Camm AJ, Slavin G. Isolated atrial amyloid contains atrial natriuretic peptide: a report of six cases. Br Heart J. 1986 Oct;56(4):317–20.

115. Kawamura S, Takahashi M, Ishihara T, Uchino F. Incidence and distribution of isolated atrial amyloid: histologic and immunohistochemical studies of 100 aging hearts. Pathol Int. 1995 May;45(5):335–42.

116. Steiner I. The prevalence of isolated atrial amyloid. J Pathol. 1987 Dec;153(4):395–8.

117. Ariyarajah V, Steiner I, Hajkova P, Khadem A, Kvasnicka J, Apiyasawat S, et al. The association of atrial tachyarrhythmias with isolated atrial amyloid disease: preliminary observations in autopsied heart specimens. Cardiology 2009;113(2):132–7.

118. Goette A, Rocken C. Atrial amyloidosis and atrial fibrillation: a gender-dependent "arrhythmogenic substrate"? Eur Heart J. 2004 Jul;25(14):1185–6.

119. Leone O, Boriani G, Chiappini B, Pacini D, Cenacchi G, Martin Suarez S, et al. Amyloid deposition as a cause of atrial remodelling in persistent valvular atrial fibrillation. Eur Heart J. 2004 Jul;25(14):1237–41.

120. Steiner I, Hajkova P. Patterns of isolated atrial amyloid: a study of 100 hearts on autopsy. Cardiovasc Pathol. 2006 Sep–Oct;15(5):287–90.

121. Rocken C, Peters B, Juenemann G, Saeger W, Klein HU, Huth C, et al. Atrial amyloidosis: an arrhythmogenic substrate for persistent atrial fibrillation. Circulation 2002 Oct 15;106(16):2091–7.

Chapter 9

Renal Amyloidosis

Laura M. Dember

Abstract The kidney is one of the most frequently affected organs in several types of systemic amyloidosis. Amyloid nephropathy is diagnosed by Congo red positivity of kidney tissue and by the presence of non-branching, randomly oriented fibrils that are 8–12 nm in diameter and evident by electron microscopy. Amyloid deposits can occur in the mesangium, glomerular capillary loops, tubulo-interstitium, and/or vasculature of the kidney. Amyloid nephropathy is typically characterized by nephrotic syndrome and progression to end-stage renal disease. The rate of decline in kidney function is variable and can be slowed by treatments that reduce the production of amyloidogenic precursor proteins or new amyloid deposits.

Keywords Renal, Nephropathy, Kidney, Glomerulus, Proteinuria, Nephrotic syndrome, End-stage renal disease, Dialysis, Acute kidney injury, Tubulo-interstitium

Introduction

The kidney is one of the most frequently affected organs in several types of systemic amyloidosis and proteinuria or elevation of serum creatinine is often the initial disease manifestation. Progressive loss of kidney function with development of end-stage renal disease is typical for patients with amyloidosis-associated kidney disease. However, as discussed in this chapter, it is becoming increasingly evident that kidney function can be preserved with treatments that eliminate production of amyloidogenic proteins or formation of amyloid deposits.

Types of Amyloidosis That Affect the Kidney

The amyloidoses are classified based on the amyloidogenic precursor protein and by the distribution of amyloid deposition as either systemic or localized. Systemic amyloidosis refers to disease in which amyloid deposits form at sites that are distant from the source of the amyloidogenic protein. In contrast, in localized amyloidosis, deposits form only at the site of synthesis of the amyloidogenic protein. The kidney is frequently involved in several of the systemic amyloidoses but not in localized amyloid disease.

The types of systemic amyloidosis that affect the kidney are shown in Table 9-1. In AL amyloidosis, the most common of the systemic amyloidoses, clonal plasma cells in the bone marrow produce amyloidogenic immunoglobulin light chains that

From: *Amyloidosis*, Contemporary Hematology,
Edited by: M.A. Gertz and S.V. Rajkumar, DOI 10.1007/978-1-60761-631-3_9,
© Springer Science+Business Media, LLC 2010

Table 9-1. Kidney involvement in the systemic amyloidoses.

Disease	Amyloidogenic protein	Organ involvement
AL amyloidosis	Monoclonal immunoglobulin light chain or fragment	Kidney, heart, liver, gastrointestinal tract, autonomic or peripheral nervous system, soft tissue, spleen, thyroid, adrenal gland
AH amyloidosis	Monoclonal immunoglobulin heavy chain or fragment	Kidney predominates in the small number of reported cases
AA amyloidosis	Proteolytic fragment (AA) of Serum Amyloid A protein	Kidney, liver, gastrointestinal tract, spleen, autonomic nervous system, thyroid, heart
Transthyretin amyloidosis (hereditary)	Transthyretin	Peripheral nervous system, heart, vitreous opacities. Kidney involvement is less common
Fibrinogen Aα amyloidosis (hereditary)	Fibrinogen Aα chain	Kidney, liver, spleen. Kidney involvement is predominantly glomerular
Apolipoprotein AI amyloidosis (hereditary)	Apolipoprotein AI	Kidney, liver, heart, skin, larynx. Kidney involvement is predominantly medullary
Apolipoprotein AII amyloidosis (hereditary)	Apolipoprotein AII	Kidney
Lysozyme amyloidosis (hereditary)	Lysozyme	Kidney, liver, GI tract, spleen, lymph nodes, lung, thyroid, salivary glands
Gelsolin amyloidosis (hereditary)	Gelsolin	Cranial nerves, lattice corneal dystrophy
Senile systemic amyloidosis	Transthyretin (wild type)	Heart, soft tissue
Dialysis-related amyloidosis	Beta-2 microglobulin	Osteoarticular tissue; less commonly involves gastrointestinal tract, blood vessels, heart

form amyloid deposits in a variety of tissues. Clinically evident kidney involvement occurs in 50–80% of patients with AL amyloidosis [1–3]. AA amyloidosis occurs in the setting of longstanding inflammation when a proteolytic fragment of serum amyloid A protein (SAA) forms amyloid. SAA is an acute phase reactant synthesized by the liver in response to inflammation. The most common inflammatory conditions underlying AA disease are rheumatoid arthritis, familial Mediterranean fever (FMF) or other auto-inflammatory disorders, inflammatory bowel disease, osteomyelitis, and bronchiectasis [4]. With the development of effective treatments for many of these conditions, the incidence of AA amyloidosis is decreasing. However, nearly all patients with AA amyloidosis have kidney involvement [4]. In hereditary amyloidoses, an amino acid substitution resulting from an inherited gene mutation renders a protein amyloidogenic. Kidney involvement is a relatively infrequent manifestation of transthyretin (TTR) amyloidosis, the most common of the hereditary forms, but the kidney is often the predominant organ affected in other forms of hereditary amyloidoses such as fibrinogen Aα, lysozyme, apolipoprotein AI and apolipoprotein AII disease. Immunoglobulin heavy chain (AH) amyloidosis can involve the kidney but is extremely rare [5]. Senile systemic amyloidosis and beta-2 microglobulin amyloidosis do not affect the kidney. Leukocyte chemotactic factor 2 (LECT2) was recently identified as the amyloidogenic protein in an individual with nephrotic syndrome, progressive renal failure, and renal cell carcinoma [6]. The absence of a mutation in the LECT2 gene led the investigators to hypothesize that LECT2 amyloidosis is an acquired form of amyloid disease [6].

The kidney is not a frequent target organ for localized forms of amyloidosis. However, localized AL amyloidosis can occur in the urinary tract when clonal plasma cells in bladder tissue produce amyloidogenic light chains. Microscopic or macroscopic hematuria is a common presenting symptom of localized AL amyloidosis of the bladder [7].

Renal Pathology

Light and Electron Microscopies

Amyloid can deposit anywhere in the kidney but glomerular changes typically predominate (see Fig. 9-1). By light microscopy, amyloid appears as an amorphous material in the mesangium and capillary walls. Mesangial cells are not increased in number, but may appear displaced peripherally by the amyloid deposits. When mesangial amyloid deposition is extensive, the glomerular lesion is nodular and can look similar to diabetic nephropathy or light chain deposition disease [8]. However, because the amyloid nodules are comprised of protein rather than extracellular matrix material, they stain weakly with periodic acid-Schiff, a feature that helps distinguish them from lesions of diabetic nephropathy or light chain deposition disease. Tubular atrophy and interstitial fibrosis without a prominent inflammatory infiltrate occur with tubulointerstitial amyloid deposition, and high-grade proteinuria can produce vacuolization of tubular epithelial cells. Amyloid infiltration of blood vessels may be seen in conjunction with glomerular or tubulointerstitial deposition or as an

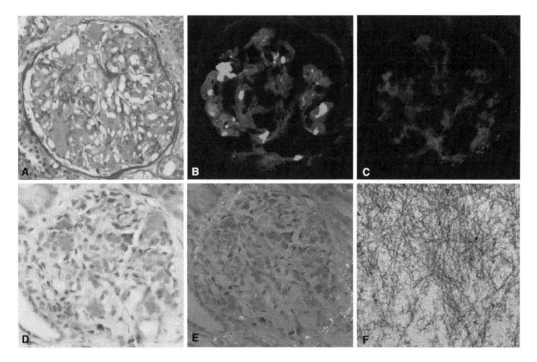

Fig. 9-1. Glomerular changes seen by kidney biopsy in AL amyloidosis. (**A**) Light microscopy shows mesangial expansion with amorphous material that stains weakly with periodic acid-Schiff dye. (**B**) Immunofluorescence shows strong reactivity for lambda light chain and (**C**) weak reactivity for kappa light chain suggesting a clonal source of light chains. (**D**) Congo red-stained material in the mesangium has an *orange-pink color* under non-polarized light and (**E**) generates *apple-green* birefringence under polarized light. (**F**) Non-branching, randomly arrayed fibrils with diameter of 12 nm can be seen by electron microscopy. Images provided by Joel Henderson and Helmut Rennke.

isolated histologic finding. Amyloid deposits isolated in the renal medulla is a feature in many patients with apoAI hereditary amyloidosis [9–11] and has been described in some individuals with AA amyloidosis [12]. Medullary limited disease can be difficult to diagnose since kidney biopsy tissue is often comprised entirely of renal cortex.

The ordered intercalation of Congo red dye into amyloid fibrils produces the amyloid-defining apple-green birefringence under polarized light. Because Congo red staining is not a routine part of the histologic evaluation of most tissues, the diagnosis of amyloidosis may be missed unless the disease is suspected. However, the likelihood of a missed diagnosis is lower with a kidney biopsy than with biopsies of other tissues because electron microscopy is a standard component of the pathologic evaluation of kidney tissue. By electron microscopy, amyloid appears as non-branching fibrils with diameters of 8–10 nm arrayed randomly without a specific orientation. The diameter of the fibrils distinguishes amyloidosis from other fibrillary kidney diseases such as fibrillary glomerulonephritis and immunotactoid glomerulopathy which have fibrils of 15–20 and 30–60 nm, respectively [13–15] (see Table 9-2). Unlike amyloid, the fibrils of immunotactoid glomerulopathy have a microtubular structure with hollow cores and are arranged in the tissue in highly ordered, parallel arrays.

Determination of Amyloid Type

The type of amyloidosis can often be determined from immunofluorescence or immunohistochemistry studies of kidney biopsy tissue using antibodies directed against amyloidogenic proteins. Reactivity for kappa and lambda light chains is assessed routinely on kidney biopsies performed for a wide array of indications in order to determine whether immune deposits are monoclonal or polyclonal. The predominance of one light chain isotype in such deposits indicates a monoclonal process, and in conjunction with Congo red positivity is diagnostic for AL amyloidosis. Because conformational changes or proteolytic cleavage of the light chain can mask or eliminate relevant epitopes, immunoreactivity for the light chain may be absent in AL amyloid deposits [16]. Most patients with AL disease will have evidence for monoclonal light chain production in the serum, urine, or bone marrow; however, because the monoclonal protein is typically present in the blood or urine in low concentrations, immunofixation electrophoresis rather than straightforward protein electrophoresis is often required for its detection. Nephelometric quantification of free light chains in the serum is also useful in establishing the presence of a monoclonal protein [16]. Because free light chains are filtered by the glomerulus, the ratio of the serum concentrations of the two light chain isotypes rather than their absolute concentrations should be assessed if the glomerular filtration rate is reduced as it often is in renal amyloidosis [17, 18]. In contrast to multiple myeloma, the monoclonal protein in AL amyloidosis is more often of the lambda than kappa isotype.

Antibodies directed against AA protein are also available and have reasonably good specificity. Loss of Congo red staining after treatment with potassium permanganate is a property of AA amyloid that can distinguish it from other types [19], but this technique is not as reliable as immunoreactivity with anti-AA antibodies. Antibodies directed against proteins underlying the hereditary amyloidoses are often not available in clinical pathology laboratories but are used by research laboratories for either immunohistochemistry or immuno-electron microscopy [20, 21].

Table 9-2. Fibrillary diseases of the kidney.

Disease	Fibril diameter and orientation	Congo red positivity	Monoclonal protein	Kidney histology	Extra-renal manifestations
Amyloidosis	8–10 nm; non-branching, randomly arrayed	Yes	Kappa or lambda light chain in AL disease; no monoclonal protein for other types	Mesangial expansion with weak PAS staining can be nodular, not hypercellular	Common
Fibrillary glomerulonephritis	15–20 nm, non-branching, randomly arrayed	No	Not usually detectable	Mesangial expansion with strong PAS staining, glomerular capillary wall thickening, double contours	Rare
Immunotactoid glomerulopathy	30–60 nm, non-branching, microtubular structure, parallel distribution	No	Monoclonal immunoglobulin may be present if there is an associated lymphoproliferative disorder	Mesangial expansion with strong PAS staining, mild mesangial hypercellularity, glomerular capillary wall thickening	Rare

Clinical Manifestations of Renal Amyloidosis

Chronic Manifestations

Most patients with renal amyloidosis have proteinuria that can range from less than 500 mg/day to greater than 30 g/day. The urinary protein is comprised mostly of albumin and many patients have the full nephrotic syndrome which is formally defined as urinary protein excretion >3.5 g/day, hypoalbuminemia, and edema. Nephrotic syndrome is often accompanied by hyperlipidemia with elevations in concentrations of both cholesterol and triglycerides. Severe hypoalbuminemia and diuretic-resistant anasarca are common. Management of fluid status can be particularly challenging in patients with heart or autonomic nervous system involvement in addition to renal amyloidosis. Marked sodium avidity by the kidney or hemodynamic instability can limit the effectiveness or tolerability of diuretics. When amyloid is confined to the tubulo-interstitium or vasculature, proteinuria is minimal. In these patients, reduced glomerular filtration rate (GFR), which is usually evident by elevated serum creatinine concentration, is the principal clinical manifestation. Unlike other causes of chronic kidney disease, renal amyloidosis is usually not accompanied by hypertension unless infiltration of the intra-renal vasculature is a prominent feature.

As in any disorder in which there is an overproduction of immunoglobulin light chains, AL amyloidosis can be accompanied by proximal tubular dysfunction. Injury to the proximal tubular cells by filtered light chains reduces the capacity of the tubules to reabsorb glucose, uric acid, bicarbonate, and amino acids from the glomerular filtrate. The alteration in proximal tubular reabsorptive function produces Fanconi syndrome, the most readily identifiable signs of which are glycosuria and metabolic acidosis. An unusual but well-documented manifestation of renal amyloidosis is nephrogenic diabetes insipidus caused by amyloid deposition in the peri-collecting duct tissue [22, 23].

Like other infiltrative diseases, amyloidosis can cause enlargement of the kidneys. However, in most patients the kidneys appear to be of normal size by ultrasound or other imaging studies [24, 25].

Although the rate of GFR decline is highly variable, gradual but progressive loss of renal function is nearly universal for all types of renal amyloidosis if deposition of new amyloid is ongoing. Renal impairment tends to progress less rapidly when tubulointerstitial rather than glomerular deposition predominates, and, on average, progression is less rapid in AA or hereditary amyloidosis than in AL disease. By reducing renal perfusion, amyloidosis-associated cardiomyopathy or autonomic neuropathy can contribute to GFR decline. Relationships between the extent of amyloid deposition evident by kidney biopsy and the severity of clinical manifestations have not been demonstrated [26]. Neither urinary protein excretion nor rate of GFR decline can be predicted based on biopsy findings.

Acute Kidney Injury

Fragile hemodynamic status present in many patients with systemic amyloidosis increases the susceptibility to acute worsening of kidney function which can occur with relatively minor alterations in intravascular volume or blood pressure. Renal amyloidosis can also increase the sensitivity to nephrotoxic agents such as intravenous radiographic contrast. As discussed later in this chapter, acute kidney injury is a frequent complication during treatment of AL amyloidosis with high-dose melphalan and autologous stem cell transplantation [27, 28].

Assessment of Kidney Function

Methods for estimating kidney function that are used in clinical practice or research may have limitations when applied to patients with systemic amyloidosis. Because many of these patients have muscle wasting the serum creatinine concentration may overestimate the GFR. For the same reason, estimating equations that are creatinine-based such as the modification of diet in renal disease (MDRD) equation for estimating GFR [29] or the Cockroft–Gault (C–G) equation for estimating creatinine clearance [30] are potentially problematic. The C–G equation incorporates weight as a proxy for muscle mass; however, for patients with nephrotic syndrome and substantial edema, the contribution of muscle to total body weight is reduced resulting in an overestimation of creatinine clearance.

Mechanisms Underlying Kidney Dysfunction

When examining biopsies of kidneys affected by amyloidosis, one can readily appreciate the deleterious effect that amyloid deposits have on the structure of the glomeruli, tubules, and vessels, and it is easy to understand why organ dysfunction accompanying amyloid deposition has long been attributed to a disruption of tissue architecture. However, relatively recent clinical and experimental observations suggest that tissue amyloid is not the sole cause of disease manifestations and that precursors to mature amyloid fibrils including precursor proteins, folding intermediates, and oligomers have important toxicities independent of the amyloid deposits [31]. Evidence supporting a role for precursor forms in disease pathogenesis includes in vitro demonstrations of toxicity of amyloidogenic precursor proteins on cultured cells or tissues [32–36], detection of amyloidogenic precursor proteins in tissue in the absence of amyloid [37], a lack of correlation between quantity of amyloid in tissue and organ dysfunction [38, 39], and alterations in disease biomarkers that occur too rapidly after precursor protein production elimination to be attributable to degradation of amyloid deposits [40, 41]. Several of these observations have been made in the context of renal amyloidosis. For example, exposure of cultured mesangial cells to amyloidogenic light chains induces phenotypic changes that do not occur if the cells are exposed to light chains without amyloidogenic potential [34], and reductions in proteinuria after treatment that eliminates or markedly reduces production of the amyloidogenic precursor protein in both AL and AA disease occur in many patients before substantial degradation of existing amyloid deposits would be expected to occur [31].

Treatment of Renal Amyloidosis

Symptomatic Management of Nephrotic Syndrome

Symptomatic management of patients with nephrotic syndrome generally includes dietary sodium and fluid restriction to prevent further edema formation. In patients with amyloidosis-associated autonomic neuropathy, compression stockings can help maintain intra-vascular fluid volume, and thereby increase the tolerability of salt restriction and diuretics. Similarly, alpha-1 agonists such as midodrine can improve blood pressure and enable diuresis. Loop diuretics such as furosemide, bumetanide, or torsemide often need to be administered in high dosages because of the marked sodium avidity that accompanies the nephrotic syndrome. When diuretic resistance is severe, the addition of a thiazide diuretic, such as metolazone, to inhibit sodium reabsorption in the distal tubule can enhance the effect of a loop diuretic. For some patients, intravenous administration of diuretics can be more effective than oral diuretics, particularly if gut absorption is impaired because of bowel wall edema. If there is marked hypoalbuminemia (e.g., serum albumin less than 1.5–2 g/dL), intravenous administration of albumin may facilitate diuresis either by increasing delivery of a loop diuretic to the tubular lumen or by increasing oncotic pressure. As in other proteinuric kidney diseases, angiotensin-converting enzyme (ACE) inhibitors or angiotensin receptor blockers (ARBs) may decrease proteinuria. The management of severely nephrotic patients always requires a balance between efforts to remove excess fluid and alterations in hemodynamics that reduce renal perfusion and GFR.

Lipid-lowering medications, particularly statins, can have some effect on nephrotic syndrome-associated hyperlipidemia; however, many patients with amyloidosis continue to have markedly elevated levels of cholesterol and triglycerides despite the use of such agents. Although patients are at risk for thromboembolic disease, anticoagulation is generally not recommended for such patients in the absence of a thrombotic event [42].

Impact of Treatment on Kidney Function

Potential targets for treating the systemic amyloidoses include production of the amyloidogenic precursor protein, formation of amyloid fibrils, deposition of amyloid into tissue, and amyloid degradation [43]. Substantial progress has been made in developing treatments directed at several of these targets; however, currently available therapies all act by reducing precursor protein production. It is now evident that improvements in organ function can occur if amyloid production is halted [2, 40, 41, 44–46]. This has been most clearly demonstrated not only for AL disease but also for AA amyloidosis and some of the hereditary types.

Treatment for AL Amyloidosis

Treatments for AL amyloidosis include the alkylating agent, melphalan, the immunomodulating agent, lenalidomide, or the proteosome-inhibitor, bortezomib, each of which may be administered in conjunction with dexamethasone. All of these treatments are directed against plasma cells, the source of the amyloidogenic light chains. Melphalan can be administered orally over many cycles or intravenously in a dose-intensive manner that requires autologous stem cell transplantation to facilitate recovery of the bone marrow. The ability to induce a hematologic remission, meaning eradication of amyloidogenic light chain production, has increased markedly over the past 15 years, first with the use of high-dose melphalan with autologous stem cell transplantation (HDM/SCT), and more recently with the use of oral melphalan and dexamethasone, lenalidomide, or bortezomib [2, 46–50]. Many patients are now offered sequential courses of treatment if there has been an inadequate response to initial therapy. Comparisons of efficacy of these treatments and approaches for selecting among them are addressed in Chapters 11 and 12.

For AL amyloidosis-associated kidney disease, the most dramatic effect of treatment is a marked reduction in proteinuria. This was initially demonstrated among patients treated with HDM/SCT. In a study of 65 patients with AL amyloidosis and kidney involvement, 12 months after treatment 71% of those with a complete hematologic response had a renal response, defined as a 50% reduction in urinary protein excretion in the absence of 25% or greater decrease in creatinine clearance. Among the hematologic responders, the median 24-h urinary protein excretion decreased from 9.6 to 1.6 g. In contrast, only 11% of patients who had ongoing production of the amyloidogenic light chain had a renal response [40]. Similar results were found by the same group after 114 patients with kidney involvement had undergone HDM/SCT [2]. This experience suggested that reduction in proteinuria is linked to hematologic response. For most patients who ultimately achieve a renal response, some reduction in proteinuria is apparent within the first 6 months, but the proteinuria reduction is progressive over time and it often takes several years before the nadir is reached [51]. Complete normalization of urinary protein excretion occurs in some patients but many continue to have mild proteinuria in the range of 150–500 mg/day. It is likely that reductions in proteinuria occur with other treatments for AL amyloidosis, such as lenalidomide- or bortezomib-based regimens, if the clonal plasma cells are eradicated; however, the early experience with these treatments has focused on assessing hematologic response rather than response of affected organs.

The effect of treatments for AL amyloidosis on GFR is more difficult to evaluate because of the long follow-up required to see differences between treatment groups or between hematologic responders and non-responders. The competing risk of death among those who have persistent hematologic disease makes comparisons of GFR decline between hematologic responders and non-responders particularly challenging. Nonetheless, there are published data and accumulated impressions suggesting that the decline in GFR is slowed when light chain amyloid production is halted. In the study of 65 patients treated with HDM/SCT described above, creatinine clearance was maintained at ≥75% of the pre-treatment value at last follow-up (12–48 months) in 90% of those with a hematologic response but only in 48% of those with persistent hematologic disease [40]. In general, stabilization of kidney function, rather than improvement, should be anticipated if amyloidogenic light chain production is halted.

Treatment for AA Amyloidosis

Reductions in proteinuria have been reported in patients with AA amyloidosis after receiving treatment for the underlying inflammatory condition, such as TNF receptor antagonists or cyclophosphamide for rheumatoid arthritis [52–55]. The proteinuria reduction is presumed to be due to suppression of SAA production and resultant reduction in AA amyloid formation. However, the authors of some of these reports suggest that these agents have additional anti-amyloid effects. For example, it has been proposed that anti-TNF therapies, by inhibiting the expression of receptors for advanced glycation end products (RAGE), might reduce interactions between AA fibrils and RAGE [32] and thereby prevent AA-mediated cell toxicity [55].

A beneficial effect on renal function decline of inhibiting new AA amyloid has been suggested by the experience with eprodisate, a small sulfonated molecule with structural similarity to heparan sulfate moieties. Unlike all of the treatments discussed above, eprodisate does not act by reducing production of the amyloidogenic precursor protein. The compound was designed to inhibit interactions between AA amyloid fibrils and glycosaminoglycans, interactions known to promote amyloid fibril formation and stability in tissue [56, 57]. In a multi-national, randomized, placebo-controlled trial of eprodisate, disease worsening (defined as doubling of serum creatinine, or 50% reduction in creatinine clearance, or progression to ESRD, or death) occurred in 27% of participants randomized to eprodisate compared to 40% of those randomized to placebo [58]. Creatinine clearance declined by 10.9 mL/min/1.73 m^2/year in the eprodisate group compared with 15.6 mL/min/1.73 m^2/year in the placebo group. Interestingly, despite the benefit on renal function, a reduction in proteinuria was not observed in the patients treated with eprodisate. This observation raises the question of whether it is the precursors to mature amyloid fibrils, which are not eliminated by eprodisate, rather than the mature amyloid fibrils that are responsible for proteinuria in amyloidosis [58, 59]. Eprodisate is not available for clinical use as additional clinical trials are required to confirm the benefit apparent in the initial trial.

Hereditary Amyloidosis

Orthotopic liver transplantation is considered the definitive treatment for transthyretin (TTR) amyloidosis, the most common of the hereditary forms [60, 61]. This approach, which has also been used in small numbers of patients with fibrinogen Aα disease [62–64] and apolipoprotein AI disease [65], removes the source of production of the amyloidogenic precursor protein. Small series of patients with TTR amyloidosis-associated kidney disease have described reductions in proteinuria after liver transplantation [66] and stable serum creatinine levels over several years [39].

Treatment-Associated Kidney Injury

Studies from two large amyloidosis treatment centers found that acute kidney injury (AKI) occurred as a complication of HDM/SCT for AL amyloidosis in approximately 20% of patients [27, 28]. In the first of these studies, dialysis was required in one-fourth of the cases of AKI which represented 5% of the entire cohort of 173 treated patients. AKI was reversible in 46% of the cases and in 44% of those who required dialysis [27]. A greater proportion (13.8% of 80 treated patients) required dialysis in the second of these studies. Only one of the patients requiring dialysis had renal recovery, and 8 of the 11 dialysis-dependent patients died [28]. AKI can develop during stem cell mobilization, during the period following administration of melphalan and infusion of stem cells, or as a later phenomenon during bone marrow recovery. The etiology of AKI appears to be multi-factorial with hemodynamic alterations and sepsis as frequent contributors. Patients with impaired renal function, heavy proteinuria, or cardiac involvement before treatment are at highest risk [27]. Based on the findings of the published studies, as well as ongoing experience with larger numbers of patients, it is appropriate to anticipate a need for dialysis during the peri-transplant period if there is significant renal impairment prior to treatment with HDM/SCT.

A small case series described five patients with plasma cell dyscrasias (three of whom had AL amyloidosis) who developed acute worsening of kidney function during treatment with lenalidomide [45]. Initiation of dialysis was necessary in four of these patients, and kidney failure was not reversible. A kidney biopsy performed in one patient showed non-specific changes of tubular atrophy and degeneration. This report as well as accumulating unpublished experience has led to concerns that lenalidomide use for AL amyloidosis may predispose some patients to AKI. Distinguishing a drug effect from progression of underlying renal amyloidosis is difficult; however, not all patients with AKI during lenalidomide use had clinically evident renal amyloid disease, and, for some patients, AKI developed despite normalization of hematologic markers of the plasma cell disease. Although further investigation is required before concluding that lenalidomide imparts risk of AKI, close monitoring of kidney function during use of this agent seems warranted.

Dose Reductions for Renal Impairment

Alterations in drug clearance as a result of renal impairment occur with several of the treatments for amyloidosis. For lenalidomide, recent pharmacokinetic studies indicate a need for dose reduction if creatinine clearance is less than 50 mL/min, and the optimal dose for patients treated with dialysis has not been established [67]. Neither melphalan nor bortezomib require dose alterations with renal impairment. For patients treated with hemodialysis, it is recommended that bortezomib be administered after a dialysis session to avoid the possibility of dialytic clearance [68]. Reductions in dosing of colchicine, which is used to prevent the development of AA amyloidosis in individuals with familial Mediterranean fever, may be required with renal impairment; development of diarrhea is an early sign of colchicine toxicity and should trigger consideration for dose reduction. Although not available outside of clinical trials, eprodisate clearance is dependent on kidney function, and dose adjustments based on creatinine clearance are required.

Dialysis and Kidney Transplantation

Despite the development of new treatments for the systemic amyloidoses, many patients with kidney involvement will have disease progression such that initiation of renal replacement therapy is needed. Both hemodialysis and peritoneal dialysis are appropriate options although specific disease manifestations may make one type preferable. For example, patients with severe autonomic neuropathy or cardiomyopathy might have difficulty tolerating the rapid fluid shifts necessitated by thrice-weekly hemodialysis and have more hemodynamic stability with peritoneal dialysis which is a continuous modality. In contrast, a patient with large pleural effusions or massive hepatomegaly might have difficulty tolerating the large intra-abdominal fluid dwells required for peritoneal dialysis. Malnutrition is a major source of morbidity for patients with ESRD from any cause and should be of particular concern for patients with amyloidosis-associated ESRD given the nutritional challenges imparted by amyloidosis itself.

Although amyloidosis-associated ESRD is irreversible, reducing or eliminating new amyloid formation may alter the course of extra-renal amyloid disease, increase life expectancy, and make possible kidney transplantation. Dialysis dependence may present certain challenges when using aggressive treatments; however, dialysis dependence, in and of itself, should not preclude aggressive treatment. In a small series of patients with AL amyloidosis and dialysis dependence who underwent treatment with HDM/SCT, a greater requirement for blood products during the period of cytopenia and mucositis of greater severity were observed; however, the hematologic response rate and treatment-associated mortality were similar for the dialysis-dependent patients and the overall population of patients undergoing this treatment [69].

Kidney transplantation is an option for selected patients with amyloidosis-associated ESRD [69]. Because of the high likelihood of recurrent disease in the allograft, transplantation should be restricted to those who have undergone treatment that has halted new amyloid production. The extent of extra-renal amyloid disease should also be considered in assessing the potential benefits of organ transplantation. The hematologic relapse rate following HDM/SCT for AL disease is sufficiently low that kidney transplantation is reasonable for those who have achieved a hematologic remission after this treatment [2]. For AA amyloidosis, suitability for kidney transplantation depends on the ability to adequately suppress the underlying inflammatory condition. Dual liver–kidney transplants have been performed in individuals with ESRD caused by TTR or fibrinogen Aα disease [63, 64]. The appropriateness of kidney transplantation is more difficult to determine when there is ongoing production of the amyloidogenic precursor protein. Proceeding with kidney transplantation might be reasonable if disease is limited to the kidney and if the progression to ESRD occurred over many years rather than rapidly. For patients who have undergone kidney transplantation before eradication of amyloid production, aggressive treatment should be considered. Treatment with HDM/SCT is possible after organ transplantation, with temporary discontinuation of those immunosuppressive agents that suppress the bone marrow (e.g., mycophenolic acid) and close monitoring for signs of allograft rejection during reconstitution of the immune system [70].

References

1. Kyle RA, Gertz MA. Primary systemic amyloidosis: clinical and laboratory features in 474 cases. Semin Hematol. 1995;32:45–59.
2. Skinner M, Sanchorawala V, Seldin DC, et al. High-dose melphalan and autologous stem-cell transplantation in patients with AL amyloidosis: an 8-year study. Ann Intern Med. 2004;140:85–93.
3. Obici L, Perfetti V, Palladini G, Moratti R, Merlini G. Clinical aspects of systemic amyloid diseases. Biochimica et Biophysica Acta 2005;1753:11–22.
4. Lachmann HJ, Goodman HJ, Gilbertson JA, et al. Natural history and outcome in systemic AA amyloidosis. N Engl J Med. 2007;356:2361–71.
5. Picken MM. Immunoglobulin light and heavy chain amyloidosis AL/AH: renal pathology and differential diagnosis. Contrib Nephrol. 2007;153:135–55.
6. Benson MD, James S, Scott K, Liepnieks JJ, Kluve-Beckerman B. Leukocyte chemotactic factor 2: a novel renal amyloid protein. Kidney Int. 2008;74:218–22.
7. Merrimen JL, Alkhudair WK, Gupta R. Localized amyloidosis of the urinary tract: case series of nine patients. Urology. 2006;67:904–9.
8. Nakamoto Y, Hamanaka S, Akihama T, Miura AB, Uesaka Y. Renal involvement patterns of amyloid nephropathy: a comparison with diabetic nephropathy. Clin Nephrol. 1984;22:188–94.
9. Vigushin DM, Gough J, Allan D, et al. Familial nephropathic systemic amyloidosis caused by apolipoprotein AI variant Arg26. Q J Med. 1994;87:149–54.
10. Booth DR, Tan SY, Booth SE, et al. Hereditary hepatic and systemic amyloidosis caused by a new deletion/insertion mutation in the apolipoprotein AI gene. J Clin Invest. 1996;97:2714–21.
11. Gregorini G, Izzi C, Obici L, et al. Renal apolipoprotein A-I amyloidosis: a rare and usually ignored cause of hereditary tubulointerstitial nephritis. J Am Soc Nephrol. 2005;16:3680–6.
12. Westermark P, Sletten K, Eriksson M. Morphologic and chemical variation of the kidney lesions in amyloidosis secondary to rheumatoid arthritis. Lab Invest. 1979;41:427–31.
13. Fogo A, Qureshi N, Horn RG. Morphologic and clinical features of fibrillary glomerulonephritis versus immunotactoid glomerulopathy. Am J Kidney Dis. 1993;22:367–77.
14. Bridoux F, Hugue V, Coldefy O, et al. Fibrillary glomerulonephritis and immunotactoid (microtubular) glomerulopathy are associated with distinct immunologic features. Kidney Int. 2002;62:1764–75.
15. Rosenstock JL, Markowitz GS, Valeri AM, Sacchi G, Appel GB, D'Agati VD. Fibrillary and immunotactoid glomerulonephritis: distinct entities with different clinical and pathologic features. Kidney Int. 2003;63:1450–61.
16. Katzmann JA, Abraham RS, Dispenzieri A, Lust JA, Kyle RA. Diagnostic performance of quantitative kappa and lambda free light chain assays in clinical practice. Clin Chem. 2005;51:878–81.
17. Akar H, Seldin DC, Magnani B, et al. Quantitative serum free light chain assay in the diagnostic evaluation of AL amyloidosis. Amyloid 2005;12:210–5.
18. Dispenzieri A, Kyle R, Merlini G, et al. International Myeloma Working Group guidelines for serum-free light chain analysis in multiple myeloma and related disorders. Leukemia. 2009;23:215–24.
19. Looi LM. An investigation of the protein components of amyloid using immunoperoxidase and permanganate methods on tissue sections. Pathology 1986;18:137–40.

20. Veeramachaneni R, Gu X, Herrera GA. Atypical amyloidosis: diagnostic challenges and the role of immunoelectron microscopy in diagnosis. Ultrastruct Pathol. 2004;28: 75–82.

21. Obici L, Palladini G, Giorgetti S, et al. Liver biopsy discloses a new apolipoprotein A-I hereditary amyloidosis in several unrelated Italian families. Gastroenterology 2004;126:1416–22.

22. Carone FA, Epstein FH. Nephrogenic diabetes insipidus caused by amyloid disease. Evidence in man of the role of the collecting ducts in concentrating urine. Am J Med. 1960;29:539–44.

23. Asmundsson P, Snaedal J. Persistent water diuresis in renal amyloidosis. A case report. Scand J Urol Nephrol. 1981;15:77–9.

24. Ekelund L. Radiologic findings in renal amyloidosis. AJR Am J Roentgenol. 1977;129:851–3.

25. Apter S, Zemer D, Terhakopian A, et al. Abdominal CT findings in nephropathic amyloidosis of familial Mediterranean fever. Amyloid 2001;8:58–64.

26. Dikman SH, Churg J, Kahn T. Morphologic and clinical correlates in renal amyloidosis. Hum Pathol. 1981;12:160–9.

27. Fadia A, Casserly LF, Sanchorawala V, et al. Incidence and outcome of acute renal failure complicating autologous stem cell transplantation for AL amyloidosis. Kidney Int. 2003;63:1868–73.

28. Leung N, Slezak JM, Bergstralh EJ, et al. Acute renal insufficiency after high-dose melphalan in patients with primary systemic amyloidosis during stem cell transplantation. Am J Kidney Dis. 2005;45:102–11.

29. Levey AS, Bosch JP, Lewis JB, Greene T, Rogers N, Roth D. A more accurate method to estimate glomerular filtration rate from serum creatinine: a new prediction equation. Modification of Diet in Renal Disease Study Group. Ann Int Med. 1999;130:461–70.

30. Cockcroft DW, Gault MH. Prediction of creatinine clearance from serum creatinine. Nephron. 1976;16:31–41.

31. Merlini G, Bellotti V. Molecular mechanisms of amyloidosis. N Engl J Med. 2003;349:583–96.

32. Yan SD, Zhu H, Zhu A, et al. Receptor-dependent cell stress and amyloid accumulation in systemic amyloidosis. Nat Med. 2000;6:643–51.

33. Sousa MM, Du Yan S, Fernandes R, Guimaraes A, Stern D, Saraiva MJ. Familial amyloid polyneuropathy: receptor for advanced glycation end products-dependent triggering of neuronal inflammatory and apoptotic pathways. J Neurosci. 2001;21:7576–86.

34. Keeling J, Teng J, Herrera GA. AL-amyloidosis and light-chain deposition disease light chains induce divergent phenotypic transformations of human mesangial cells. Lab Invest. 2004;84:1322–38.

35. Brenner DA, Jain M, Pimentel DR, et al. Human amyloidogenic light chains directly impair cardiomyocyte function through an increase in cellular oxidant stress. Circ Res. 2004;94:1008–10.

36. Liao R, Jain M, Teller P, et al. Infusion of light chains from patients with cardiac amyloidosis causes diastolic dysfunction in isolated mouse hearts. Circulation. 2001;104: 1594–97.

37. Sousa MM, Cardoso I, Fernandes R, Guimaraes A, Saraiva MJ. Deposition of transthyretin in early stages of familial amyloidotic polyneuropathy: evidence for toxicity of nonfibrillar aggregates. Am J Pathol. 2001;159:1993–2000.

38. Lobato L, Beirao I, Guimaraes SM, et al. Familial amyloid polyneuropathy type I (Portuguese): distribution and characterization of renal amyloid deposits. Am J Kidney Dis. 1998;31:940–46.

39. Snanoudj R, Durrbach A, Gauthier E, et al. Changes in renal function in patients with familial amyloid polyneuropathy treated with orthotopic liver transplantation. Nephrol Dial Transplant. 2004;19:1779–85.

40. Dember LM, Sanchorawala V, Seldin DC, et al. Effect of dose-intensive intravenous melphalan and autologous blood stem-cell transplantation on al amyloidosis-associated renal disease. Ann Int Med. 2001;134:746–53.

41. Palladini G, Lavatelli F, Russo P, et al. Circulating amyloidogenic free light chains and serum N-terminal natriuretic peptide type B decrease simultaneously in association with improvement of survival in AL. Blood. 2006;107:3854–8.

42. Glassock RJ. Prophylactic anticoagulation in nephrotic syndrome: a clinical conundrum. J Am Soc Nephrol. 2007;18:2221–5.

43. Dember LM. Emerging treatment approaches for the systemic amyloidoses. Kidney Int. 2005;68:1377–90.

44. Girnius S, Seldin DC, Skinner M, et al. Hepatic response after high-dose melphalan and stem cell transplantation in patients with AL amyloidosis associated liver disease. Haematologica 2009;94:1029–32.

45. Batts ED, Sanchorawala V, Hegerfeldt Y, Lazarus HM. Azotemia associated with use of lenalidomide in plasma cell dyscrasias. Leuk Lymphoma 2008;49:1108–15.

46. Sanchorawala V, Wright DG, Rosenzweig M, et al. Lenalidomide and dexamethasone in the treatment of AL amyloidosis: results of a phase 2 trial. Blood 2007;109:492–6.

47. Palladini G, Perfetti V, Obici L, et al. Association of melphalan and high-dose dexamethasone is effective and well tolerated in patients with AL (primary) amyloidosis who are ineligible for stem cell transplantation. Blood 2004;103:2936–8.

48. Jaccard A, Moreau P, Leblond V, et al. High-dose melphalan versus melphalan plus dexamethasone for AL amyloidosis. N Engl J Med. 2007;357:1083–93.

49. Dispenzieri A, Lacy MQ, Zeldenrust SR, et al. The activity of lenalidomide with or without dexamethasone in patients with primary systemic amyloidosis. Blood. 2007;109:465–70.

50. Comenzo RL. Managing systemic light-chain amyloidosis. J Natl Compr Canc Netw. 2007;5:179–87.

51. Leung N, Dispenzieri A, Fervenza FC, et al. Renal response after high-dose melphalan and stem cell transplantation is a favorable marker in patients with primary systemic amyloidosis. Am J Kidney Dis. 2005;46:270–7.

52. Elkayam O, Hawkins PN, Lachmann H, Yaron M, Caspi D. Rapid and complete resolution of proteinuria due to renal amyloidosis in a patient with rheumatoid arthritis treated with infliximab. Arthritis Rheum. 2002;46:2571–3.

53. Mpofu S, Teh LS, Smith PJ, Moots RJ, Hawkins PN. Cytostatic therapy for AA amyloidosis complicating psoriatic spondyloarthropathy. Rheumatology (Oxford) 2003;42:362–6.

54. Ravindran J, Shenker N, Bhalla AK, Lachmann H, Hawkins P. Case report: response in proteinuria due to AA amyloidosis but not Felty's syndrome in a patient with rheumatoid arthritis treated with TNF-alpha blockade. Rheumatology (Oxford) 2004;43:669–72.

55. Gottenberg JE, Merle-Vincent F, Bentaberry F, et al. Anti-tumor necrosis factor alpha therapy in fifteen patients with AA amyloidosis secondary to inflammatory arthritis: a followup report of tolerability and efficacy. Arthritis Rheum. 2003;48:2019–24.

56. Kisilevsky R, Lemieux LJ, Fraser PE, Kong X, Hultin PG, Szarek WA. Arresting amyloidosis in vivo using small-molecule anionic sulphonates or sulphates: implications for Alzheimer's disease. Nat Med. 1995;1:143–8.

57. Kisilevsky R. The relation of proteoglycans, serum amyloid P and apo E to amyloidosis current status, 2000. Amyloid 2000;7:23–5.

58. Dember LM, Hawkins PN, Hazenberg BP, et al. Eprodisate for the treatment of renal disease in AA amyloidosis. N Engl J Med. 2007;356:2349–60.

59. Dember LM. Modern treatment of amyloidosis: unresolved questions. J Am Soc Nephrol. 2009;20:469–72.

60. Ericzon BG, Larsson M, Herlenius G, Wilczek HE. Report from the Familial Amyloidotic Polyneuropathy World Transplant Registry (FAPWTR) and the Domino Liver Transplant Registry (DLTR). Amyloid 2003;10 Suppl 1:67–76.

61. Holmgren G, Ericzon BG, Groth CG, et al. Clinical improvement and amyloid regression after liver transplantation in hereditary transthyretin amyloidosis. Lancet 1993;341:1113–6.

62. Zeldenrust S, Gertz M, Uemichi T, et al. Orthotopic liver transplantation for hereditary fibrinogen amyloidosis. Transplantation 2003;75:560–61.

63. Mousson C, Heyd B, Justrabo E, et al. Successful hepatorenal transplantation in hereditary amyloidosis caused by a frame-shift mutation in fibrinogen Aalpha-chain gene. Am J Transplant. 2006;6:632–5.

64. Gillmore JD, Booth DR, Rela M, et al. Curative hepatorenal transplantation in systemic amyloidosis caused by the Glu526Val fibrinogen alpha-chain variant in an English family. QJM. 2000;93:269–75.

65. Gillmore JD, Stangou AJ, Tennent GA, et al. Clinical and biochemical outcome of hepatorenal transplantation for hereditary systemic amyloidosis associated with apolipoprotein AI Gly26Arg. Transplantation 2001;71:986–92.

66. Carvalho MJ, Lobato L, Ventura A, et al. Remission of proteinuria following liver transplantation for familial amyloid polyneuropathy TTR met30. Transplant Proc. 2000;32:2664–6.

67. Chen N, Lau H, Kong L, et al. Pharmacokinetics of lenalidomide in subjects with various degrees of renal impairment and in subjects on hemodialysis. J Clin Pharmacol. 2007;47:1466–75.

68. Chanan-Khan AA, Kaufman JL, Mehta J, et al. Activity and safety of bortezomib in multiple myeloma patients with advanced renal failure: a multicenter retrospective study. Blood. 2007;109:2604–6.

69. Casserly LF, Fadia A, Sanchorawala V, et al. High-dose intravenous melphalan with autologous stem cell transplantation in AL amyloidosis-associated end-stage renal disease. Kidney Int. 2003;63:1051–7.

70. Leung N, Griffin MD, Dispenzieri A, et al. Living donor kidney and autologous stem cell transplantation for primary systemic amyloidosis (AL) with predominant renal involvement. Am J Transplant. 2005;5:1660–70.

Chapter 10

Primary Systemic Amyloid Neuropathy

Harman P.S. Bajwa and John J. Kelly

Abstract Primary systemic amyloidosis (PSA) is a plasma cell dyscrasia. Organ damage is caused by deposition of amyloid, derived from monoclonal light chains, in tissues including nerves. PSA damages tissues and leads to combinations of neuropathy and renal, cardiac, and liver failure. The neuropathy of PSA is relatively stereotyped with damage to small and autonomic nerve fibers and superimposed carpal tunnel syndrome. The disease is progressive and mortality is high, especially when there is early involvement of vital organs. Treatment in the past was relatively ineffective. However, with the advent of peripheral blood stem cell transplantation and chemotherapy in selected patients, prolonged survival is possible if the weight of organ damage at onset of treatment is not too high. Thus, early detection is paramount.

Keywords Amyloid, Peripheral neuropathy, Amyloidosis, Primary systemic amyloid, Primary systemic amyloid neuropathy, Familial amyloid neuropathy

Introduction

The peripheral nervous system is frequently affected in amyloidosis. In some studies, peripheral neuropathy (PN) is the presenting sign of primary systemic amyloidosis (PSA) or multiple myeloma (MM) in about 15% of patients [1, 2] and may be the cardinal manifestation. Hence, understanding the clinical presentation of PN is important in early diagnosis of PSA. This chapter will focus on primary systemic amyloidosis neuropathy (PSAN), but will also briefly discuss familial amyloid polyneuropathy (FAP), which often enters into the differential diagnosis of PSAN.

Case Vignette

A 67-year-old man presented with a 6-month history of pain and numbness in his lower extremities. He described the pain as burning in his distal legs and feet that kept him awake at night. The burning was interspersed with sharp, shooting pains "like needle pricks" in his legs and other parts of his body, including his trunk. He denied any associated weakness or ataxia. He also complained of the recent onset of intermittent numbness of his hands that bothered him at night and continued to be present in the morning upon awakening. He would often rub and shake his hands with some sensation recovery. More recently, he had developed diarrhea after eating and had lost 10% in weight despite a good appetite. He also noted that he felt light-headed

From: *Amyloidosis*, Contemporary Hematology,
Edited by: M.A. Gertz and S.V. Rajkumar, DOI 10.1007/978-1-60761-631-3_10,

after rapidly rising from a chair or when he got out of bed in the morning. On one occasion, a week prior to examination, he nearly fainted while taking a prolonged hot shower.

Examination disclosed distal loss of pain and temperature sensations. Vibration sense was mildly impaired, and position sense was intact. Sensation was also diminished in the median nerve distribution of both hands. Strength was intact, but he had atrophy of distal calf and foot muscles in addition to mild atrophy of the thenar muscles. Ankle reflexes were absent, knee reflexes 1/4, and arm reflexes 2/4 bilaterally. Gait was antalgic and cautious. He looked pale and gaunt with bruises on his trunk and eyelids. Peripheral nerves were not palpably enlarged. On orthostatic testing, supine blood pressure was 146/77, with a regular pulse of 87. After 5 min of standing, blood pressure dropped to 117/57, with a relatively unchanged pulse of 90. He felt slightly light-headed, which eased when he sat down.

Laboratory tests showed a mild normocytic anemia. The erythrocyte sedimentation rate was elevated at 56 mm/h. Serum protein electrophoresis (SPEP) revealed a slightly low albumin level (3.2 g/dL) with a normal gamma globulin level. The other routine chemical tests were normal, including a fasting blood glucose, a hemoglobin A1C level, and a subsequent 2-h glucose tolerance test. Serum immunofixation electrophoresis (SIFE) showed a small IgG kappa monoclonal protein (MP). Urinalysis was normal. Urine immunofixation electrophoresis (UIFE) showed a monoclonal kappa light chain despite a negative test for Bence-Jones proteins.

Nerve conduction studies showed a distal axonal neuropathy with absent sural nerve action potentials and mild slowing of leg motor nerve conduction velocities with a low-amplitude tibial compound muscle action potential (CMAP). In the upper extremities, studies showed evidence of carpal tunnel syndrome (CTS), worse on the right. Electromyography (EMG) showed active and chronic changes of denervation in distal leg and foot muscles. Cardiac R–R interval variation study showed evidence of autonomic involvement. A fat pad aspirate and sural nerve biopsy were both positive for amyloid which proved to be kappa light chain-type PSA. Despite treatment with melphalan and prednisone in addition to supportive measures, the disease progressed, and the patient died approximately 1 year later.

Clinical Manifestations

PN is the most common initial neurological manifestation of PSA [1, 2]. PSAN is typically distal, symmetrical, and progressive. Sensory symptoms usually dominate the initial presentation. In most patients, there is a clear dissociation of sensory signs with temperature and pain perception affected earlier and to a greater degree than vibration sense and proprioception. The typical patient presents with painful dysesthesias of the distal legs with the involvement of the hands and arms soon after. Distal weakness and muscle atrophy, although typically present, are not as prominent and rarely become severe in PSAN [1].

Less common presentations include initial median neuropathy at the wrist (CTS) due to amyloid deposition in the carpal tunnel, followed by generalized symptoms. If tissues resected in carpal tunnel surgeries are regularly stained for amyloid, occasional patients are found to have PSA before presenting with more common symptoms. About a quarter of patients also present with cardiac failure, slightly more commonly than presentation with generalized PN and autonomic failure [3]. Rarely, cranial neuropathies can herald PSA that eventually becomes generalized [1, 4]. Amyloid deposits have occasionally been noted in unusual locations such as trigeminal ganglia [5–7]. PSAN can infrequently present as a relatively pure autonomic neuropathy due to amyloid deposition in autonomic fibers and ganglia [8, 9]. On rare occasions, typical PSAN can present with signs of more diffuse upper and lower extremity motor involvement [10]. In addition, asymmetric presentation of chronically progressive peripheral motor and sensory neuropathies has been associated with amyloid deposition in the lumbosacral plexus and nerve roots with distal axonal degeneration [11].

Since the onset of amyloid neuropathy is so variable, a careful search for involvement of small myelinated and unmyelinated sensory and autonomic fibers is helpful in diagnosis. The finding of selective loss of temperature and pain perceptions in the distal legs with relative retention of touch sense and proprioception can suggest amyloidosis. Less commonly, patients may have equal involvement of all sensory modalities, or even predominant large fiber sensory loss [1]. Motor examination usually reveals mild to moderate distal weakness with atrophy of intrinsic foot muscles, which is typically overshadowed by the sensory loss. Deep tendon reflexes are usually decreased or absent distally. Skin trophic changes and reduced sweating are often noted. As in our patient, despite amyloid deposition, palpably enlarged nerves are uncommon [1]. Autonomic dysfunction with frequent sweating and gastrointestinal or renal involvement, with or without other motor or sensory changes, should suggest the diagnosis of amyloid neuropathy [9].

Differential Diagnosis

Even with careful neurological examination, PSAN can be difficult to differentiate from other axonal neuropathies of late life. All of these can present initially with small fiber sensory loss (pain and temperature), with considerable spontaneous neuropathic pain and relative sparing of motor and discriminative functions. Though clinically difficult to differentiate, most of these late-life axonal peripheral neuropathies can be separated by laboratory testing and biopsy.

However, the disorder that most closely mimics primary PSAN is hereditary or familial amyloid polyneuropathy [12]. FAP is not a single disease entity but an umbrella term for several distinctive clinical syndromes due to specific genetic abnormalities. Of the various types, FAP types I and II represent the bulk of the cases, and thus their peripheral neurological involvement will be briefly discussed. Both are most commonly caused by a point mutation in the transthyretin gene on chromosome 18. The most frequent mutation is a substitution of methionine for valine at position 40 (met 40).

Clinically, FAP type I typically presents with loss of pain and temperature sensation in the lower extremities, which frequently results in painless ulcers and amputations. Later, paresthesias and dysesthesias become prominent with defects of proprioception and touch. Over the years, these symptoms spread to the upper extremities [13]. Muscle weakness generally developed much later and is accompanied by prominent distal muscle wasting with associated decreased or absent deep tendon reflexes. In one study of FAP, autonomic neuropathy ultimately developed in 70% of patients [14] and impotence is frequent and early. Type II FAP was first described in a Swiss family living in Indiana [15]. These patients did not develop symptoms until the fourth or fifth decade of their lives. In these patients, carpal tunnel symptoms due to deposition of amyloid in the flexor retinaculum were the earliest, and often the sole manifestations for many years. A sensorimotor peripheral neuropathy eventually developed in the arms and later in the legs. This disease has a more benign course and usually spares the autonomic nervous system. Vitreous opacities are prominent and can lead to blindness. Even with this clinical and genetic heterogeneity, the diagnosis of familial amyloid polyneuropathy can be relatively straightforward when there is a positive family history and a compatible clinical picture [16].

Pathophysiology

In PSA, the amyloid fibrils are derived from monoclonal light chain immunoglobulins. Lambda light chains are twice as common as kappa [17–19]. The monoclonal light chains are processed by macrophages producing amyloid fibrils that are insoluble, resistant to proteolysis, and form protein aggregates [20]. Older theories of neuropathy pathogenesis, mostly discarded now, have included mechanical compression and ischemia. It is now thought that the protein aggregates are directly toxic to nerves and other tissues, similar to the effects of amyloid aggregates in the brain, as seen in degenerative disorders, such as Alzheimer's. The anatomic locale of these deposits vary greatly, ranging from the dorsal root ganglion to the peripheral nerve, thus possibly accounting for the diverse and complicated presentation of amyloid neuropathy. Moreover, research has also implicated a potential humoral immune role in explaining the pathogenesis of amyloid neuropathy. For example, rare patients with IgM-derived PSA have been shown to display antibodies against myelin-associated glycoprotein (anti-MAG antibodies), similar to patients with the neuropathy associated with IgM monoclonal gammopathy without amyloidosis. However, unlike the latter patients, the neuropathy in the IgM PSA patients does not show the histopathological demyelinating features that are seen in IgM anti-MAG neuropathy. This suggests that the anti-MAG antibody is an epiphenomenon, and not likely the primary pathologic factor [20]. Thus, although there may be other pathologic processes affecting patients with PSAN, the main factor is a direct toxic effect of local amyloid deposits on nerves and other organs.

Histopathology of the sural nerve shows predominant axonal degeneration preferentially affecting small myelinated and unmyelinated fibers [1, 21]. Large myelinated fibers are also affected to a lesser extent. Electron microscopy confirms the striking loss of unmyelinated fibers with amyloid deposits in a beta-pleated sheet appearance. Amyloid deposits typically form a cuff around, and are deposited in, the walls of endoneural and epineural vessels, which appear thickened on H and E staining. Also, diffuse or linear streaks of amyloid can be seen in the epineurium with globular-shaped deposits noted in the endoneurium [1, 21]. These deposits may contribute to the local structural distortion of the nerve fibers, which originally led to the compression theory of pathogenesis, now mostly discarded, except in conditions like CTS [21]. In addition, neuron cell counts in the intermediolateral column are reduced by 50–75% in patients with orthostatic hypotension, possibly explaining the prevalence and early onset of autonomic disturbances seen in PSA [22].

Diagnosis

With knowledge of the spectrum of the clinical presentation of PSAN complemented with appropriate testing, the diagnosis of PSAN is no longer elusive. In particular, nerve conduction studies (NCS) and electromyography (EMG) are useful in documenting findings in PSAN. NCS are usually minimally slowed despite reduction in motor responses, with sensory nerve responses often being absent [23, 24]. When sensory nerve action potentials are present, distal latencies are only mildly delayed, proportional to the slowing of conduction velocities if temperature is well controlled, except for patients with superimposed CTS. However, routine nerve conduction studies early in the disease may not show clear sensory findings, since small myelinated and unmyelinated sensory fibers, not testable by conventional nerve conduction techniques, are affected first. In these patients, autonomic testing may detect dysfunction early in the disease, as documented in asymptomatic familial amyloidosis carriers [9, 25, 26]. Typical EMG findings in PSAN show a symmetrical, primarily axonal neuropathy affecting the longest axons with findings of distal and symmetric active and chronic denervation with reinnervation potentials. The longest nerves are maximally impacted, so distal lower limbs are affected more than upper, with the exception of CTS.

In addition to these neurophysiological findings, other abnormal laboratory findings and evidence of organ dysfunction outside the peripheral nervous system can suggest the diagnosis of PSAN (Table 10-1). Anemia is seen in about 50% of the patients [27], secondary to gastrointestinal bleeding, multiple myeloma, or renal insufficiency. About 80% of the patients have proteinuria [1, 2, 28], but Bence-Jones proteins are usually undetectable in patients without MM. Serum creatinine levels are above 1.3 mg/dL in half of patients. SPEP is usually abnormal, showing hypogammaglobulinemia in about 15% of patients with MM and 33% of those with PSA [27]. A narrow monoclonal peak in the gamma region, usually of moderate size (less than 3 g/dL), can be seen in about 40% of patients with PSA. Patients with a monoclonal spike of more than 3.0 g/dL are more likely to have MM. The gamma globulin peak can be small, however, and immunoelectrophoresis or immunofixation may be necessary to identify the monoclonal protein in some patients. Therefore, all patients with idiopathic peripheral neuropathy should undergo SIFE, even if SPEP is negative. Immunoelectrophoresis or immunofixation electrophoresis, however, is usually necessary to reveal a monoclonal light chain, which is seen in approximately 75% of patients. Electrophoresis of an adequately concentrated urine specimen usually shows a large albumin peak. As in the serum, a localized monoclonal band can be seen in urine in almost two-thirds of patients with multiple myeloma. Immunofixation of urine in a patient with unexplained nephrotic syndrome can sometimes help establish a diagnosis of amyloidosis by detecting a monoclonal light chain [2, 28]. Other tests that can be helpful include serum light chain assay and levels of beta-2 microglobulin [29].

The diagnosis of PSAN ultimately depends on the demonstration of amyloid in the tissue, either in a sural nerve biopsy or in other tissue. Amyloid appears pink with hematoxylin and eosin stains. Congo red is the most commonly used stain to identify amyloid, producing a reddish color routinely, but an apple-green birefringence under polarized light, diagnostic of all types of amyloid. This stain, however, is not 100% reliable, since some neural structures, bony trabeculae, and connective tissues can

Table 10-1. Organ involvement with PSA.

Organ	Percentage involved	Syndrome
Kidney	32	Nephrotic
Heart	23	Congestive heart failure, cardiomyopathy
Autonomic neuropathy	14	Orthostatic hypotension, impotence, etc.
Median nerve	24	Carpal tunnel
Peripheral nerves	17	Peripheral neuropathy

Adapted with permission from Kyle and Gertz [3]

display green birefringence as well [30]. Metachromatic stains such as cresyl violet or methyl violet can be useful, especially in sural nerve biopsies, where metachromasia stands out from the background. In occasional cases, all these stains are negative and electron microscopy is needed to demonstrate the diagnostic amyloid fibrils that appear as beta-pleated sheets. However, this is a tedious process best restricted to suspicious areas seen under light microscopy. High-resolution scintigraphic studies, using 123-I labeled purified human serum amyloid P component, can reveal focal deposits of all varieties of amyloid [31]. Identification of specific types requires staining with anti-sera to the abnormal constituent proteins such as kappa or gamma light chains, beta-2 microglobulin, and transthyretin.

The diagnosis of PSA should be considered in any patient with a sensorimotor peripheral neuropathy who has an abnormal monoclonal protein in serum or urine or a suggestive clinical picture. Diagnosis can be confirmed by obtaining appropriate tissue for histological investigation. We generally recommend biopsy of at least two sites, either at the same time or sequentially, since any individual site, including sural nerve even in neuropathy, can be negative. Abdominal fat aspirate or biopsy is an uncomplicated procedure that is positive in about 70–80% of patients [2, 28, 32, 33]. Bone marrow biopsy is positive in only half of patients with amyloidosis, but is safe and easy to do, and can reveal an abnormal proliferation of monoclonal plasma cells with appropriate histochemical staining. The presence of more than 20% plasma cells in the bone marrow, especially if atypical and nucleated, is associated with MM [2]. Sural nerve and rectal biopsies are both positive in over 80% of patients with PSAPN, and should be considered when other biopsies are negative. Care should be taken to include submucosa in the rectal specimen (2). If these tissues are negative and the diagnosis is strongly suspected, tissue should be obtained from involved organs (renal, liver, carpal tunnel, small intestine, heart, etc.), which have a high rate of positivity when clinically affected, but involve more risk. The relatively new technique of skin biopsies to diagnose small fiber neuropathy can reveal amyloid in blood vessels of subcutaneous tissues when properly stained [34].

Management

As a general principle, patients with a low burden of amyloid in a non-vital organ survive longer than patients with advanced multi-organ disease. The median survival of all patients with primary amyloidosis is about 2 years [28]. In a review of prognosis and treatment in PSA, several clinical and laboratory features were found to predict survival [35]. Patients with PN as the sole manifestation of PSA had the longest survival, ranging from 40 to 56 months [1, 28, 35, 36]. These patients eventually died from involvement of other organs [1]. Conversely, patients with congestive heart failure or orthostatic hypotension had the shortest survival, usually less than 1 year [28, 35]. Nephrotic syndrome and MM have a detrimental impact on survival in PSA as well [28].

The treatment of PSA has had minimal success until recently, partly due to the relative resistance of the amyloidogenic clone to chemotherapy, the insolubility of deposited amyloid and the delay in diagnosis in many cases. Unfortunately, even with somewhat successful treatment, the symptoms and findings of PN persist or even may continue to worsen despite improvement in other organs. Dysesthesias tend to disappear or spread proximally as the disease progresses and distal analgesia increases. Treatment of symptoms with analgesics, tricyclic antidepressants, and newer anticonvulsants may be helpful in supportive management. In some cases, low-dose narcotics at bedtime can be helpful, either alone, or combined with other medications.

Side effects can be troublesome in these patients, however, and include worsening of orthostatic hypotension and gastrointestinal and genitourinary functions. Orthostatic hypotension can be helped with fitted, supportive elastic stockings that extend up to the waist, although patients frequently refuse to wear them. Drugs that promote sodium retention and increase alpha-adrenergic tone can be helpful in the early stages, but lose their effectiveness as patients develop cardiac, kidney, and autonomic failure. These interventions are only symptomatic treatments, with long term efficacy at best anecdotal.

With the introduction of quantitative scintigraphic and turnover studies with radiolabeled serum amyloid P component [31], amyloid deposits have been shown to regress rapidly when the supply of the amyloid protein precursor is substantially reduced [37]. This constitutes the rationale for alkylating therapy in primary amyloidosis, with the hope of controlling plasma cell proliferation and production of light chains. Melphalan and prednisone, with or without colchicine and other chemotherapeutic agents, have been tried in multiple prospective trials [35, 37–40]. Overall, melphalan and prednisone treatment, continued for at least 1 year, has resulted in increased survival rates. The highest response rate (39%) was obtained in patients with nephrotic syndrome with normal serum creatinine levels, and no echocardiographic evidence of cardiac amyloidosis. Fifteen percent of patients with cardiac amyloidosis also responded [39, 40]. However, peripheral neuropathy did not respond [1, 2, 37, 40]. The combination of melphalan and prednisone has been proved superior to colchicine [39], and the addition of colchicine to the above regimen did not add any benefit in one randomized trial [41]. Thus, a trial of alkylating agents and prednisone is warranted in most patients.

More recent reports suggest benefit from high dose chemotherapy with melphalan and steroids followed by peripheral blood stem cell transplantation (PBSCT) [42–44]. PBSCT requires adequate renal, pulmonary, hepatic, and cardiac function that may be absent in many PSA patients [45]. Small numbers of transplants have been reported to date with encouraging results. In one study, neurological improvement occurred in four of five neuropathy patients [42]. Another group reported improved organ function in 12 of 20 patients [43]. Gertz, and colleagues at the Mayo Clinic, presented a series of 66 patients treated with PBSCT [46]. Of the 66 patients, seven died during the follow-up period. The 2-year actuarial survival was 70%. Patients with limited disease did the best (91% survived for 2 years), whereas those with multiple organ involvement did the worst (33% of patients with three organ involvement and 0% of four organ involvement survived 2 years). Thus, early PBSCT in the first year for those with minimal organ involvement is now the treatment of choice if the patient qualifies [44, 46, 47]. Unfortunately, many patients do not qualify for this new treatment. Dispenzieri and colleagues found that only 234 of 1,228 patients with amyloidosis satisfied eligibility criteria for transplantation [34]. Diagnosis is delayed most (median 26 months) in patients with relatively pure neuropathies without significant organ failure, who are the most likely to benefit from peripheral blood stem cell transplantation [1, 48, 49]. Without modern therapy, the disease has a dismal prognosis [1, 35, 50]. Neurologists are uniquely situated to identify patients with early PSAN when they are most likely to benefit from PBSCT.

Since for most patients there is no cure, supportive care is important. Cardiac transplantation, hemodialysis, continual peritoneal dialysis, and renal transplantation can improve survival in highly selected patients with primary amyloidosis, although amyloid can accumulate in transplanted organs [35, 37]. Recognition of presentation of amyloid neuropathy can be vital to early diagnosis and thus management of an otherwise relentless, generally progressive, terminal course of amyloidosis.

References

1. Kelly JJ, Kyle RA, O'Brien PC, Dyck PJ. The natural history of peripheral neuropathy in primary systemic amyloidosis. Ann Neurol. 1979;6:1–7.
2. Kyle RA, Greipp PR. Amyloidosis (AL): clinical and laboratory features. Mayo Clinic Proc. 1983;58:665–83.
3. Kyle RA, Gertz MA. Systemic amyloidosis. Crit Rev Oncol/Hematol. 1990;10:49–87.
4. Traynor AE, Gertz MA, Kyle RA. Cranial neuropathy associated with primary amyloidosis. Ann Neurol. 1991;29:451–54.
5. Gottfried ON, Chin S, Davidson HC, et al. Trigeminal amyloidoma: case report and review of the literature. Skull Base. 2007 Sep;17(5):317–24.
6. Bookland MJ, Bagley CA, Schwarz J, et al. Intracavernous trigeminal ganglion amyloidoma: case report. Neurosurgery. 2007 Mar;60(3):E574.
7. Yu E, de Tilly LN. Amyloidoma of Meckel's cave: a rare cause of trigeminal neuralgia. AJR Am J Roentgenol. 2004 Jun;182(6):1605–6.
8. Lingenfelser T, Linke RP, Dette S, Roggendorf W, Wietholter H. Amyloidosis mimicking a preferentially autonomic chronic Guillain-Barre syndrome. Clin invest. 1992;70: 159–62.
9. Wang AK, Fealey RD, Gehrking TL, et al. Patterns of neuropathy and autonomic failure in patients with amyloidosis. Mayo Clin Proc. 2008 Nov;83(11):1226–30.
10. Abarbanel JM, Frisher S, Osimani A. Primary amyloidosis with peripheral neuropathy and signs of motor neuron disease. Neurology. 1986;36:1125–27.
11. Antoine JC, Baril A, Guittier C, et al. Unusual amyloid polyneuropathy with predominant lumbosacral nerve roots and plexus involvement. Neurology. 1991;41:206–08.
12. Buxbaum JN, Tagoe CE. The genetics of the amyloidosis. Ann Rev Med. 2000;51: 543–69.
13. Ikeda S, Yanagisawa N, Hongo M, Ito N. Vagus nerve and celiac ganglion lesions in generalized amyloidosis: a correlative study of familial polyneuropathy and AL-amyloidosis. J Neurol Sci. 1987;79:129–39.
14. Gertz MA, Kyle RA, Thibodeau SN. Familial amyloidosis: a study of 52 north American-born patients examined during a 30-year period. Mayo Clin Proc. 1992;67: 428–40.
15. Rukavina JG, Block WD, Curtis AC. Familial primary systemic amyloidosis: an experimental, genetic and clinical study. J Invest Dermatol – Symp Proc. 1956;27:111.
16. Benson MD, Kincaid JC. The molecular biology and clinical features of amyloid neuropathy. Muscle Nerve. 2007 Oct;36(4):411–23.
17. Dalakas MC, Engel WK. Amyloid in hereditary amyloid polyneuropathy is related to prealbumin. Arch Neurol. 1981;38:420–22.
18. Chalk CH, Dyck PJ. Application of immunohistochemical techniques to sural nerve biopsies. Neurol Clin. 1992;10:601–13.
19. Vital C, Vital A, Bouillot-Eimer S, Brechenmacher C, Ferrer X, Lagueny A. Amyloid neuropathy: a retrospective study of 35 peripheral nerve biopsies. J Peripher Nerv Syst. 2004;9(4):232–41.
20. Garces-Sanchez M, Dyck PJ, Kyle RA, et al. Antibodies to myelin-associated glycoprotein (anti Mag) in IgM amyloidosis may influence expression of neuropathy in rare patients. Muscle Nerve. 2008 Apr;37(4):490–95.
21. Dyck PJ, Lambert EH. Dissociated sensation in amyloidosis: compound action potential, quantitative histologic and teased-fiber, and electron microscopic studies of sural nerve biopsies. Arc Neurol. 1969;20:490–507.
22. Low PA, Dyck PJ, Okasaki H, Kyle R, Fealet RD. The splanchnic autonomic outflow in amyloid neuropathy and Tangier disease. Neurology. 1981;31:461–63.
23. Melgaard B, Nielsen B. Electromyographic findings in amyloid neuropathy. Electromyogr Clin Neurophysiol. 1977;17:31–34.
24. Kelly JJ Jr.. The electrodiagnostic findings in peripheral neuropathy associated with monoclonal gammopathy. Muscle Nerve. 1983;6:504–09.

25. Ando Y, Ikegawa S, Miyazaki A, Inoue M, Morino Y, Araki S. Role of variant prealbumin in the pathogenesis of familial amyloidotic polyneuropathy: fate of normal and variant prealbumin in the circulation. Arch Biochem Biophys. 1989;274:87–93.

26. McLeod JG. Invited review: autonomic dysfunction in peripheral nerve disease. Muscle Nerve. 1992;15:3–13.

27. Kyle RA, Garton JP. Laboratory monitoring of myeloma proteins. Sem Oncol. 1986;13:310–17.

28. Kyle RA, Bayrd ED. Amyloidosis: review of 236 cases. Medicine. 1975;54(4):271–99.

29. Disperienzi A, Kyle R, Mertini JS, et al. International myeloma working group guidelines for serum-free light chain analysis in multiple myeloma and related disorders. Leukemia. 2009;23(2):215–24.

30. Klatskin G. Nonspecific green birefringence in Congo red-stained tissues. Am J Pathol. 1969;56:1–13.

31. Hawkins PN, Lavender JP, Pepys MB. Evaluation of systemic amyloidosis by scintigraphy with 123I-labeled serum amyloid -P component. N Engl J Med. 1990;323:508–13.

32. Gertz MA, Li CT, Shirahama T, Kyle RA. Utility of subcutaneous fat aspiration for the diagnosis of systemic amyloidosis (immunoglobulin light chain). Arch Intern Med. 1988;148:929–33.

33. Ansari-Lari MA, Ali SZ. Fine-needle aspiration of abdominal fat pad for amyloid detection: a clinically useful test?. Diagn Cytopathol. 2004;30(3):178–81.

34. Huang CY, Wang WJ, Wong CK. Skin biopsy gives the potential benefit in the diagnosis of systemic amyloidosis associated with cardiac involvement. Arch Dermatol. 1998;134:643.

35. Gertz MA, Kyle RA. Amyloidosis: prognosis and treatment. Sem Arthritis Rheum. 1994;24(2):124–38.

36. Duston M, Skinner M, Anderson J, Cohen AS. Peripheral neuropathy as an early marker of AL amyloidosis. Arch Intern Med. 1989;149:358–60.

37. Merlini G. Treatment of primary amyloidosis. Semin Hematol. 1995;32:60–79.

38. Ravid M, Robson M, Kedar I. Prolonged colchicine treatment in four patients with amyloidosis. Ann Intern Med. 1977;87:568–70.

39. Kyle RA, Greipp PR, Garton JP, Gertz MA. Primary systemic amyloidosis: comparison of melphalan/prednisone versus colchicine. Am J Med. 1985;79:708–.

40. Cohen AS, Rubinow A, Anderson JJ, et al. Survival of patients with primary amyloidosis: colchicine-treated cases from 1976 to 1983 compared with cases seen in previous years (1961 to 1973). Am J Med. 1987;82:1182–90.

41. Gertz MA, Kyle RA. Amyloidosis: prognosis and treatment. Sem Arthritis Rheum. 1994;24(2):124–38.

42. Comenzo RL. Primary systemic amyloidosis. Curr Treat Options Oncol. 2000;1(1):83–89.

43. Gertz MA, Lacy MQ, Gastineau DA, et al. Blood stem cell transplantation as therapy for primary systemic amyloidosis (AL). Bone Marrow Transplant. 2000;26(9):963–69.

44. Dispenzieri A, Kyle RA, Lacy MQ, et al. Superior survival in primary systemic amyloidosis patients undergoing peripheral blood stem cell transplantation: a case-control study. Blood. 2004;103(10):3960–63.

45. Gertz MA, Lacy MQ, Dispenzieri A, Hayman SR. Amyloidosis: diagnosis and management. Clin Lymphoma Myeloma. 2005;6(3):208–19.

46. Gertz MA, Lacy MQ, Dispenzieri A, et al. Stem cell transplantation for the management of primary systemic amyloidosis. Am J Med. 2002;113(7):549–55.

47. Rajkumar SV, Dispenzieri A, Kyle RA. Monoclonal gammopathy of undetermined significance, Waldenstrom macroglobulinemia, AL amyloidosis, and related plasma cell disorders: diagnosis and treatment. Mayo Clin Proc. 2006;81(5):693–703.

48. Spuler S, Emslie-Smith A, Engel AG. Amyloid myopathy: an underdiagnosed entity. Ann Neurol. 1998;43:719–28.

49. Rajkumar SV, Gertz MA, Kyle RZ. Prognosis of patients with primary systemic amyloidosis who present with dominant neuropathy. Am J Med. 1998;104:232–37.

50. Gertz MA, Kyle RZ, Greipp PR. Response rates and survival in primary systemic amyloidosis. Blood. 1991;77:257–62.
51. Durie BG, Persky B, Soenlen BJ, Grogan TM, Salmon SE. Amyloid production in human myeloma stem-cell culture, with morphologic evidence of amyloid secretion by associated macrophages. N Engl J Med. 1982;307:1689–92.

Chapter 11

Conventional Treatment of Amyloidosis

Morie A. Gertz and Francis Buadi

Abstract All patients with proven light chain amyloidosis deserve a trial of therapy. Although high dose therapy has been shown to be highly effective, only a quarter of patients are actually eligible for this technique. Lower intensity treatments are required for the majority of patients. We review the history of treatment of amyloidosis beginning with the use of conventional alkylating agent chemotherapy, the role of the novel agents bortezomib, lenalidomide, and thalidomide in the treatment of amyloidosis. A suggested treatment algorithm is given to help guide decisions regarding therapy.

Keywords Melphalan, Dexamethasone, Chemotherapy, Treatment of amyloidosis, Thalidomide, Lenalidomide, Bortezomib

Introduction

By definition, immunoglobulin light chain amyloidosis is associated with a plasma cell dyscrasia [1]. The current pathophysiology, as it is understood, is that the plasma cells synthesize immunoglobulin light chains or immunoglobulin light and heavy chains, or heavy chain fragments [2] that, due to their primary sequence, cannot be either catabolized completely or undergo misfolding so that catabolic enzymes are incapable of breaking the protein down to constituent amino acids [3]. These light chain subunits, which range from 6,000 to 20,000 molecular weight, in other words half the usual size of a light chain, represent the amyloid fibril subunit. These assemble into protofibrils [4], which undergo winding to form the amyloid fibril, which has an x-ray diffraction pattern of the beta-pleated sheet and binds Congo red with its tinctorial properties of green birefringence under polarized light. The actual mechanism whereby amyloid deposits produce organ dysfunction remains unclear. Whether the finally formed amyloid deposit is responsible for the dysfunction or whether soluble, toxic intermediates mediate the dysfunction that is seen remains a subject of controversy [5].

In theory, there would be two ways to interfere with amyloidosis. One would be to interfere with the misfolding of the amyloid fibril, thereby rendering it soluble. Although research is underway with transthyretin amyloid [6], no published studies exist on attempts to "dissolve" or solubilize amyloid.

It has been demonstrated using I [123]-SAP that amyloid deposits are in dynamic equilibrium with a soluble pool and that if precursor production is interrupted, deposits can regress [7]. The equilibrium constant likely varies among light chains,

From: *Amyloidosis*, Contemporary Hematology,
Edited by: M.A. Gertz and S.V. Rajkumar, DOI 10.1007/978-1-60761-631-3_11,
© Springer Science+Business Media, LLC 2010

and how much of a reduction in precursor protein production must occur in order to resorb amyloid deposits remains unknown and is not currently measurable. All current strategies to manage amyloidosis involve systemic therapies designed to destroy the plasma cell responsible for the synthesis of the immunoglobulin light chain [8]. Initial studies of colchicine to treat amyloidosis were published [9], but subsequent studies demonstrated that colchicine is ineffective therapy and, with greater understanding of the pathophysiology of the disease, should not be expected to benefit patients with amyloidosis other than those patients with familial Mediterranean fever [10].

Every therapy that has been attempted in the management of amyloidosis has been derived from favorable results obtained in comparable multiple myeloma populations. In every instance from original alkylator-based therapy [11] to the current use of novel agents in amyloidosis, efficacy is first demonstrated in a multiple myeloma population and subsequently applied to amyloidosis patients with generally, similarly successful results excepting for the fact that patients with amyloidosis have unique organ dysfunction that tends to increase the toxicity associated with systemic therapy.

High-dose chemotherapy with stem cell reconstitution has been a validated technique in the treatment of patients with multiple myeloma for over a decade [12]. Unfortunately, only the minority of patients with amyloidosis would be eligible for safe stem cell transplantation. The majority of patients with multiple myeloma have excellent performance status and normal organ function with the exception of creatinine elevation, which is present in 12% of patients after 4 months of induction therapy [13]. Amyloidosis patients, on the contrary, have a 50% prevalence of echocardiographic evidence of cardiac involvement, 15% clinically significant liver involvement, 15% debilitating peripheral neuropathy, and 20% serum creatinine elevation [14]. By virtue of these issues, no more than 25% of patients seen at Mayo Clinic ultimately are offered stem cell transplantation [15]. The majority of patients require alternatives to high-dose therapy. It is not clear that high-dose therapy is a consistently preferred alternative. The single, prospective, randomized study did not favor transplantation [16], although high-risk patients poorly suited for high-dose therapy were enrolled and were included in this paper so that further studies need to be done [17]. The majority of patients with amyloidosis need to be treated conventionally.

Alkylator-Based Therapy

The first reports on the use of alkylator agent chemotherapy for AL were first published nearly 35 years ago [18]. Melphalan/prednisone was demonstrated to be an effective therapy [19]. Disadvantages of alkylator-based therapy include low response rate and a long time for a response to be recognized. When patients are on alkylator therapy, it is difficult to know whether they are destined to fail therapy or whether additional therapy is appropriate and too early to abandon. The median time to detect a response for melphalan-treated patients is nearly 1 year. Moreover, melphalan therapy can result in late myelodysplasia. Originally, 7% of exposed patients developed MDS after melphalan exposure for amyloidosis [20]. With the introduction of improved supportive care and better salvage regimens, the median survival has been steadily improving, and the number of patients at risk for developing MDS is increasing. The most recent updates suggest that the actuarial risk of MDS/ANLL at 10 years is approaching 20% [21]. Response rates to melphalan-based therapy, when combined with prednisone, are generally not greater than 30% [22]. One must keep in mind that the immunoglobulin-free light chain assay, which is currently used to assess response, was not available for those studies and prior response rates may be an underestimate. The key point is that melphalan and prednisone can be administered to virtually any patient with amyloidosis regardless of performance status, serum creatinine level (with dose adjustment), or the extent of cardiac failure. Therefore, if the patient is willing to undergo a trial of melphalan and prednisone and accepts the risks, there is not a good reason to withhold therapy [23].

The best responses to melphalan and prednisone occur in patients with single-organ nephrotic syndrome without renal insufficiency. The response rate looking at all patients treated with melphalan and prednisone is 18% if the definition is organ based [24]. However, if the alkaline phosphatase level is four times normal or the serum creatinine is >3 mg/dL, responses are rare, and the development of dialysis-dependent renal failure is likely. Although uncommon, clinically important responses have been reported with melphalan even in advanced cardiomyopathy, and in prospective studies, a modest prolongation of survival has been demonstrated in the presence of amyloid heart failure [25]. In a retrospective analysis of 153 patients treated with melphalan/prednisone, the 5-year survival of responders was 78% [24]. In a cohort of 810 patients, the 10-year survival was 4.7%, and all 10-year survivors received melphalan/prednisone [26]. Of the 30 ten-year survivors, 14 exhibited a complete hematologic response. Two prospective randomized studies have demonstrated a survival advantage with melphalan-based therapy. One 3-arm study accrued 219 patients and randomly assigned them to colchicine 0.6 mg twice daily, standard melphalan/prednisone, or melphalan plus prednisone and colchicine. Half of the patients had proteinuria in the nephrotic range and 20% had overt clinical heart failure. The median survival for both melphalan-containing regimens was 17 months compared with 8.5 months for colchicine alone [27]. A second prospective randomized study of 100 patients, 50 receiving colchicine and 50 receiving melphalan and prednisone and colchicine, showed a median survival of 6.7 months in the colchicine group versus 12 months in the three-drug group [28]. Because there is a survival advantage in the melphalan-based group, withholding therapy is not justified, but the short median survival reflects the necessity for better therapies.

In patients whose cardiac status makes anything other than the gentlest therapy impractical, continuous oral daily melphalan has been used. In a report of 30 treated patients, 7 of the 13 evaluable after 4 months of therapy achieved partial hematologic response, in 3 a complete hematologic response. This suggests that melphalan can provide significant palliation even in patients with advanced disease [29].

Dexamethasone-Based Regimens

Vincristine, doxorubicin, and dexamethasone therapy were reported in eight patients with AL. Four fulfilled criteria for an objective hematologic response [30]. Vincristine use is contraindicated in those patients with amyloid peripheral neuropathy, and doxorubicin is a poor choice with the high prevalence of amyloid cardiomyopathy. When four patients with amyloid nephrotic syndrome were treated with VAD, three responded and were alive and in remission for 4–9 years [31]. VAD has been used as an induction to reduce the plasma cell burden prior to stem cell transplantation, but clinical improvement associated with VAD did not reduce the transplant-related mortality [32]. Ninety-two patients treated in Great Britain received four cycles of VAD with an organ response in 42% and a treatment-related mortality of 7% [33]. Nine consecutive patients with AL were treated with pulse dexamethasone for three to six cycles, days 1–4, 9–12, and 17–20, followed by maintenance interferon 3–6 million

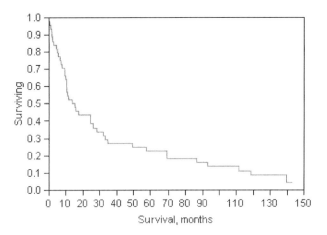

Fig. 11-1. Overall survival of 44 amyloidosis patients treated with high-dose dexamethasone.

units three times per week [34]. Improvement in organ involvement was seen in eight of the nine patients, and six of the seven patients with nephrotic syndrome had a 50% reduction in proteinuria. We have reported on 44 patients with amyloidosis, a high proportion of whom had cardiac involvement [35, 36]. The survival of these patients is shown in Fig. 11-1. A modified, lower dose and lower frequency of dexamethasone can produce a response in 35% of patients with a median time to response of 4 months [37]. Ninety-three patients with AL were enrolled in a multicenter cooperative group trial of dexamethasone and interferon. Hematologic complete responses were seen in 24% and improvement in organ dysfunction was seen in 45% of evaluable patients with a median survival of 31 months and an overall 2-year survival of 60% [38]. Heart failure and serum beta 2 microglobulin levels were predictors of adverse outcome. In a subset of patients eligible for stem cell transplantation, the estimated 2-year overall survival was 78%. Dexamethasone toxicity in amyloidosis patients is substantial. Fluid retention occurs in patients with nephrotic syndrome and heart failure, and dose reductions are common. In the Southwest Oncology Group Study, 24 patients with cardiomyopathy had a significantly lower response rate. The median time to hematologic response was 103 days. Toxicity from dexamethasone is related to the number of organs involved. Statistically, only heart failure predicted excessive toxicity.

Melphalan with Dexamethasone

The use of melphalan plus high-dose dexamethasone has been reported in the management of amyloidosis. Patients were selected on the basis of their ineligibility for high-dose melphalan plus transplant therapy. Of 46 patients, a hematologic response was seen in 31, and a hematologic complete response was seen in 15 (33%). Improvement in organ dysfunction was seen in 22 patients (48%). Advantages of this regimen included a 100-day mortality of 4%, resolution of cardiac failure in 6 of 32 patients with a median time to response of 4.5 months, and only 11% adverse effects [39]. These results were updated with 5-year follow-up. The actuarial survival at 6 years was approximately 50%, and the progression-free survival was 40% [40]. Patients who relapse could be re-induced successfully with melphalan and dexamethasone. Of 41 evaluable patients, there were ultimately 30 responders and 11 nonresponders with the responders' median survival not having been reached and nonresponders' median survival of just over 2 years. Boston University Medical Center has used pulsed low-dose melphalan in patients ineligible for stem cell transplant because of severe cardiac involvement or poor performance status [29]. All patients received growth factor support, and the melphalan dose was adjusted to produce mid-cycle myelosuppression. Fifteen patients, median age 55, received a median of three cycles. Eight of ten evaluable patients had a hematologic response and two of the eight were complete. Of 15 patients treated, 2 survived 6 months, and 24 months after treatment, 13 have died. Median survival was 2 months. Ten patients died within 5 weeks of starting treatment.

One hundred and forty-four patients in Great Britain received melphalan IV 25 mg/m^2 with dexamethasone 20 mg for 4 days every 21–28 days. Median number of cycles was three. Fifty-one patients did not receive dexamethasone. Treatment-related mortality was 2%; 23% had normalization of free light chains; 31% had a 50% decrease in serum-free light chain; and 46% were nonresponders. The response rate was higher in patients who received dexamethasone [41]. Most clinical responses were evidenced within two cycles. Median survival for responders was 44 months, and amyloid organ dysfunction improved in 14% of patients.

Thalidomide

Sixteen patients were enrolled in a study of thalidomide. The median maximum tolerated dose was 300 mg. Fifty percent of the patients experienced grade 3–4 toxicity; 25% had to discontinue taking the medication; 25% had a reduction in light chain proteinuria but not in total urinary protein [42]. In a Mayo Clinic report on 12 patients with thalidomide therapy, 75% had drug-related toxicity [43]. Progressive renal insufficiency developed in five and deep vein thrombosis and syncope in two. The median time of thalidomide treatment was a mere 72 days due to intolerance. The Italian amyloidosis group reported on thalidomide and dexamethasone therapy in 31 patients. Only 11 patients tolerated 400 mg a day for a median of 5.7 months [44]. Twenty experienced grade 3 or greater toxicity. In Great Britain, thalidomide [45] was administered at a median dose of 100 mg/day but was discontinued in 31% of patients. The hematologic response rate was 55%. Thalidomide and dexamethasone appear to be active. However, the toxicity is substantial, and the thalidomide dose is best started at 50 mg and should not exceed 100 mg. In the Mayo Clinic experience, the median dose of thalidomide is only 50 mg a day, which might limit its efficacy. Symptomatic bradycardia has been seen in as many as 26%. Melphalan, thalidomide, and dexamethasone were administered to 22 patients with advanced cardiac amyloidosis. Eight hematologic responses and four organ responses were reported. Six patients died due to their advanced cardiac amyloidosis before cycle 3, a common outcome in patients with cardiac amyloidosis [46].

Lenalidomide

Lenalidomide has been combined with dexamethasone in the treatment of amyloidosis [47]. In a phase II trial as a single agent in combination with dexamethasone, 34 patients received lenalidomide 25 mg/day. This dose was poorly tolerated, but at a reduced dose of 15 mg a day, it was well tolerated. Of 24 evaluable patients, 7 or 29% achieved a hematologic response and 8 or 38% achieved a partial hematologic response for an overall hematologic response rate of 67%. Fatigue and myelosuppression were the most common treatment-related adverse events (35%), while thromboembolic complications were seen in 9%. In a second trial, single-agent lenalidomide was administered, and after three cycles, dexamethasone was added if a response had not been achieved. Twenty-three patients were enrolled, 13 previously treated. Cardiac, renal, hepatic, and peripheral nerve amyloidosis was present in 64, 73, 23, and 14%, respectively. Ten patients discontinued treatment within the first three cycles of therapy either due to rapid progression, death, or intolerance of treatment [48]. There were ten patients who responded: nine required dexamethasone, one without dexamethasone. The responses were hematologic in nine, renal in four, cardiac in two, and hepatic in two. Neutropenia, thrombocytopenia, rash, and fatigue were the most common side effects.

When these data were updated to 37 patients, 22 received 25 mg/day and 15 received 15 mg/day. As of July 11, 2008, five patients remained on active therapy. The overall hematologic response rate was 41%: one complete and 14 partial. With a median follow-up of 33.6 months, 22 patients died; only two were possibly related to treatment. The median response duration and overall survival were 19.2 and 31 months. Overall survival from diagnosis was 48 months. Outcomes were dependent on underlying risk stratification. High-risk patients, based on cardiac biomarkers, were more likely to drop out early and were less likely to respond; high-risk patients had shorter progression-free and overall survival.

In patients with amyloidosis treated with lenalidomide, 43% will develop a rash [49]. In certain instances, severe rashes required permanent discontinuation of lenalidomide. A late-onset rash has occurred in 28%. The incidence of dermatologic adverse effects is higher in amyloidosis than in multiple myeloma. The concurrent use of dexamethasone did not reduce the risk of a skin rash. Progressive azotemia has been reported in AL patients treated with lenalidomide and dexamethasone. The onset of azotemia can range anywhere from 2 weeks to several months and was irreversible in four. This is an uncommon but serious complication of lenalidomide therapy, and careful monitoring in AL is required [50].

Bortezomib Treatment of Amyloidosis

By inhibiting proteasome function in multiple myeloma cells, bortezomib activates stress-activated protein kinase and mitochondrial apoptotic signaling [51]. Bortezomib can induce rapid renal improvement targeting NF κB activation and result in improved kidney function [52]. Amyloid forming light chains can produce a load for the endoplasmic reticulum that makes these cells more sensitive to proteasome inhibition [53]. The first case report described a patient with hepatic AL, previously treated with melphalan, dexamethasone, and thalidomide who received bortezomib with a reduction in hepatic size from 20 to 10 cm with disappearance of the monoclonal protein [54]. The National Amyloidosis Center in Britain reported 18 patients treated with bortezomib, half of whom received dexamethasone, all of whom had received prior thalidomide. A hematologic response was seen in 77% of patients, 16% complete, 27% organ responses [55]. This experience was updated to 20 patients with a response rate to bortezomib of 80% with 15% complete responses; 40% had to discontinue therapy due to treatment-related toxicity [56]. In 2007, an abstract from a phase I–II study of single-agent bortezomib was reported. There were seven cohorts using two schedules of bortezomib weekly on a 5-week cycle, weekly for 4 weeks out of five, or biweekly 2 weeks out of three [57]. The dose in the weekly schedules was 1.6 mg/m^2; biweekly dose was 1.3 mg/m^2. Toxicities included ileus, constipation, nausea, vomiting, and diarrhea. Grade II and IV adverse events were seen in 42%

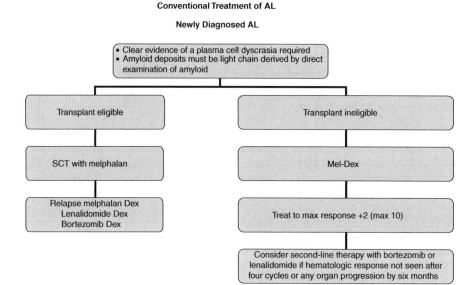

Fig. 11-2. Therapy algorithm for AL.

of patients. Of 13 patients in cohorts 3–6, there were eight responses (62%). Organ responses were seen in three cardiac, five renal, and two peripheral nervous system patients.

Eighteen patients, including seven that had relapsed or progressed after prior therapy, were treated with bortezomib and dexamethasone. Sixteen of the 18 were evaluable. Eleven or 61% had two or more organs involved. The serum creatinine was elevated in six. The bortezomib was administered on a biweekly schedule, 2 weeks of three with dexamethasone 40 mg 4 days every 21. A median of five cycles was administered. The hematologic response was 94%, and hematologic complete response was 44% including patients who had failed prior high-dose dexamethasone. Twenty-five percent of patients had an organ response. These responses were achieved at a median of 0.9 months. The median time to organ response was 4 months. Neurotoxicity, fatigue, edema, and postural hypotension were seen, and dose modification or a cessation of therapy was required in 11. The optimal duration, the durability, and the tolerability of the drug remain undefined [58].

Immunologic Therapy

The development of murine amyloid reactive monoclonal antibodies has provided a passive immunotherapy approach to the management of AL [59]. Antibodies against human light chain-related fibrils recognize an epitope common to the beta-pleated sheet structure of AL and have produced regression in amyloidomas administered to mice injected with human AL extracts. A chimeric prototype antibody has been developed [60]. Immunotherapy might benefit individuals with AL amyloidosis.

Conclusion

The optimal therapy for AL amyloidosis is unknown. Virtually all patients receive some form of cytotoxic chemotherapy. High-dose chemotherapy is widely used but is applicable to the minority. Dexamethasone-based therapies including alkylating agents, immunomodulatory drugs, bortezomib, and antibody therapy are all important considerations for the management of patients. In Fig. 11-2, a possible schema for the initiation of therapy in amyloidosis patients is given.

References

1. Comenzo RL. Managing systemic light-chain amyloidosis. J Natl Compr Canc Netw. 2007;5:179–87.
2. Miyazaki D, Yazaki M, Gono T, et al. AH amyloidosis associated with an immunoglobulin heavy chain variable region (VH1) fragment: a case report. Amyloid. 2008;15:125–28.
3. Obici L, Perfetti V, Palladini G, Moratti R, Merlini G. Clinical aspects of systemic amyloid diseases. Biochim Biophys Acta. 2005;1753:11–22.
4. Ionescu-Zanetti C, Khurana R, Gillespie JR, et al. Monitoring the assembly of Ig light-chain amyloid fibrils by atomic force microscopy. Proc Natl Acad Sci USA. 1999;96:13175–79.
5. Brenner DA, Jain M, Pimentel DR, et al. Human amyloidogenic light chains directly impair cardiomyocyte function through an increase in cellular oxidant stress. Circ Res. 2004;94:1008–10.
6. Kingsbury JS, Laue TM, Klimtchuk ES, Theberge R, Costello CE, Connors LH. The modulation of transthyretin tetramer stability by cysteine 10 adducts and the drug diflunisal. Direct analysis by fluorescence-detected analytical ultracentrifugation. J Biol Chem. 2008;283:11887–96.
7. Hazenberg BP, van Rijswijk MH, Lub-de Hooge MN, et al. Diagnostic performance and prognostic value of extravascular retention of 123I-labeled serum amyloid P component in systemic amyloidosis. J Nucl Med. 2007;48:865–72.
8. Buxbaum J. Aberrant immunoglobulin synthesis in light chain amyloidosis. Free light chain and light chain fragment production by human bone marrow cells in short-term tissue culture. J Clin Invest. 1986;78:798–806.
9. Cohen AS, Rubinow A, Anderson JJ, et al. Survival of patients with primary (AL) amyloidosis. Colchicine-treated cases from 1976 to 1983 compared with cases seen in previous years (1961 to 1973). Am J Med. 1987;82:1182–90.
10. Brandwein SR, Sipe JD, Skinner M, Cohen AS. Effect of colchicine on experimental amyloidosis in two CBA/J mouse models. Chronic inflammatory stimulation and administration of amyloid-enhancing factor during acute inflammation. Lab Invest. 1985;52: 319–25.
11. Schwartz RS, Cohen JR, Schrier SL. Therapy of primary amyloidosis with melphalan and prednisone. Arch Intern Med. 1979;139:1144–47.
12. Gertz MA, Lacy MQ, Dispenzieri A, et al. Effect of hematologic response on outcome of patients undergoing transplantation for primary amyloidosis: importance of achieving a complete response. Haematologica. 2007;92:1415–18.
13. Gertz MA, Lacy MQ, Dispenzieri A, et al. Impact of age and serum creatinine value on outcome after autologous blood stem cell transplantation for patients with multiple myeloma. Bone Marrow Transplant. 2007;39:605–11.
14. Comenzo RL. Systemic immunoglobulin light-chain amyloidosis. Clin Lymphoma Myeloma. 2006;7:182–85.
15. Gertz MA, Lacy MQ, Dispenzieri A, Hayman SR, Kumar S. Transplantation for amyloidosis. Curr Opin Oncol. 2007;19:136–41.
16. Jaccard A, Moreau P, Leblond V, et al. High-dose melphalan versus melphalan plus dexamethasone for AL amyloidosis. N Engl J Med. 2007;357:1083–93.
17. Kumar S, Dispenzieri A, Gertz MA. High-dose melphalan versus melphalan plus dexamethasone for AL amyloidosis. N Engl J Med. 2008;358:91, author reply 92–93.
18. Horne MK III.. Letter: improvement in amyloidosis. Ann Intern Med. 1975;83:281–282.
19. Corkery J, Bern MM, Tullis JL. Resolution of amyloidosis and plasma-cell dyscrasia with combination chemotherapy. Lancet. 1978;2:425–426.

20. Gertz MA, Kyle RA. Acute leukemia and cytogenetic abnormalities complicating melphalan treatment of primary systemic amyloidosis. Arch Intern Med. 1990;150:629–33.

21. Gertz MA, Lacy MQ, Lust JA, Greipp PR, Witzig TE, Kyle RA. Long-term risk of myelodysplasia in melphalan-treated patients with immunoglobulin light-chain amyloidosis. Haematologica. 2008;93:1402–6.

22. Kyle RA, Greipp PR. Primary systemic amyloidosis: comparison of melphalan and prednisone versus placebo. Blood. 1978;52:818–27.

23. Kyle RA, Greipp PR. Amyloidosis (AL). Clinical and laboratory features in 229 cases. Mayo Clin Proc. 1983;58:665–83.

24. Gertz MA, Kyle RA, Greipp PR. Response rates and survival in primary systemic amyloidosis. Blood. 1991;77:257–62.

25. Grogan M, Gertz MA, Kyle RA, Tajik AJ. Five or more years of survival in patients with primary systemic amyloidosis and biopsy-proven cardiac involvement. Am J Cardiol. 2000;85(664–665):A611.

26. Kyle RA, Gertz MA, Greipp PR, et al. Long-term survival (10 years or more) in 30 patients with primary amyloidosis. Blood. 1999;93:1062–66.

27. Kyle RA, Gertz MA, Greipp PR, et al. A trial of three regimens for primary amyloidosis: colchicine alone, melphalan and prednisone, and melphalan, prednisone, and colchicine. N Engl J Med. 1997;336:1202–07.

28. Skinner M, Anderson J, Simms R, et al. Treatment of 100 patients with primary amyloidosis: a randomized trial of melphalan, prednisone, and colchicine versus colchicine only. Am J Med. 1996;100:290–98.

29. Sanchorawala V, Wright DG, Seldin DC, et al. Low-dose continuous oral melphalan for the treatment of primary systemic (AL) amyloidosis. Br J Haematol. 2002;117:886–89.

30. Tazawa K, Matsuda M, Yoshida T, et al. Therapeutic outcome of cyclic VAD (vincristine, doxorubicin and dexamethasone) therapy in primary systemic AL amyloidosis patients. Intern Med. 2008;47:1517–22.

31. Sezer O, Schmid P, Shweigert M, et al. Rapid reversal of nephrotic syndrome due to primary systemic AL amyloidosis after VAD and subsequent high-dose chemotherapy with autologous stem cell support. Bone Marrow Transplant. 1999;23:967–69.

32. van G II, Hazenberg BP, Jager PL, Smit JW, Vellenga E. AL amyloidosis treated with induction chemotherapy with VAD followed by high dose melphalan and autologous stem cell transplantation. Amyloid. 2002;9:165–74.

33. Lachmann HJ, Gallimore R, Gillmore JD, et al. Outcome in systemic AL amyloidosis in relation to changes in concentration of circulating free immunoglobulin light chains following chemotherapy. Br J Haematol. 2003;122:78–84.

34. Dhodapkar MV, Jagannath S, Vesole D, et al. Treatment of AL-amyloidosis with dexamethasone plus alpha interferon. Leuk Lymphoma. 1997;27:351–56.

35. Gertz MA, Lacy MQ, Lust JA, Greipp PR, Witzig TE, Kyle RA. Phase II trial of high-dose dexamethasone for untreated patients with primary systemic amyloidosis. Med Oncol. 1999;16:104–09.

36. Gertz MA, Lacy MQ, Lust JA, Greipp PR, Witzig TE, Kyle RA. Phase II trial of high-dose dexamethasone for previously treated immunoglobulin light-chain amyloidosis. Am J Hematol. 1999;61:115–19.

37. Palladini G, Anesi E, Perfetti V, et al. A modified high-dose dexamethasone regimen for primary systemic (AL) amyloidosis. Br J Haematol. 2001;113:1044–46.

38. Dhodapkar MV, Hussein MA, Rasmussen E, et al. Clinical efficacy of high-dose dexamethasone with maintenance dexamethasone/alpha interferon in patients with primary systemic amyloidosis: results of United States Intergroup Trial Southwest Oncology Group (SWOG) S9628. Blood. 2004;104:3520–26.

39. Palladini G, Perfetti V, Obici L, et al. Association of melphalan and high-dose dexamethasone is effective and well tolerated in patients with AL (primary) amyloidosis who are ineligible for stem cell transplantation. Blood. 2004;103:2936–38.

40. Palladini G, Russo P, Nuvolone M, et al. Treatment with oral melphalan plus dexamethasone produces long-term remissions in AL amyloidosis. Blood. 2007;110:787–788.

41. Goodman HJB, Lachmann HJ, Bradwell AR, Hawkins PN. Intermediate dose intravenous melphalan and dexamethasone treatment in 144 patients with systemic AL amyloidosis (abstract 755). Blood. 2004;104:755.

42. Seldin DC, Choufani EB, Dember LM, et al. Tolerability and efficacy of thalidomide for the treatment of patients with light chain-associated (AL) amyloidosis. Clin Lymphoma. 2003;3:241–46.

43. Dispenzieri A, Lacy MQ, Rajkumar SV, et al. Poor tolerance to high doses of thalidomide in patients with primary systemic amyloidosis. Amyloid. 2003;10:257–61.

44. Palladini G, Perfetti V, Perlini S, et al. The combination of thalidomide and intermediate-dose dexamethasone is an effective but toxic treatment for patients with primary amyloidosis (AL). Blood. 2005;105:2949–51.

45. Wechalekar AD, Goodman HJ, Lachmann HJ, Offer M, Hawkins PN, Gillmore JD. Safety and efficacy of risk-adapted cyclophosphamide, thalidomide, and dexamethasone in systemic AL amyloidosis. Blood. 2007;109:457–64.

46. Palladini G, Russo P, Lavatelli F, et al. Treatment of patients with advanced cardiac AL amyloidosis with oral melphalan, dexamethasone, and thalidomide. Ann Hematol. 2009 Apr; 88(4):347–50.

47. Sanchorawala V, Wright DG, Rosenzweig M, et al. Lenalidomide and dexamethasone in the treatment of AL amyloidosis: results of a phase 2 trial. Blood. 2007;109:492–96.

48. Dispenzieri A, Lacy MQ, Zeldenrust SR, et al. The activity of lenalidomide with or without dexamethasone in patients with primary systemic amyloidosis. Blood. 2007;109: 465–70.

49. Sviggum HP, Davis MD, Rajkumar SV, Dispenzieri A. Dermatologic adverse effects of lenalidomide therapy for amyloidosis and multiple myeloma. Arch Dermatol. 2006;142:1298–302.

50. Batts ED, Sanchorawala V, Hegerfeldt Y, Lazarus HM. Azotemia associated with use of lenalidomide in plasma cell dyscrasias. Leuk Lymphoma. 2008;49:1108–15.

51. Sterz J, von Metzler I, Hahne JC, et al. The potential of proteasome inhibitors in cancer therapy. Expert Opin Invest Drugs. 2008;17:879–95.

52. Dimopoulos MA, Kastritis E, Rosinol L, Blade J, Ludwig H. Pathogenesis and treatment of renal failure in multiple myeloma. Leukemia. 2008;22:1485–93.

53. Sitia R, Palladini G, Merlini G. Bortezomib in the treatment of AL amyloidosis: targeted therapy? Haematologica. 2007;92:1302–7.

54. Fauble VS, Shah-Reddy I. Primary amyloidosis treated with bortezomib with a clinical and radiological response (abstract 5111). Blood. 2006;108:5111.

55. Wechalekar AD, Gillmore JD, Lachmann HJ, Offer M, Hawkins PN. Efficacy and safety of bortezomib in systemic AL amyloidosis – a preliminary report (abstract 129). Blood. 2006;108:129.

56. Wechalekar AD, Lachmann HJ, Offer M, Hawkins PN, Gillmore JD. Efficacy of bortezomib in systemic AL amyloidosis with relapsed/refractory clonal disease. Haematologica. 2008;93:295–98.

57. Reece DESV, Hegenbart U, Merlini G, et al. Phase I/II study of bortezomib (B) in patients with systemic AL-amyloidosis (AL). J Clin Oncol. 2007;25:453s.

58. Kastritis E, Anagnostopoulos A, Roussou M, et al. Treatment of light chain (AL) amyloidosis with the combination of bortezomib and dexamethasone. Haematologica. 2007;92:1351–58.

59. Wall JS, Kennel SJ, Paulus M, et al. Radioimaging of light chain amyloid with a fibril-reactive monoclonal antibody. J Nucl Med. 2006;47:2016–24.

60. Solomon A, Weiss DT, Wall JS. Immunotherapy in systemic primary (AL) amyloidosis using amyloid-reactive monoclonal antibodies. Cancer Biother Radiopharm. 2003;18:853–60.

Chapter 12

High-Dose Therapy in Amyloidosis

Adam D. Cohen and Raymond L. Comenzo

Abstract High-dose melphalan with autologous stem cell support (SCT) has improved outcomes for patients with systemic AL amyloidosis. A significantly greater proportion of patients remain alive and progression-free 5 or 10 years post-therapy than with historical traditional regimens. However, at most only one-third of newly diagnosed AL patients are eligible for SCT and, as attempts to minimize morbidity and mortality lead to refined patient selection, fewer AL patients may ultimately have SCT made available to them. Standard oral melphalan and dexamethasone, as well as combinations that include the novel agents lenalidomide and bortezomib, may allow for rapid elimination of circulating light chains and achieve response rates similar to SCT. In addition, as more data are obtained about complete response frequency, response duration, and tolerability of the novel agents in AL patients, it is possible that the risk-to-benefit ratio of high-dose therapy as initial treatment will become less favorable and that SCT may become more appropriate as second-line therapy. Indeed, the central challenge of the upcoming decade will be how and when to best incorporate the novel agents, either alone or in combination with both conventional and high-dose chemotherapeutic regimens, into our armamentarium against AL. Certainly, more randomized clinical trials will be needed to answer these questions, requiring cooperative group involvement and cooperation among amyloidosis treatment centers. Fortunately, risk-adapted high-dose therapy and the novel agents have greatly expanded the options for AL patients compared with a decade ago and the future continues to look bright.

Keywords Stem cell transplant, Melphalan, Thalidomide, Bortezomib

Background and Rationale

The rationale for high-dose chemotherapy in the treatment of AL amyloidosis is derived from studies in multiple myeloma and stems from initial observations made in the 1980s that high doses of intravenous melphalan ($100–200$ mg/m^2) could overcome plasma cell chemo-resistance in relapsed and refractory myeloma patients [1, 2]. These observations eventually led to phase III myeloma clinical trials in the 1990s, demonstrating the superiority of high-dose melphalan (HDM) with autologous hematopoietic stem cell support over continued conventional chemotherapy [3, 4] and establishing melphalan 200 mg/m^2 as the optimal conditioning regimen [5].

Around this time, the treatment of choice for AL amyloidosis patients had become oral melphalan and prednisone (MP) based on superior response rates and overall

From: *Amyloidosis*, Contemporary Hematology,
Edited by: M.A. Gertz and S.V. Rajkumar, DOI 10.1007/978-1-60761-631-3_12,
© Springer Science+Business Media, LLC 2010

survival for MP with or without colchicine over colchicine alone in two random-ized phase III trials [6, 7]. Colchicine had been chosen based on activity in treating "secondary" AA amyloidosis associated with familial Mediterranean fever, but was shown to be ineffective for AL amyloidosis in these trials. Despite this superior-ity, oral MP was associated with response rates of 20–30% with rare complete responses (CR) and median survival of 12–18 months (compared with 6–8 months for colchicine), with cardiac AL patients surviving less than 6 months. Only 5% of patients survived 10 years or more [8], with a significant risk of myelodyspla-sia/AML in long-term survivors, estimated as high as 20% in some studies [6, 7, 9]. As with myeloma, combining additional cytotoxic agents with MP (e.g., the VBMCP regimen—vincristine, carmustine, melphalan, cyclophosphamide, and prednisone) failed to improve long-term outcomes [10]. Thus, by the mid- to late 1990s there remained a need for novel therapeutic approaches to AL amyloidosis. The impressive response rates and survival in the myeloma high-dose melphalan trials made this an attractive strategy to appropriate for AL patients.

Initial High-Dose Therapy Studies

Several case series and phase II studies first demonstrated the feasibility of treat-ing AL patients with high-dose melphalan and autologous stem cell transplant (HDM/ASCT) [11–15]. Hematologic responses, including complete responses, were seen in 50–60% of patients, significantly higher than those reported for oral MP, and improvement in involved organ function was observed in 40–50%, confirming the clinical activity of this approach. The most striking observation of these initial studies, however, was the higher-than-expected treatment-related mortality (TRM), averaging 21% in early single-center trials [11–13, 16] and as high as 43% in a retro-spective multi-center series [17]. Frequent causes of death included gastrointestinal hemorrhage, intractable hypotension, sepsis, arrhythmias/sudden cardiac death, and multi-organ failure. In addition, growth factor-mediated stem cell mobilization was associated with morbidity (e.g., volume overload, congestive failure, hypotension, and tachyarrhythmias) and mortality in a significant minority of patients [11, 12]. More stringent patient selection, risk-adapted melphalan dosing, and better support-ive care (as described in the next section) have decreased TRM to 5–15% in more recently reported studies [18–21], though this remains significantly higher than TRM for other indications (e.g., lymphoma, myeloma) for which high-dose therapy is fre-quently used.

Despite this high TRM, the impressive hematologic and organ response rates seen in initial trials and the generally poor outlook for most AL patients led to continued clinical studies refining the high-dose therapy approach. Recently, retrospective, long-term outcomes data on over 800 AL patients treated with high dose therapy have been published [19, 22–25] (summarized in Table 12-1). The transplant patients described in these historical series represent the era before the availability of the serum free light chain assay and cardiac biomarkers; therefore, response data were based on serum immunofixation results and assessment of cardiac amyloidosis was usually based on history, exam, echocardiogram, and electrocardiogram. With these caveats in mind, the results of the initial decade's work in HDM/SCT for AL remain substantial and positive.

The largest of these series, from Boston Medical Center (BMC), describes 312 patients treated on sequential high-dose therapy protocols from 1994 to 2002. TRM was 15.7% (including deaths during mobilization), and median overall survival was

Table 12-1. High-dose therapy outcomes: large retrospective series.

Center (references)	n	TRM[a] (%)	Heme RR (CR)[b]	Organ RR[b]	Med OS	Conditioning[c] full/reduced
Boston [19]	312	16	n/a (27%)	26%[d]	4.6 years	56%/44%
Mayo [23]	282	11	71%(33%)	n/a	NR at 5 years	67%/33%
Pavia [20]	22	14	55%(36%)	45%	5.7 years	68%/32%
UK [24] (multi-center)	92	23	37%(20%)	n/a[e]	5.3 years	69%/31%
CIBMTR [25] (multi-center)	107	27	32%(16%)	26%	3.9 years	46%/54%

n=number; TRM=treatment-related mortality; Heme=hematologic; RR=response rate; CR=complete response; OS=overall survival; NR=not reached
[a]Includes deaths during stem cell mobilization, when reported
[b]Intent-to-treat analysis
[c]Full conditioning = melphalan 200 mg/m^2 or melphalan 140 mg/m^2 + total body irradiation; reduced conditioning = melphalan 140 or 100 mg/m^2
[d]Organ response rate of 44% in 181 evaluable patients
[e]Organ response rate of 48% in 51 evaluable patients

4.6 years, with 47% alive at 5 years. Median survival for patients with cardiac involvement was 1.6 years, with 29% alive at 5 years. Complete hematologic responses (CR) were seen in 27% of patients by intention-to-treat (40% in 181 evaluable patients), and organ responses were seen in 44% of evaluable patients [19]. Similar overall survival was seen for patients older or younger than age 65, though the attenuated melphalan dosing used in the majority of the older cohort led to a non-significant decrease in hematologic complete response rate (44% versus 32%, p=0.19) [26]. An updated analysis focusing on the first 80 patients treated at BMC (1994–1997; minimum 10 years follow-up) showed a median survival of 57 months (4.75 years), with 24% of patients surviving over 10 years. For patients achieving a hematologic CR (n=32, 40%), median survival was not reached and 10-year survival was 53%, compared with 50-month median survival and 6% 10-year survival for patients without hematologic CR. Deaths amongst CR patients were related to progressive organ dysfunction (n=12: 6 with hematologic relapse, 6 despite sustained CR), metastatic solid tumors (n=2), and therapy-related MDS/AML (n=1) [22]. Importantly, objective improvements in quality of life measures were reported for AL patients undergoing dose-intensive therapy [27].

A similar analysis of 282 consecutive AL patients treated with high-dose therapy at Mayo Clinic showed a day 100 mortality of 11% and hematologic response rate of 71%, with 33% CR rate. In a landmark analysis of 213 patients who survived at least 6 months, hematologic response was significantly associated with overall survival (CR>PR>no response, Fig. 12-1), both for the entire cohort as well as those with echocardiographic evidence of cardiac involvement. Median survival was not reached in the CR and PR subsets, with 5-year survival over 85% in the CR group [23].

Similar overall survival has been reported in one other single-center [20] and two multi-center series [24, 25], though treatment-related mortality was higher in the multi-center setting (Table 12-1). Importantly, in two of the latter series, undergoing HDM/ASCT more recently was independently associated with improved survival, implying a learning curve associated with center experience, more stringent patient selection, and better supportive care. Finally, two studies examined the role of induction therapy (either MP [28] or VAD [29] (vincristine, adriamycin, dexamethasone)) prior to HDM/ASCT and did not find any significant benefit. Therefore, unlike in

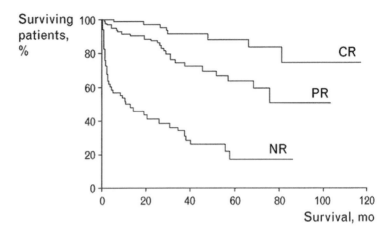

Fig. 12-1. Survival following high-dose therapy is related to hematologic response. Kaplan–Meier analysis of overall survival as a function of response for 270 patients who underwent high-dose therapy and autologous stem cell transplant at Mayo Clinic. Hematologic response was scored by the current consensus criteria [30]. Reprinted with permission from Gertz et al. [66]. CR, complete response ($n = 94$); NR, no response ($n = 71$); PR, partial response ($n = 105$). *Tick marks* indicate censored patients (alive).

myeloma, the standard has been to go directly to high-dose therapy for ASCT-eligible AL amyloidosis patients.

The take-home message from these initial experiences is that high-dose therapy with autologous stem cell support has resulted in unprecedented rates of hematologic response (especially CR), organ response, and overall survival for patients with AL amyloidosis, but that the high treatment-related morbidity and mortality continues to necessitate refinement in patient selection criteria, melphalan dosing, and supportive care.

In addition, the association of hematologic response, especially CR, with organ responses and long-term survival following high-dose therapy has now been demonstrated in multiple studies [19, 21–23], suggesting that additional strategies aimed at eliminating residual clonal plasma cell disease (e.g., combining high-dose melphalan with novel agents) are warranted. Moreover, the availability of the serum free light chain assay (FLC) has enabled a more effective definition of CR to be implemented (i.e., one that includes negative serum and urine immunofixation as well as normalization of the FLC ratio) [30], allowing greater accuracy in assessing response and identifying patients who may benefit from further therapy.

Toward a Risk-Adapted Approach to Decreasing Mortality

Analyses of these early studies identified several risk factors associated with increased treatment-related mortality, including higher number of involved organs (usually >2), advanced age, poor performance status, and presence of advanced cardiac involvement (e.g., uncompensated congestive failure, syncope, recurrent pleural effusions, ventricular tachyarrhythmias) [11–13]. In addition, both frequency and grade of treatment-related toxicities (especially GI toxicity, edema and bleeding) were associated with renal function and the dose of intravenous melphalan and were significantly higher at 200 mg/m^2 compared with 100 mg/m^2. These observations led to a proposal for a risk-adapted approach to high-dose therapy [31], excluding patients

Table 12-2. Risk-adapted approach to high-dose therapy for AL amyloidosis.

Good risk (any age; all criteria met)
- One or two organs involved
- No cardiac involvement
- Creatinine clearance $\geq$ 51 mL/min

Intermediate risk (age < 71; either criteria)
- One or two organs involved (must include cardiac or renal with creatinine clearance < 51 mL/min)
- Asymptomatic or compensated cardiac

Poor risk (either criteria)
- Three organs involved
- Advanced cardiac involvement

Melphalan dosing: based on risk group and age

Good risk	Intermediate risk	Poor risk
200 mg/m^2 if $\leq$ 60	140 mg/m^2 if $\leq$ 60	Standard therapy
140 mg/m^2 if 61–70	100 mg/m^2 if 61–70	Clinical trials
100 mg/m^2 if $\geq$ 71		

This research was originally published in Comenzo and Gertz [31]. © the American Society of Hematology [30]

most likely to have treatment-related mortality (i.e., those with three or more involved organs or advanced cardiac involvement) and modifying the dose of melphalan based on age, renal function, and presence or absence of any cardiac amyloid (Table 12-2). The de facto adaptation of this approach in several centers has contributed greatly to the decreased treatment-related mortality (TRM) reported in recent retrospective series (11–16%) [18–20], and the strict application of this strategy in a prospective phase II study led to a TRM of 4.4% (2/45 patients), the lowest yet reported for an amyloidosis high-dose therapy trial [21].

The trade-off, of course, for reducing the dose of melphalan is a potentially lower hematologic response rate. In the Mayo Clinic series, hematologic responses were seen in 53% of patients receiving melphalan 100 or 140 mg/m^2 (n=51), compared with 75% receiving melphalan 200 mg/m^2 (n=120). In the BMC series, complete hematologic responses at 1 year were seen in 45 and 33% of patients getting melphalan 200 mg/m^2 (n=113) and 100/140 mg/m^2 (n=68), respectively [19]. These lower response rates may be overcome, however, by the addition of adjuvant therapy with novel agents, such as thalidomide [21] or bortezomib [32], for patients with residual clonal plasma cell disease post-ASCT. This sequential administration of risk-adapted melphalan followed by additional drugs with non-overlapping mechanisms of activity may therefore allow the greatest number of AL patients to benefit safely from high-dose therapy, without compromising the hematologic response rates which appear critical for long-term survival.

Another important risk-reduction strategy has been the implementation of aggressive supportive care measures during the mobilization and peri-SCT period. Most of these are admittedly empiric, without formalized measures of their impact on patient outcomes. Nonetheless, they likely have contributed significantly to improved treatment-related mortality reported in recent years. To minimize the risk of the rare but sometimes fatal fluid retention, hypoxia, and hypotension seen with high-dose G-CSF during stem cell mobilization, we recommend using a twice daily, lower dose regimen (6 mcg/kg q12 h for 5 days) [33], and we often monitor patients with significant cardiac involvement or orthostatic hypotension on telemetry during the mobilization period and during stem cell re-infusion. In addition, some centers do not use G-CSF post-SCT because of the fluid retention associated with its use [34], though this was associated with a delayed median time to neutrophil engraftment (14 days until ANC > 500/μL compared with 10 days at most centers), which may increase the risk of infection. Whether pegylated filgrastim (Neulasta®) is as effective and better tolerated is currently under investigation [35]. GI bleeding is a significant contributor to early treatment-related mortality and can occur as frequently as 20% of AL patients undergoing HDM/ASCT. This is likely from occult amyloid deposition in the submucosa which can exacerbate chemotherapy-induced mucositis and lead to hemorrhage [36]. All patients should be screened with fecal occult blood testing before and during the SCT period, with positive screening tests prompting endoscopic evaluation for potentially treatable causes. Patients should receive proton pump inhibition during the peri-SCT period, with maintenance of platelets over 50,000/μL and hemoglobin over 9 g/dL should occult or obvious GI bleeding become manifest. Other important supportive measures include use of aggressive immediate- and delayed-emesis regimens, supporting intravascular oncotic pressure in nephrotic patients through albumin infusions to keep albumin>2 g/dL, maintaining euvolemia through judicious but not overaggressive use of diuretics, and maintaining normal electrolyte levels, especially in cardiac patients.

Finally, several reports have documented the feasibility of performing organ transplantation, particularly heart transplantation, prior to high-dose therapy and stem cell transplant [37–39]. This sequential approach allows AL patients with advanced cardiac involvement to become eligible for high-dose therapy and theoretically decreases their risk of peri-SCT cardiac complications. The use of extended donor criteria to increase the likelihood of obtaining a donor heart should increase the number of AL patients who can benefit from this approach and merits further study [38].

High-Dose Therapy Versus Conventional Chemotherapy

A criticism of the improved long-term outcomes reported for high-dose therapy compared with prior conventional therapy studies has been that they reflect a selection bias, in that only the fittest AL patients undergo SCT. In fact, a retrospective Mayo Clinic study of 229 AL patients who met SCT eligibility criteria but did not undergo SCT found that this cohort had a median survival of 42 months, with 5- and 10-year survivals of 36 and 15%, respectively. These numbers were significantly higher than those reported in historic series of AL patients or in the oral MP trials, demonstrating that these were, indeed, a good-risk subset of patients [40]. However, these same investigators then performed a case-control study examining 126 SCT-eligible AL patients, 63 of whom underwent high-dose therapy, and 63 who were matched for age, sex, and clinical variables but were treated conventionally (83% received MP). Overall survival at 2 years (81 versus 55%) and 4 years (71 versus 41%) significantly favored the high-dose therapy cohort, suggesting that even within this good-risk population, there was a benefit to high-dose therapy [41].

More recently, however, therapy for AL patients not undergoing SCT has migrated from oral MP to dexamethasone-based regimens. A SWOG multi-center study of pulse dexamethasone (40 mg orally daily on days 1–4, 9–12, 17–20 every 35 days) for three cycles, followed by maintenance for responders with interferon-alpha and dexamethasone days 1–4 every 28 days, led to hematologic responses in 53%, organ responses in 45%, and median survival of 31 months [42]. Toxicity was significant, however, with 7% treatment-related mortality. More promising was the phase II trial from the Pavia group using oral melphalan and dexamethasone (Mel/Dex) for 4 days every month. In 46 SCT-ineligible patients, hematologic responses were seen in 67% (including 33% CR) and organ responses in 48%, with no treatment-related mortality. Updated follow-up data showed median progression-free and overall survival of 3.8 and 5.1 years, respectively [43, 44]. This regimen has become widely used for non-SCT-eligible patients.

Based on these promising results, the French Myélome Autogreffe Groupe (MAG) conducted a multi-center phase III trial randomizing newly diagnosed AL patients ($n=100$) to high-dose melphalan and autologous SCT or oral Mel/Dex for up to 18 months. There were no significant differences observed for hematologic (68% for Mel/Dex versus 66% for HDM/ASCT) or organ responses (39 versus 45%), but median overall survival was significantly longer in the oral Mel/Dex arm (56.9 versus 22.2 months, $p=0.04$) [45]. Several aspects of this trial merit cautious interpretation, however. First, 13 (26%) of the 50 patients assigned to HDM/ASCT never received melphalan, due largely to death or early progression during stem cell mobilization. Another nine patients died within 100 days after SCT (transplant-related mortality of 24%). Thus, only 56% of HDM/ASCT patients were evaluable for response or long-term survival. This high early death rate was likely related to three factors: (1) inclusion of patients who may not have been considered SCT eligible at other treatment centers (e.g., 36% of patients assigned to the high-dose therapy arm had three or more organs involved with amyloid; 12% had poor LV ejection fraction); (2) the relative infrequent use of dose-adjusted melphalan despite these high-risk features (10/37 (27%) patients received MEL 140 mg/m^2; the remainder MEL 200 mg/m^2); and (3) treatment in multiple centers, many of which may have had limited experience with SCT for amyloidosis patients. Nonetheless, a landmark analysis examining only patients surviving at least 6 months after randomization still showed no advantage in overall survival for high-dose therapy [45]. Therefore, while the high response rates and prolonged survival with oral Mel/Dex confirm its place in the treatment of AL patients, a disparity remains apparent between the outcomes in the SCT arm in this study compared with recent studies at amyloidosis referral centers, suggesting that high-dose therapy may best be performed at specialty centers with experience using SCT for AL amyloidosis patients.

Improving upon High-Dose Therapy

Recently, there have been two separate but complementary approaches for improving upon current outcomes with high-dose therapy: (1) incorporate new prognostic factors which can further refine patient selection by identifying patients at high risk of treatment-related mortality and (2) incorporate novel therapeutic approaches into high-dose treatment platforms. The former has been led by groups at Mayo Clinic and Pavia, who first identified cardiac biomarkers such as serum N-terminal pro-brain natriuretic peptide (NT-proBNP) and troponin I or T as predictive not only of cardiac involvement but of clinical outcomes in general for AL patients, even in those without echocardiographic or clinical evidence of cardiac amyloid [46–49]. A staging system incorporating NT-proBNP and troponin T has been proposed and was able to identify a high-risk group of patients with poor outcomes following SCT (median OS 8.4 months if both markers were elevated at baseline versus not reached if 0 or 1 marker was elevated) [48]. Another retrospective study found that elevated troponin T (> 0.06 μg/L) was predictive of treatment-related mortality in patients undergoing high-dose therapy (28 versus 7% for troponin T < 0.06 μg/L) [50]. Other baseline characteristics that have been associated with poor outcome in patients undergoing high-dose therapy include elevated uric acid, excessive fluid retention during stem cell mobilization, and the absolute value of the involved serum free light chain [51–53]. In addition, expression of calreticulin, as measured by gene expression profiling, quantitative RT-PCR, and immunohistochemistry in plasma cells obtained pre-treatment from AL patients, was significantly higher in patients achieving a CR post-SCT compared to those with no response, suggesting that this protein may have value in predicting sensitivity to high-dose melphalan [54]. While these prognostic factors need to be validated at other centers and in prospective studies, they provide a framework toward further refining patient selection to reserve high-dose therapy for those AL patients most likely to have long-term benefit (and least likely to have treatment-related mortality).

Other approaches for improving upon current outcomes with high-dose therapy include tandem autologous SCT, use of allogeneic or syngeneic stem cell donors, and incorporation of novel agents. A single-institution study of tandem SCT for AL amyloidosis enrolled 62 patients with plans for melphalan 200 mg/m^2 and autologous SCT, followed by melphalan 140 mg/m^2 and a second autologous SCT for patients not in hematologic CR at 6 months after the first SCT. Overall, 32 patients (50%) achieved a CR (27 after the first, and 5 after the second SCT), with a 50% organ response rate and median survival not reached after median follow-up of 43 months. Seven patients were unable to collect enough stem cells for tandem SCT, and TRM was 9% [55]. Thus, while this approach was feasible, it is unclear whether the added benefit is worth the morbidity of a second SCT. Allogeneic or syngeneic SCT has been used only rarely in AL patients, predominantly in previously treated patients, with durable complete responses reported, but with high rates of acute and chronic graft-versus-host-disease and high TRM (40%) that make adoption of this approach outside of a clinical trial not recommended at this time [56].

The novel immunomodulatory agents thalidomide and lenalidomide, as well as the proteosome inhibitor bortezomib, have now all been shown to have significant activity in AL amyloidosis, either alone or in combination with other therapies such as dexamethasone or cyclophosphamide [57–65]. The first study incorporating these novel agents into a high-dose therapy platform was a phase II trial for newly diagnosed AL patients [21] in which 45 patients received risk-adapted high-dose melphalan and autologous stem cell support. Those who did not achieve a hematologic CR at 3 months received 9 months of adjuvant dexamethasone and thalidomide (or dexamethasone alone if there was a history of deep venous thrombosis or neuropathy). Complete response in this trial was strictly defined, employing serum free light chain as well immunofixation results. Organ involvement was kidney (67%), heart (24%), liver/GI (22%), and peripheral nervous system (18%), with 31% having two organ systems involved. Based on age, creatinine clearance, and cardiac involvement (as per Table 12-2), six patients were assigned to melphalan 100 mg/m^2, 24–140 mg/m^2, and 15–200 mg/m^2. TRM was 4.4%, and 31 patients began adjuvant therapy because of persistent clonal plasma cell disease at 3 months. Median dose of thalidomide tolerated was 150 mg daily, and only 52% ($n=16$) completed all 9 months of therapy, with 16 and 32% discontinuing for disease progression and toxicity, respectively. Despite this, 42% of patients getting adjuvant therapy improved their hematologic response by 12 months post-SCT, with overall and complete response rates of 71 and 36%, respectively, and organ responses of 44%. With median follow-up of 31 months, 2-year progression-free and overall survival was 74 and 84%, respectively. Overall survival was 63% at 2 years for patients with cardiac involvement. This study showed prospectively how risk-adapted dosing could decrease treatment-related mortality and demonstrated that sequential therapy with a novel regimen post-SCT can deepen hematologic responses, potentially making organ improvement and long-term disease control more likely.

Because of the poor tolerability of thalidomide seen in this and other studies of AL patients [58, 60], a subsequent high-dose therapy trial uses the same risk-adapted trial design but substitutes bortezomib for thalidomide during adjuvant therapy. Of 21 patients evaluable post-SCT, 5 achieved CR and 16 had persistent clonal plasma cell disease. Fifteen patients received adjuvant therapy. At 1-year post-SCT, the overall response rate was 92% with 67% achieving CR. Fifty percent of patients had organ improvement. Adjuvant therapy was tolerated and resulted in improved responses in 88% of patients [32].

While longer follow-up of this approach is obviously needed, the ability to upgrade responses and achieve a higher percentage of complete responses makes this a rational strategy to enhance the balance of tolerability and efficacy needed to obtain better long-term outcomes for AL patients.

Future Directions

High-dose melphalan with autologous stem cell support has improved outcomes for patients with AL amyloidosis, with a significantly greater proportion remaining alive and progression-free 5 or 10 years post-therapy than with historical traditional regimens. Unfortunately, only one-third of newly diagnosed AL patients are eligible for SCT and, as patient selection becomes even more refined to minimize morbidity and mortality, fewer AL patients may ultimately have this option made available. On the other hand, the promising activity of oral Mel/Dex, lenalidomide, and bortezomib may allow for rapid elimination of circulating light chains and sufficient improvement in performance status and organ function to make previously ineligible patients eligible for SCT. Thus, it is appropriate to re-explore the question of brief induction therapy prior to SCT now that more active agents and regimens are available. In addition, as more data are obtained about complete response frequency, response duration, and tolerability of the novel agents in AL patients, it is possible that the risk-to-benefit ratio of high-dose therapy as initial treatment will become less favorable and that HDM/SCT may become more appropriate as second-line therapy. Indeed, the central challenge of the upcoming decade will be how and when to best incorporate these agents, either alone or in combination with both conventional and high-dose chemotherapeutic regimens, into our armamentarium against amyloidosis. Certainly, more randomized clinical trials will be needed to answer these questions, requiring cooperative group involvement and cooperation among amyloidosis treatment centers. Fortunately, risk-adapted high-dose therapy and the novel agents have greatly expanded the options for AL patients compared with a decade ago and the future continues to look bright.

References

1. Barlogie B, Hall R, Zander A, Dicke K, Alexanian R. High-dose melphalan with autologous bone marrow transplantation for multiple myeloma. Blood 1986;67:1298–301.
2. McElwain TJ, Powles RL. High-dose intravenous melphalan for plasma-cell leukaemia and myeloma. Lancet 1983;2:822–4.
3. Attal M, Harousseau JL, Stoppa AM, et al. A prospective, randomized trial of autologous bone marrow transplantation and chemotherapy in multiple myeloma. Intergroupe Francais du Myelome. N Engl J Med. 1996;335:91–7.

4. Child JA, Morgan GJ, Davies FE, et al. High-dose chemotherapy with hematopoietic stem-cell rescue for multiple myeloma. N Engl J Med. 2003;348:1875–83.
5. Moreau P, Facon T, Attal M, et al. Comparison of 200 mg/m(2) melphalan and 8 Gy total body irradiation plus 140 mg/m(2) melphalan as conditioning regimens for peripheral blood stem cell transplantation in patients with newly diagnosed multiple myeloma: final analysis of the Intergroupe Francophone du Myelome 9502 randomized trial. Blood 2002;99:731–5.
6. Kyle RA, Gertz MA, Greipp PR, et al. A trial of three regimens for primary amyloidosis: colchicine alone, melphalan and prednisone, and melphalan, prednisone, and colchicine. N Engl J Med. 1997;336:1202–7.
7. Skinner M, Anderson J, Simms R, et al. Treatment of 100 patients with primary amyloidosis: a randomized trial of melphalan, prednisone, and colchicine versus colchicine only. Am J Med. 1996;100:290–8.
8. Kyle RA, Gertz MA, Greipp PR, et al. Long-term survival (10 years or more) in 30 patients with primary amyloidosis. Blood 1999;93:1062–6.
9. Gertz MA, Kyle RA. Acute leukemia and cytogenetic abnormalities complicating melphalan treatment of primary systemic amyloidosis. Arch Intern Med. 1990;150:629–33.
10. Gertz MA, Lacy MQ, Lust JA, Greipp PR, Witzig TE, Kyle RA. Prospective randomized trial of melphalan and prednisone versus vincristine, carmustine, melphalan, cyclophosphamide, and prednisone in the treatment of primary systemic amyloidosis. J Clin Oncol. 1999;17:262–7.
11. Comenzo RL, Sanchorawala V, Fisher C, et al. Intermediate-dose intravenous melphalan and blood stem cells mobilized with sequential GM+G-CSF or G-CSF alone to treat AL (amyloid light chain) amyloidosis. Br J Haematol. 1999;104:553–9.
12. Comenzo RL, Vosburgh E, Falk RH, et al. Dose-intensive melphalan with blood stem-cell support for the treatment of AL (amyloid light-chain) amyloidosis: survival and responses in 25 patients. Blood 1998;91:3662–70.
13. Gertz MA, Lacy MQ, Gastineau DA, et al. Blood stem cell transplantation as therapy for primary systemic amyloidosis (AL). Bone Marrow Transplant. 2000;26:963–9.
14. van Buren M, Hene RJ, Verdonck LF, Verzijlbergen FJ, Lokhorst HM. Clinical remission after syngeneic bone marrow transplantation in a patient with AL amyloidosis. Ann Intern Med. 1995;122:508–10.
15. Moreau P, Milpied N, de Faucal P, et al. High-dose melphalan and autologous bone marrow transplantation for systemic AL amyloidosis with cardiac involvement. Blood 1996;87:3063–4.
16. Saba N, Sutton D, Ross H, et al. High treatment-related mortality in cardiac amyloid patients undergoing autologous stem cell transplant. Bone Marrow Transplant. 1999;24:853–5.
17. Moreau P, Leblond V, Bourquelot P, et al. Prognostic factors for survival and response after high-dose therapy and autologous stem cell transplantation in systemic AL amyloidosis: a report on 21 patients. Br J Haematol. 1998;101:766–9.
18. Gertz MA, Lacy MQ, Dispenzieri A, et al. Risk-adjusted manipulation of melphalan dose before stem cell transplantation in patients with amyloidosis is associated with a lower response rate. Bone Marrow Transplant. 2004;34:1025–31.
19. Skinner M, Sanchorawala V, Seldin DC, et al. High-dose melphalan and autologous stem-cell transplantation in patients with AL amyloidosis: an 8-year study. Ann Intern Med. 2004;140:85–93.
20. Perfetti V, Siena S, Palladini G, et al. Long-term results of a risk-adapted approach to melphalan conditioning in autologous peripheral blood stem cell transplantation for primary (AL) amyloidosis. Haematologica. 2006;91:1635–43.
21. Cohen AD, Zhou P, Chou J, et al. Risk-adapted autologous stem cell transplantation with adjuvant dexamethasone +/– thalidomide for systemic light-chain amyloidosis: results of a phase II trial. Br J Haematol. 2007;139:224–33.
22. Sanchorawala V, Skinner M, Quillen K, Finn KT, Doros G, Seldin DC. Long-term outcome of patients with AL amyloidosis treated with high-dose melphalan and stem-cell transplantation. Blood 2007;110:3561–3.

23. Gertz MA, Lacy MQ, Dispenzieri A, et al. Effect of hematologic response on outcome of patients undergoing transplantation for primary amyloidosis: importance of achieving a complete response. Haematologica. 2007;92:1415–8.

24. Goodman HJ, Gillmore JD, Lachmann HJ, Wechalekar AD, Bradwell AR, Hawkins PN. Outcome of autologous stem cell transplantation for AL amyloidosis in the UK. Br J Haematol. 2006;134:417–25.

25. Vesole DH, PÃ©rez WS, Akasheh M, Boudreau C, Reece DE, Bredeson CN. High-dose therapy and autologous hematopoietic stem cell transplantation for patients with primary systemic amyloidosis: a center for international blood and marrow transplant research study. Mayo Clinic Proc. 2006;81:880–8.

26. Seldin DC, Anderson JJ, Skinner M, et al. Successful treatment of AL amyloidosis with high-dose melphalan and autologous stem cell transplantation in patients over age 65. Blood 2006;108:3945–7.

27. Seldin DC, Anderson JJ, Sanchorawala V, et al. Improvement in quality of life of patients with AL amyloidosis treated with high-dose melphalan and autologous stem cell transplantation. Blood 2004;104:1888–93.

28. Sanchorawala V, Wright DG, Seldin DC, et al. High-dose intravenous melphalan and autologous stem cell transplantation as initial therapy or following two cycles of oral chemotherapy for the treatment of AL amyloidosis: results of a prospective randomized trial. Bone Marrow Transplant. 2004;33:381–8.

29. Perz JB, Schonland SO, Hundemer M, et al. High-dose melphalan with autologous stem cell transplantation after VAD induction chemotherapy for treatment of amyloid light chain amyloidosis: a single centre prospective phase II study. Br J Haematol. 2004;127:543–51.

30. Gertz MA, Comenzo R, Falk RH, et al. Definition of organ involvement and treatment response in immunoglobulin light chain amyloidosis (AL): a consensus opinion from the 10th International Symposium on Amyloid and Amyloidosis, Tours, France, 18–22 April 2004. Am J Hematol. 2005;79:319–28.

31. Comenzo RL, Gertz MA. Autologous stem cell transplantation for primary systemic amyloidosis. Blood 2002;99:4276–82.

32. Landau H, Hassoun H, Bello C, Hoover E, Ciminiello J, McCullagh E, Riedel E, Cohen A, Nimer SD, Comenzo RL. Adjuvant bortezomib and dexamethasone following risk-adapted melphalan and stem cell transplant in systemic light-chain amyloidosis (AL): a phase II study. Blood 2009;114:533a.

33. Arbona C, Prosper F, Benet I, Mena F, Solano C, Garcia-Conde J. Comparison between once a day vs twice a day G-CSF for mobilization of peripheral blood progenitor cells (PBPC) in normal donors for allogeneic PBPC transplantation. Bone Marrow Transplant. 1998;22:39–45.

34. Gertz MA, Lacy MQ, Dispenzieri A, et al. Transplantation without growth factor: engraftment kinetics after stem cell transplantation for primary systemic amyloidosis (AL). Bone Marrow Transplant. 2007;40:989–93.

35. Rice RD, Baker LB, Moskowitz CH. 95: Neulasta(TM) as growth factor support after autologous stem cell transplantation. Biol Blood Marrow Transplant. 2008;14:37.

36. Kumar S, Dispenzieri A, Lacy MQ, Litzow MR, Gertz MA. High incidence of gastrointestinal tract bleeding after autologous stem cell transplant for primary systemic amyloidosis. Bone Marrow Transplant. 2001;28:381–5.

37. Gillmore JD, Goodman HJ, Lachmann HJ, et al. Sequential heart and autologous stem cell transplantation for systemic AL amyloidosis. Blood 2006;107:1227–9.

38. Maurer MS, Raina A, Hesdorffer C, et al. Cardiac transplantation using extended-donor criteria organs for systemic amyloidosis complicated by heart failure. Transplantation 2007;83:539–45.

39. Mignot A, Varnous S, Redonnet M, et al. Heart transplantation in systemic (AL) amyloidosis: a retrospective study of eight French patients. Arch Cardiovasc Dis. 2008;101:523–32.

40. Dispenzieri A, Lacy MQ, Kyle RA, et al. Eligibility for hematopoietic stem-cell transplantation for primary systemic amyloidosis is a favorable prognostic factor for survival. J Clin Oncol. 2001;19:3350–6.

41. Dispenzieri A, Kyle RA, Lacy MQ, et al. Superior survival in primary systemic amyloidosis patients undergoing peripheral blood stem cell transplantation: a case-control study. Blood 2004;103:3960–3.

42. Dhodapkar MV, Hussein MA, Rasmussen E, et al. Clinical efficacy of high-dose dexamethasone with maintenance dexamethasone/alpha interferon in patients with primary systemic amyloidosis: results of United States Intergroup Trial Southwest Oncology Group (SWOG) S9628. Blood 2004;104:3520–6.

43. Palladini G, Perfetti V, Obici L, et al. Association of melphalan and high-dose dexamethasone is effective and well tolerated in patients with AL (primary) amyloidosis who are ineligible for stem cell transplantation. Blood 2004;103:2936–8.

44. Palladini G, Russo P, Nuvolone M, et al. Treatment with oral melphalan plus dexamethasone produces long-term remissions in AL amyloidosis. Blood 2007;110:787–8.

45. Jaccard A, Moreau P, Leblond V, et al. High-dose melphalan versus melphalan plus dexamethasone for AL amyloidosis. N Engl J Med. 2007;357:1083–93.

46. Palladini G, Campana C, Klersy C, et al. Serum N-terminal pro-brain natriuretic peptide is a sensitive marker of myocardial dysfunction in AL amyloidosis. Circulation 2003;107:2440–5.

47. Dispenzieri A, Gertz MA, Kyle RA, et al. Serum cardiac troponins and N-terminal pro-brain natriuretic peptide: a staging system for primary systemic amyloidosis. J Clin Oncol. 2004;22:3751–7.

48. Dispenzieri A, Gertz MA, Kyle RA, et al. Prognostication of survival using cardiac troponins and N-terminal pro-brain natriuretic peptide in patients with primary systemic amyloidosis undergoing peripheral blood stem cell transplantation. Blood 2004;104:1881–7.

49. Dispenzieri A, Kyle RA, Gertz MA, et al. Survival in patients with primary systemic amyloidosis and raised serum cardiac troponins. Lancet 2003;361:1787–9.

50. Gertz M, Lacy M, Dispenzieri A, et al. Troponin T level as an exclusion criterion for stem cell transplantation in light-chain amyloidosis. Leukemia Lymphoma. 2008;49:36–41.

51. Kumar S, Dispenzieri A, Lacy MQ, et al. Serum uric acid: novel prognostic factor in primary systemic amyloidosis. Mayo Clin Proc. 2008;83:297–303.

52. Leung N, Leung TR, Cha SS, Dispenzieri A, Lacy MQ, Gertz MA. Excessive fluid accumulation during stem cell mobilization: a novel prognostic factor of first-year survival after stem cell transplantation in AL amyloidosis patients. Blood 2005;106:3353–7.

53. Dispenzieri A, Lacy MQ, Katzmann JA, et al. Absolute values of immunoglobulin free light chains are prognostic in patients with primary systemic amyloidosis undergoing peripheral blood stem cell transplantation. Blood 2006;107:3378–83.

54. Zhou P, Teruya-Feldstein J, Lu P, Fleisher M, Olshen A, Comenzo RL. Calreticulin expression in the clonal plasma cells of patients with systemic light-chain (AL–) amyloidosis is associated with response to high-dose melphalan. Blood 2008;111:549–57.

55. Sanchorawala V, Wright DG, Quillen K, et al. Tandem cycles of high-dose melphalan and autologous stem cell transplantation increases the response rate in AL amyloidosis. Bone Marrow Transplant. 2007;40:557–62.

56. Schonland SO, Lokhorst H, Buzyn A, et al. Allogeneic and syngeneic hematopoietic cell transplantation in patients with amyloid light-chain amyloidosis: a report from the European Group for Blood and Marrow Transplantation. Blood 2006;107:2578–84.

57. Palladini G, Perfetti V, Perlini S, et al. The combination of thalidomide and intermediate-dose dexamethasone is an effective but toxic treatment for patients with primary amyloidosis (AL). Blood 2005;105:2949–51.

58. Seldin DC, Choufani EB, Dember LM, et al. Tolerability and efficacy of thalidomide for the treatment of patients with light chain-associated (AL) amyloidosis. Clinical Lymphoma. 2003;3:241–6.

59. Sanchorawala V, Wright DG, Rosenzweig M, et al. Lenalidomide and dexamethasone in the treatment of AL amyloidosis: results of a phase 2 trial. Blood 2007;109:492–6.

60. Dispenzieri A, Lacy MQ, Rajkumar SV, et al. Poor tolerance to high doses of thalidomide in patients with primary systemic amyloidosis. Amyloid 2003;10:257–61.

61. Dispenzieri A, Lacy MQ, Zeldenrust SR, et al. The activity of lenalidomide with or without dexamethasone in patients with primary systemic amyloidosis. Blood 2007;109: 465–70.

62. Wechalekar AD, Goodman HJ, Lachmann HJ, Offer M, Hawkins PN, Gillmore JD. Safety and efficacy of risk-adapted cyclophosphamide, thalidomide, and dexamethasone in systemic AL amyloidosis. Blood 2007;109:457–64.

63. Wechalekar AD, Lachmann HJ, Offer M, Hawkins PN, Gillmore JD. Efficacy of bortezomib in systemic AL amyloidosis with relapsed/refractory clonal disease. Haematologica 2008;93:295–8.

64. Kastritis E, Anagnostopoulos A, Roussou M, et al. Treatment of light chain (AL) amyloidosis with the combination of bortezomib and dexamethasone. Haematologica 2007;92:1351–8.

65. Reece DE, Sanchorawala V, Hegenbart U, et al. Phase I/II study of bortezomib (B) in patients with systemic AL-amyloidosis (AL). J Clin Oncol (2007 ASCO Annual Meeting Proceedings). 2007;25:8050.

66. Gertz MA, Lacy MQ, Dispenzieri A, Hayman SR, Kumar S. Transplantation for amyloidosis. Curr Opin Oncol. 2007;19:136–41.

Chapter 13

Secondary, AA, Amyloidosis

Helen J. Lachmann

Abstract AA amyloidosis, otherwise known as secondary amyloidosis, is a complication of chronic inflammation. The amyloid fibrils are derived from the hepatic acute phase reactant, serum amyloid A protein. Clinically AA amyloidosis has a predominantly renal presentation with proteinuria and renal impairment. Untreated disease will progress to end-stage renal failure. Treatment depends on complete control of the underlying chronic inflammatory condition, and if this can be achieved long-term outcomes are favourable. Median survival in patients with AA amyloidosis now exceeds 12 years although renal failure eventually develops in more than 40%.

Keywords AA amyloidosis, Serum amyloid A protein (SAA), Cytokines, Inflammation, Arthritis, Renal, Proteinuria

Introduction

AA amyloidosis, otherwise known as secondary amyloidosis, is a complication of chronic inflammation and is the third commonest type of systemic amyloidosis seen in the United Kingdom. It has a predominantly renal presentation and is responsible for approximately 15% of the new cases of systemic amyloidosis in the United Kingdom each year.

Pathology

In AA amyloidosis the amyloid fibrils are derived from the acute phase reactant, serum amyloid A protein (SAA) [1]. SAA is an apolipoprotein of high-density lipoprotein, which, like C-reactive protein (CRP), is synthesized by hepatocytes under the transcriptional regulation of proinflammatory cytokines, particularly tumour necrosis factor (TNF) alpha, interleukin-1 (IL-1) and interleukin-6 (IL-6) [2]. The median plasma concentration of SAA in healthy blood donors is 3 mg/L [3], but this can increase rapidly to over 2,000 mg/L during a brisk acute phase response. AA amyloidosis can complicate any chronic disorder that stimulates a frequent or prolonged acute phase response. Although sustained overproduction of SAA is a necessary prerequisite for the development of AA amyloidosis it is not sufficient as AA amyloid deposition occurs in a minority of patients with inflammatory diseases [4–6]. The factors beyond supply of SAA, the amyloid fibril precursor protein, which predispose to development of AA amyloidosis, are largely still unclear but one important contributor appears to be the SAA gene isotype. There are four SAA genes in man, all

From: *Amyloidosis*, Contemporary Hematology,
Edited by: M.A. Gertz and S.V. Rajkumar, DOI 10.1007/978-1-60761-631-3_13,
© Springer Science+Business Media, LLC 2010

on chromosome 11. SAA_1 and SAA_2 are responsible for the acute phase response; SAA_4 is expressed constitutively; and SAA_3 is a pseudogene. There are a number of isoforms at the SAA_1 and SAA_2 loci [7]. Susceptibility to AA amyloidosis is increased among individuals who are homozygous for their SAA_1 allele [8, 9], and studies in Japan suggest that $SAA_{1\gamma}$ is more inherently amyloidogenic than the α and β isotypes [10, 11]. Similar results have been reported in SAA_2 where the allele $SAA_{2\alpha2}$ is significantly overrepresented in Caucasian patients with AA amyloidosis complicating juvenile inflammatory arthritis [12].

Epidemiology

The exact prevalence of AA amyloidosis is unclear as diagnosis is difficult and it is almost certainly underreported. Biopsy and post-mortem series suggest that the prevalence of AA amyloidosis in patients with chronic arthritides is between 3.6 and 5.8% [4, 5, 13]. Extrapolating from published data on the prevalence and lifetime incidence of amyloidosis in rheumatoid arthritis, ankylosing spondylitis and juvenile idiopathic arthritis patients and on the prevalence of these chronic arthritides, an upper limit for the community prevalence of AA amyloidosis in the general European population can be estimated at 1.8/10,000 people. An observation that remains unexplained is that the incidence of AA amyloid is lower in the United States and much higher in parts of central Europe and Scandinavia [14, 15] and, perhaps by the same, as yet unknown, mechanisms, its prevalence in Europe is believed to have decreased substantially over the past 40 years [16].

The list of chronic inflammatory, infective and neoplastic disorders that can lead to AA amyloidosis is almost without limit (Table 13-1), and the predominant aetiology varies among different populations [17]. In the Western world the commonest predisposing conditions are the chronic inflammatory arthritides which account for 60% of cases. Chronic infections are the major underlying cause in the developing world but account for only 15% of cases in the United Kingdom [18] (Table 13-2). Amyloidosis occurs exceptionally rarely in systemic lupus erythematosus and ulcerative colitis reflecting the unusually modest acute phase response evoked by these particular conditions. AA amyloidosis can complicate cytokine-producing tumours, particularly localised Castleman's disease which secretes IL-6. The inherited fever syndromes, which are significant causes of amyloid in affected populations, carry an exceptionally high risk of complication by AA amyloid deposition. These diseases include familial Mediterranean fever (FMF), TNF receptor-associated periodic syndrome (TRAPS) [19], cryopyrin-associated periodic syndrome (CAPS) and mevalonate kinase deficiency (MKD) [20]. All present early in life, and clinical attacks are accompanied by a very striking acute phase response in which the peak SAA level may exceed 2,000 mg/L. The pattern of lifelong recurrent attacks accompanied by a massive increase in the supply of a potential amyloid precursor protein probably provides the explanation for the striking relative risk of AA amyloidosis in these diseases, and there are data to suggest that the availability of effective disease control in the form of colchicine in FMF has reduced the risk of developing amyloidosis from 60 to 13% [21].

The median latency between onset of inflammation and diagnosis of amyloid is approximately 17 years for all of the major underlying disease groups, although some individuals develop clinically significant amyloid in less than 12 months and others only after many decades. The median age at diagnosis is 50 years but presentation in childhood, although becoming less common, is still well recognised, and at the other extreme patients may not develop clinical amyloidosis until their ninth decade.

Table 13-1. Conditions reported to be complicated by AA amyloidosis.

Conditions associated with systemic AA (secondary) amyloidosis	
Inflammatory arthritides Adult Still's disease [41] Ankylosing spondilitis [6] Juvenile idiopathic arthritis [5] Psoriatic arthropathy [42] Reiter's syndrome [43] Rheumatoid arthritis [44]	*Neoplasia* Adenocarcinoma of the lung, gut, urogenital tract [64] Basal cell carcinoma [65] Carcinoid tumour [66] Castleman's disease [34] Gastrointestinal stromal tumour Hairy cell leukaemia [67] Hepatic adenoma [68] Hodgkin's disease [69] Mesothelioma Renal cell carcinoma [70] Sarcoma [71] Peritoneal pseudomyxoma
Systemic vasculitis Giant cell arteritis [45] Polyarteritis nodosa [46] Polymyalgia rheumatica [47] Systemic lupus erythematosis [48] Takayasu's arteritis [49]	
Autoinflammatory disorders Cryopyrin-associated periodic fever syndrome [50] Familial Mediterranean fever [51] Mevalonate kinase deficiency [52] SAPHO syndrome [53] TNF receptor-associated periodic syndrome [54]	*Immunodeficiency states* Common variable immunodeficiency [72] Cyclic neutropenia [73] Hyperimmunoglobulin M syndrome [74] Hypogammaglobulinaemia [75] Sex-linked agammaglobulinaemia [76] HIV/AIDS
Chronic infections Bronchiectasis [30] Chronic cutaneous ulcers [55] Chronic pyelonephritis [56] HIV [57] Leprosy [58] Osteomyelitis [31] Q fever [59] Subacute bacterial endocarditis [60] Tuberculosis [17] Whipple's disease [61]	*Other conditions predisposing to chronic infections* Cystic fibrosis [77] Epidermolysis bullosa [78] Intravenous and subcutaneous drug abuse [32] Kartagener's syndrome [79] Paraplegia [80] Sickle-cell anaemia [81]
Inflammatory bowel disease Crohn's disease [62] Ulcerative colitis [63]	*Other* Atrial myxoma [82, 83] Behcet's disease [84] Inflammatory aortic aneurism [85] Retroperitoneal fibrosis [86] Sarcoidosis [87] Sinus histiocystosis with massive lymphadenopathy [88]

As with all types of amyloidosis, AA appears slightly commoner in men who account for 56% of the largest characterised series [18]. This is particularly striking when it is remembered that rheumatoid arthritis is a disease with a marked female predominance. In the large series from the United Kingdom there was significant overrepresentation of ethnic groups originating from the eastern Mediterranean and an underrepresentation of people of African origin. The relative paucity of AA amyloidosis in Americans of African origin has previously been noted [22]. This does not appear to be due to protection from amyloidosis in general and may be due to the relatively low number of patients of African origin who suffer from rheumatoid arthritis or to the lack of other factors predisposing to AA amyloidosis in general such as SAA type.

Table 13-2. Major underlying causes of AA amyloidosis in the United Kingdom.

Underlying disease	Percentage of cases
Chronic inflammatory arthritis	60
Rheumatoid arthritis	33
Juvenile idiopathic arthritis	17
Other chronic inflammatory arthritides	10
Chronic sepsis	15
Bronchiectasis	5
Injected drug abuse	4
Complications of paraplegia	2
Other chronic sepsis	4
Periodic fever syndromes	9
Familial Mediterranean fever	5
TNF receptor-associated periodic fever syndrome	2
Cryopyrin-associated periodic syndrome	1
Mevalonate kinase deficiency	0.5
Crohn's disease	5
Miscellaneous	6
Castleman's disease	2
Neoplasia	1
Vasculitis	1
Other	1.5
Unknown	6
No diagnosis made despite extensive investigation	

Clinical Features

Extensive AA amyloid deposition can occur without causing symptoms [23]. The predominant clinical manifestations of AA amyloidosis are renal and more than 95% of patients present with proteinuric kidney dysfunction. Approximately 5% of cases will not have proteinuria despite extensive renal amyloid deposition. Haematuria, tubular defects and diffuse renal calcification occur rarely [24]. Just over 50% of patients have nephrotic syndrome at presentation and 75% of cases present with an estimated glomerular filtration rate of more than 30 mL/min, i.e. chronic kidney disease stage 1, 2 or 3. Approximately 10% of patients are at end-stage renal failure when the diagnosis is made, and progression to dialysis dependence is eventually seen in almost 50%. The spleen is infiltrated in almost all cases and the adrenal glands in at least a third, although clinical hypoadrenalism is not common. The liver and gut are also frequent sites of AA amyloid deposition, and hepatosplenomegaly is present in 9% of cases at presentation. Hepatic failure due to AA amyloidosis is exceptionally rare, and gut dysfunction causing motility disorders and malabsorption does occur but generally only in exceptionally advanced disease. Cardiac amyloidosis is also not usually a clinical problem. Suggestive echocardiographic and electrocardiographic abnormalities are seen in about 2% of cases, and biopsy evidence of cardiac amyloid deposition has been reported at post-mortem or in patients with generally advanced disease and established renal failure. Neurological involvement is also not typical. Autonomic neuropathy does not appear to be a common feature. Mild peripheral neuropathy is occasionally seen, mostly in patients with long-standing end-stage renal failure, and there are likely to be multiple other metabolic factors contributing to the neuropathic symptoms.

Treatment

It is now well recognised that the outcome in systemic amyloidosis of all types is related to the supply of fibril precursor protein [25, 26]. If the supply precursor can be reduced sufficiently this can alter the equilibrium between amyloid deposition and turnover in favour of amyloid regression. As the fibril precursor protein in AA-type amyloid is the acute phase reactant SAA the aim of treatment must be sustained and complete control of the underlying inflammatory disease process [25, 27–30]. Clearly the choice of therapy depends on the nature of the underlying disease process but therapeutic success must always be assessed by the long-term control of SAA production or, if this is not available, CRP measurements, performed frequently—in our practice monthly.

Most patients with inflammatory arthritis have previously failed to respond to conventional disease modifying anti-rheumatoid drugs such as methotrexate and many do well with anti-TNF therapies or other biologics such as anti-CD20 antibodies or anti-IL-1 or IL-6 therapies. In patients who fail to respond to these agents there may still be a role for therapy with alkylating agents such as chlorambucil or cyclophosphamide [27]. Treatment of chronic sepsis is based on long-term appropriate antimicrobials and may need to be combined with surgical debridement or excision of infected tissue [31]. In patients with long-term drug addiction this must be combined with support to enable them to stop self-injecting with contaminated apparatus or drugs [32]. Treatment of the periodic fever syndromes is highly specific. Excellent disease control can be achieved in the majority of patients with FMF with long-term colchicine prophylaxis. In CAPS anti-IL-1 therapies have proven remarkably effective [33]. TRAPS and MVK have proven to be more difficult to treat but many patients respond to anti-TNF or anti-IL-1 therapies. Crohn's disease often responds to conventional immunosuppression or anti-TNF therapies. Some patients do require surgical bowel excision as well. Castleman's disease, a rare IL-6-secreting tumour, can sometimes be completely excised [34], and in those cases where surgery is not feasible or curative there is evidence for benefit for anti-IL-6 therapies [35]. The 6% of patients in whom the underlying inflammatory disease cannot be identified are a serious management challenge, and therapy in these cases has to be empirical—guided by frequent assays of SAA.

Specific therapies tailored to control the underlying inflammatory state must be combined with general supportive measures. Kidneys extensively infiltrated by amyloid are exquisitely vulnerable to intercurrent insults such as hypoperfusion, hypertension, nephrotoxic drugs and surgery, all of which should be avoided.

Many patients will eventually require renal replacement therapy. Survival on dialysis is now comparable with that of non-diabetic-associated end-stage renal failure [36], although earlier series reported less good outcomes [37]. Recent experience of renal transplantation in selected patients has been encouraging with long-term graft and patient survival exceeding that set by British and American standards. Recurrent amyloidosis is surprisingly infrequent. The encouraging outcomes in patients whose underlying disease can be controlled has resulted in some cases receiving living donor renal transplants [38].

As SAA production can be modified by medical management it is absolutely vital that levels are measured serially and management changes tailor according to the results. Nonetheless for many clinicians measurement of CRP is often more useful as SAA measurement is available only in a relatively limited number of research laboratories. Median CRP also predicts clinical outcome and can be used as a surrogate marker of SAA provided its values are interpreted with some caution. CRP and SAA rise and fall in parallel but some patients may have 5- or even 10-fold SAA bias, and as a result although elevated levels of median CRP are strongly associated with a poor outcome levels of less than 10 mg/L will include some patients with significantly higher SAA concentrations, and consequently low CRP levels may sometimes be falsely reassuring.

Outcome

The prognosis in AA amyloidosis has improved significantly and median survival is now just under 12 years, which compares very favourably with median survival in AL amyloidosis [39]. Prognosis is related to the degree of renal involvement. Without treatment the outlook was bleak. Almost three-quarters of patients reached end-stage renal failure within 5 years of diagnosis, and once the serum creatinine was elevated beyond the normal range half the patients were dead within 18 months. Although AA amyloid is a relatively unusual complication of juvenile idiopathic arthritis it has been reported to be responsible for 40–50% of all deaths in these patients. Fifty per cent of juvenile idiopathic arthritis patients with amyloidosis have been reported to die within 5 years and a further 25% within the following 10 years.

Factors at presentation that are associated with a worse prognosis in this type of amyloidosis included older age, reduced serum albumin concentration and end-stage renal failure [18]. There is little difference in outcome between different groups of underlying diseases, although multivariate analysis in one study has suggested patients with periodic fever syndromes have slightly better survival. Increased production of SAA is the most powerful risk factor for death with evidence of an almost 18-fold increased relative risk between patients with completely normal levels of SAA production (median of $\leq$ 4 mg/L) compared to patients with a median SAA of $\geq$ 155 mg/L. SAA production also predicts the risk of development of end-stage renal failure and median SAA levels in patients whose renal function improved has been reported as 6 mg/L compared to 28 mg/L in patients whose renal function worsened by consensus criteria. Renal failure is more likely to supervene in patients with chronic sepsis or Crohn's disease perhaps reflecting the increased risks from surgery in patients with Crohn's and additional comorbidity burdens in patients with chronic sepsis—particularly the injecting drug users who have particularly poor outcomes. AA amyloid deposits gradually regress in the majority of patients whose inflammatory disease remains in remission, but the rate varies substantially between different individuals [40]. These differences suggest that the amyloid deposits are either more stable in some patients than in others or that individuals simply differ in their capacity to mobilise amyloid. Renal function, however, especially proteinuria, often improves even when the amyloid deposits only remain stable, and equally, in a minority of cases, amyloid regression may be seen on SAP scintigraphy (a nuclear medicine technique for imaging amyloid deposits) without improvement in renal function. Residual amyloid deposits may be present to a substantial extent in some patients who appear to have been in complete clinical remission for decades. This is very relevant in terms of patient management as the presence of even a small amount of amyloid may serve as a template for further rapid amyloid accumulation should there be a recrudescence of inflammatory activity.

Conclusion

The causes of AA amyloidosis have changed in line with the predominant causes of refractory and chronic inflammation in the general population. That amyloidosis now presents at an older age is likely to be due to both the increasing predominance of inflammatory arthritis as the underlying cause and the improvements in its medical care. The longer latency between onset of inflammation and presentation of amyloidosis suggests that many of these patients may have less florid inflammation than in the past. Although almost 30% of patients still present with established or incipient end-stage renal failure, AA amyloidosis is a potentially reversible disease and rigorous control of the underlying inflammatory disease can result in improvement in renal function and prolonged survival. In this disease every effort should be made to establish the aetiology of the underlying inflammation and to provide treatment aimed at producing sustained complete normalisation of the inflammatory response. It is hoped that in the near future these management options will be combined with specific anti-amyloid therapies.

References

1. Parmelee DC, Titani K, Ericsson LH, Eriksen N, Benditt EP, Walsh KA. Amino acid sequence of amyloid-related apoprotein (apoSAA$_1$) from human high density lipoprotein. Biochemistry. 1982;21:3298–303.
2. Urieli-Shoval S, Linke RP, Matzner Y. Expression and function of serum amyloid A, a major acute-phase protein, in normal and disease states. Curr Opin Hematol. 2000;7: 64–69.
3. Ledue TB, Weiner DL, Sipe JD, Poulin SE, Collins MF, Rifai N. Analytical evaluation of particle-enhanced immunonephelometric assays for C-reactive protein, serum amyloid A and mannose-binding protein in human serum. Ann Clin Biochem. 1998;35:745–53.
4. de Beer FC, Mallya RK, Fagan EA, Lanham JG, Hughes GRV, Pepys MB. Serum amyloid A protein (SAA) concentration in inflammatory diseases and its relationship to the incidence of reactive systemic amyloidosis. Lancet. 1982;ii:231–34.
5. Schnitzer TJ, Ansell BM. Amyloidosis in juvenile chronic polyarthritis. Arthritis Rheum. 1977;20:245–52.
6. Gratacos J, Orellana C, Sanmarti R, et al. Secondary amyloidosis in ankylosing spondylitis. A systematic survey of 137 patients using abdominal fat aspiration. J Rheumatol. 1997;24:912–15.
7. Faulkes DJ, Betts JC, Woo P. Characterization of five human serum amyloid A$_1$ alleles. Amyloid: Int J Exp Clin Invest. 1994;1:255–62.
8. Booth DR, Booth SE, Gillmore JD, Hawkins PN, Pepys MB. SAA$_1$ alleles as risk factors in reactive systemic AA amyloidosis. Amyloid: Int J Exp Clin Invest. 1998;5:262–65.
9. Cazeneuve C, Ajrapetyan H, Papin S, et al. Identification of *MEFV*-independent modifying genetic factors for familial Mediterranean fever. Am J Hum Genet. 2000;67:1136–43.
10. Baba S, Masago SA, Takahashi T, et al. A novel allelic variant of serum amyloid A, SAA1g: genomic evidence, evolution, frequency, and implication as a risk factor for reactive systemic AA-amyloidosis. Hum Med Genet. 1995;4:1083–87.
11. Yamada S, Gotoh T, Nakashima Y, et al. Distribution of serum C-reactive protein and its association with atherosclerotic risk factors in a Japanese population: Jichi Medical School Cohort Study. Am J Epidemiol. 2001;153:1183–90.
12. Faulkes DJ, Woo P. Do alleles at the serum amyloid A locus influence susceptibility to reactive amyloidosis in systemic onset juvenile chronic arthritis? Amyloid: Int J Exp Clin Invest. 1997;4:75–79.
13. Myllykangas-Luosujärvi R, Aho K, Kautiainen H, Hakala M. Amyloidosis in a nationwide series of 1666 subjects with rheumatoid arthritis who died during 1989 in Finland. Rheumatology. 1999;38:499–503.

14. Filipowicz-Sosnowska AM, Roztropowicz-Denisiewicz K, Rosenthal CJ, Baum J. The amyloidosis of juvenile rheumatoid arthritis—comparative studies in Polish and American children. I. Levels of serum SAA protein. Arthritis Rheum. 1978;21:699–703.

15. Svantesson H, Akesson A, Eberhardt K, Elborgh R. Prognosis in juvenile rheumatoid arthritis with systemic onset. A follow-up study. Scand J Rheumatol. 1983;12:139–44.

16. Laiho K, Tiitinen S, Kaarela K, Helin H, Isomaki H. Secondary amyloidosis has decreased in patients with inflammatory joint disease in Finland. Clin Rheumatol. 1999;18:122–23.

17. Mehta HJ, Talwalkar NC, Merchant MR, et al. Pattern of renal amyloidosis in western India. A study of 104 cases. J Assoc Physicians India. 1990;38:407–10.

18. Lachmann HJ, Goodman HJ, Gilbertson JA, et al. Natural history and outcome in systemic AA amyloidosis. N Engl J Med. 2007;356(23):2361–71.

19. McDermott MF. Autosomal dominant recurrent fevers. Clinical and genetic aspects. Rev Rhum [Engl Ed]. 1999;66:484–91.

20. Hawkins PN, Booth DR. Familial Mediterranean fever and other inherited periodic fever syndromes. In: Warrell DA, Cox TM, Firth JD, Benz EJ Jr, editors. Oxford textbook of medicine. 4th ed. Oxford: Oxford University Press; 2003. pp. 158–62.

21. Tunca M, Akar S, Onen F, et al. Familial Mediterranean fever (FMF) in Turkey: results of a nationwide multicenter study. Medicine (Baltimore). 2005;84:1–11.

22. Buck FS, Koss MN, Sherrod AE, Wu A, Takahashi M. Ethnic distribution of amyloidosis: an autopsy study. Mod Pathol. 1989;2:372–77.

23. Hawkins PN, Richardson S, Vigushin DM, et al. Serum amyloid P component scintigraphy and turnover studies for diagnosis and quantitative monitoring of AA amyloidosis in juvenile rheumatoid arthritis. Arthritis Rheum. 1993;36:842–51.

24. Luke RG, Allison ME, Davidson JF, Duguid WP. Hyperkalemia and renal tubular acidosis due to renal amyloidosis. Ann Intern Med. 1969;70:1211–17.

25. Gillmore JD, Lovat LB, Persey MR, Pepys MB, Hawkins PN. Amyloid load and clinical outcome in AA amyloidosis in relation to circulating concentration of serum amyloid A protein. Lancet. 2001;358:24–29.

26. Lachmann HJ, Goodman HJB, Gilbertson JA, et al. Natural history and outcome in systemic AA amyloidosis. N Engl J Med. 2007;356:2361–71.

27. Berglund K, Thysell H, Keller C. Results, principles and pitfalls in the management of renal AA-amyloidosis; a 10–21 year followup of 16 patients with rheumatic disease treated with alkylating cytostatics. J Rheumatol. 1993;20:2051–57.

28. Livneh A, Zemer D, Langevitz P, Laor A, Sohar E, Pras M. Colchicine treatment of AA amyloidosis of familial Mediterranean fever. An analysis of factors affecting outcome. Arthritis Rheum. 1994;37:1804–11.

29. Keven K, Nergizoglu G, Ates K, et al. Remission of nephrotic syndrome after removal of localized Castleman's disease. Am J Kidney Dis. 2000;35:1207–11.

30. Goldsmith DJA, Roberts ISP, Short CD, Mallick NP. Complete clinical remission and subsequent relapse of bronchiectasis-related (AA) amyloid induced nephrotic syndrome. Nephron. 1996;74:572–76.

31. Gertz MA, Kyle RA. Secondary systemic amyloidosis: response and survival in 64 patients. Medicine. 1991;70:246–56.

32. Connolly JO, Gillmore JD, Lachmann HJ, Davenport A, Hawkins PN, Woolfson RG. Renal amyloidosis in intravenous drug users. Q J Med. 2006;99:737–42.

33. Leslie KS, Lachmann HJ, Bruning E, et al. Phenotype, genotype, and sustained response to anakinra in 22 patients with autoinflammatory disease associated with CIAS-1/NALP3 mutations. Arch Dermatol. 2006;142(12):1591–97.

34. Lachmann HJ, Gilbertson JA, Gillmore JD, Hawkins PN, Pepys MB. Unicentric Castleman's disease complicated by systemic AA amyloidosis: a curable disease. Q J Med. 2002;95:211–18.

35. Nishimoto N, Sasai M, Shima Y, et al. Improvement in Castleman's disease by humanized anti-interleukin-6 receptor antibody therapy. Blood. 2000;95:56–61.

36. UK Renal Registry Report. 2003. UK Renal Registry, Bristol.

37. Sengul S, Arat Z, Ozdemir FN. Renal amyloidosis is associated with increased mortality in hemodialysis patients. Artif Organs. 2004;28:846–52.

38. Sherif AM, Refaie AF, Sobh MA, Mohamed NA, Sheashaa HA, Ghoneim MA. Long-term outcome of live donor kidney transplantation for renal amyloidosis. Am J Kidney Dis. 2003;42:370–75.
39. Kyle RA, Gertz MA. Primary systemic amyloidosis: clinical and laboratory features in 474 cases. Semin Hematol. 1995;32:45–59.
40. Hawkins PN. Studies with radiolabelled serum amyloid P component provide evidence for turnover and regression of amyloid deposits in vivo. Clin Sci. 1994;87:289–95.
41. Rivera F, Gil CM, Gil MT, Batlle-Gualda E, Trigueros M, Olivares J. Vascular renal AA amyloidosis in adult Still's disease. Nephrol Dial Transplant. 1997;12:1714–16.
42. Ahmed Q, Chung-Park M, Mustafa K, Khan MA. Psoriatic spondyloarthropathy with secondary amyloidosis. J Rheumatol. 1996;23:1107–10.
43. Wakefield D, Charlesworth J, Pussell B, Wenman J. Reiter's syndrome and amyloidosis. Br J Rheumatol. 1987;26:156–58.
44. Ahlmen M, Ahlmen J, Svalander C, Bucht H. Cytotoxic drug treatment of reactive amyloidosis in rheumatoid arthritis with special reference to renal insufficiency. Clin Rheumatol. 1987;6:27–38.
45. Moraga SJJ, Blanco J, Ubeda I. Giant cell arteritis and renal amyloidosis: report of a case. Clin Nephrol. 2001;56:402–6.
46. Yorioka N, Taniguchi Y, Okushin S, Amimoto D, Kataoka K, Taguchi T. Classic polyarteritis nodosa associated with renal amyloidosis. Nephron. 1999;82:93–94.
47. Escriba A, Morales E, Albizua E, et al. Secondary (AA-type) amyloidosis in patients with polymyalgia rheumatica. Am J Kidney Dis. 2000;35:137–40.
48. Aktas Yilmaz B, Duzgun N, Mete T, et al. AA amyloidosis associated with systemic lupus erythematosus: impact on clinical course and outcome. Rheumatol Int. 2008;28:367–70.
49. Nonoguchi H, Kohda Y, Fukutomi R, et al. A case with acute renal failure and subsequent nephrotic syndrome. Ren Fail. 2009;31:162–66.
50. Muckle TJ, Wells MV. Urticaria, deafness and amyloidosis: a new heredo-familial syndrome. Q J Med. 1962;31:235–48.
51. Ben-Chetrit E, Levy M. Familial Mediterranean fever. Lancet. 1998;351:659–64.
52. Lachmann HJ, Goodman HJ, Andrews PA, et al. AA amyloidosis complicating hyperimmunoglobulinemia D with periodic fever syndrome: a report of two cases. Arthritis Rheum. 2006;54:2010–14.
53. Valentin R, Gurtler KF, Schaker A. Renal amyloidosis and renal failure–a novel complication of the SAPHO syndrome. Nephrol Dial Transplant. 1997;12:2420–23.
54. Aganna E, Hammond L, Hawkins PN, et al. Heterogeneity among patients with tumor necrosis factor receptor-associated periodic syndrome phenotypes. Arthritis Rheum. 2003;48:2632–44.
55. Landau M, Ophir J, Gal R, Pras M, Brenner S. Systemic amyloidosis secondary to chronic leg ulcers. Cutis. 1992;50:47–49.
56. Islek I, Baris S, Albayrak D, Buyukalpelli R, Sancak R. Chronic nephrotic syndrome and chronic renal failure by amyloidosis secondary to xanthogranulomatous pyelonephritis. Clin Nephrol. 1998;49:62–65.
57. de Valliere S, Mary C, Joneberg JE, et al. AA-amyloidosis caused by visceral leishmaniasis in a human immunodeficiency virus-infected patient. Am J Trop Med Hyg. 2009;81:209–12.
58. Nakayama EE, Ura S, Fleury RN, Soares V. Renal lesions in leprosy: a retrospective study of 199 autopsies. Am J Kidney Dis. 2001;38:26–30.
59. Kayser K, Wiebel M, Schulz V, Gabius HJ. Necrotizing bronchitis, angiitis, and amyloidosis associated with chronic Q fever. Respiration. 1995;62:114–16.
60. Herbert MA, Milford DV, Silove ED, Raafat F. Secondary amyloidosis from long-standing bacterial endocarditis. Pediatr Nephrol. 1995;9:33–35.
61. Farr M, Hollywell CA, Walton KW, Morris C, Scott DL, Bacon PA. Amyloidosis in Whipple's arthritis. J Royal Soc Med. 1983;76:963–66.
62. Lovat LB, Madhoo S, Pepys MB, Hawkins PN. Long term survival in systemic AA amyloidosis complicating Crohn's disease. Gastroenterology. 1997;112:1362–65.

63. Wester AL, Vatn MH, Fausa O. Secondary amyloidosis in inflammatory bowel disease: a study of 18 patients admitted to Rikshospitalet University Hospital, Oslo, from 1962 to 1998. Inflamm Bowel Dis. 2001;7:295–300.

64. Melato M, Manconi R, Falconieri G. Amyloidosis and lung cancer. A morphological and histochemical study. Morphol Embryol (Bucur). 1981;27:137–42.

65. Cox NH, Nicoll JJ, Popple AW. Amyloid deposition in basal cell carcinoma: a cause of apparent lack of sensitivity to radiotherapy. Clin Exp Dermatol. 2001;26:499–500.

66. Vigushin DM, Gough J, Allan D, et al. Familial nephropathic systemic amyloidosis caused by apolipoprotein AI variant Arg26. Q J Med. 1994;87:149–54.

67. Linder J, Silberman HR, Croher BP. Amyloidosis complicating hairy cell leukaemia. Am J Clin Pathol. 1982;78:864–67.

68. Cosme A, Horcajada JP, Vidaur F, Ojeda E, Torrado J, Arenas JI. Systemic AA amyloidosis induced by oral contraceptive-associated hepatocellular adenoma: a 13-year follow up. Liver. 1995;15:164–67.

69. Perez Equiza E, Arguinano JM, Gastearena J. Successful treatment of AA amyloidosis secondary to Hodgkin's disease with 4'-iodo-4'-deoxydoxorubicin. Haematologica. 1999;84:93–94.

70. Pras M, Franklin EC, Shibolet S, Frangione B. Amyloidosis associated with renal cell carcinoma of the AA type. Am J Med. 1982;73:426–28.

71. Agha I, Mahoney R, Beardslee M, Liapis H, Cowart RG, Juknevicius I. Systemic amyloidosis associated with pleomorphic sarcoma of the spleen and remission of nephrotic syndrome after removal of the tumor. Am J Kidney Dis. 2002;40:411–15.

72. Celik AF, Altiparmak MR, Pamuk GE, Pamuk ON, Tabak F. Association of secondary amyloidosis with common variable immune deficiency and tuberculosis. Yonsei Med J. 2005;46:847–50.

73. Metin A, Ersoy F, Tinaztepe K, Besbas N, Tezcan I, Sanal O. Cyclic neutropenia complicated by renal AA amyloidosis. Turk J Pediatr. 2000;42:61–64.

74. Oner A, Demircin G, Erdogan O, et al. A family with hyperimmunoglobulin M syndrome and systemic amyloidosis. Nephrol Dial Transplant. 2000;15:1480–82.

75. Kotilainen P, Vuori K, Kainulainen L, et al. Systemic amyloidosis in a patient with hypogammaglobulinaemia. J Intern Med. 1996;240:103–6.

76. Tezcan I, Ersoy F, Sanal O, Gonc EN, Arici M, Berkel I. A case of X linked agammaglobulinaemia complicated with systemic amyloidosis. Arch Dis Child. 1998;79:94.

77. Yahiaoui Y, Jablonski M, Hubert D, et al. Renal involvement in cystic fibrosis: diseases spectrum and clinical relevance. Clin J Am Soc Nephrol. 2009;4:921–28.

78. Csikos M, Orosz Z, Bottlik G, et al. Dystrophic epidermolysis bullosa complicated by cutaneous squamous cell carcinoma and pulmonary and renal amyloidosis. Clin Exp Dermatol. 2003;28:163–66.

79. Osman EM, Abboud OI, Sulaiman SM, Musa AR, Beleil OM, Sharfi AA. End-stage renal failure in Kartagener's syndrome. Nephrol Dial Transplant. 1991;6:747.

80. Barton CH, Vaziri ND, Gordon S, Tilles S. Renal pathology in end-stage renal disease associated with paraplegia. Paraplegia. 1984;22:31–41.

81. Win N, Brozovic M, Gabriel R. Secondary amyloidosis accompanying multiple sickle cell crises. Trop Doct. 1993;23:45–46.

82. Wens R, Goffin Y, Pepys MB, et al. Left atrial myxoma associated with systemic AA amyloidosis. Arch Intern Med. 1989;149:453–54.

83. Navas-Parejo A, Moreno E, Riera M, Garcia-Orta R, Correa C. Left atrial myxoma associated with systemic AA amyloidosis. Clin Nephrol. 2003;60:441–43.

84. Skhiri H, Mahjoub S, Harzallah O, et al. Secondary amyloidosis, a fatal complication of Behcet's disease: three case reports. Saudi J Kidney Dis Transpl. 2004;15:57–60.

85. Odabas AR, Cetinkaya R, Selcuk Y, et al. AA amyloidosis complicating an inflammatory abdominal aortic aneurysm. Nephrol Dial Transplant. 2002;17:281–82.

86. Hosaka N, Ito M, Taki Y, Iwai H, Toki J, Ikehara S. Amyloid A gastrointestinal amyloidosis associated with idiopathic retroperitoneal fibrosis. Report of a rare autopsy case and review of the literature. Arch Pathol Lab Med. 2003;127:735–38.

87. Levasseur R, Le Goff C, Richer C, Hurault de Ligny B, Marcelli C, Ryckelynck JP. AA amyloidosis complicating sarcoidosis. Rev Med Interne. 1999;20:168–70.
88. Rocken C, Wieker K, Grote HJ, Muller G, Franke A, Roessner A. Rosai-Dorfman disease and generalized AA amyloidosis: a case report. Hum Pathol. 2000;31:621–24.

Chapter 14

ATTR: Diagnosis, Prognosis, and Treatment

Steven R. Zeldenrust

Abstract ATTR is the most common form of inherited systemic amyloidosis. The signs and symptoms of ATTR are often subtle and overlap with more common diseases, including AL. Treatment for ATTR is most effective early in the course of the disease, making timely diagnosis critical. Orthotopic liver transplantation is the only proven effective therapy. Recent reports have suggested that amyloid deposition may progress after liver transplantation in some cases. Emerging therapies designed to prevent circulating TTR from forming amyloid are currently being tested and hold promise for patients not eligible for solid organ transplant and for those with progressive symptoms after transplant.

Keywords Transthyretin, Prealbumin, Hereditary, Liver transplantation, ATTR

Transthyretin-associated systemic amyloidosis (ATTR) is the most common form of hereditary systemic amyloidosis worldwide. The clinical manifestations of ATTR are indistinguishable from those of the more common immunoglobulin light chain associated form of amyloidosis (AL), making accurate diagnosis difficult. New proteomic technologies have aided in establishing the diagnosis, but are not widely available. The aggressive use of chemotherapy for AL and the availability of new treatment options for ATTR have made it even more critical to identify ATTR in newly diagnosed systemic amyloidosis.

Background

Over 100 different mutations of the TTR gene have been reported to date, most associated with the development of amyloidosis [1]. Considerable heterogeneity is seen in the clinical manifestations of the disease, depending on which organs are predominantly affected. Specific clinical syndromes are associated with each mutation, although some variation occurs even in patients with the same mutation (Table 14-1). The prognosis for individual patients varies according to which organs are predominantly affected.

Diagnosis

The most crucial step in establishing a diagnosis of amyloidosis is considering it in the differential diagnosis in the first place. It is not uncommon that patients will have been evaluated for a specific symptom for years before amyloidosis is recognized as

From: *Amyloidosis*, Contemporary Hematology,
Edited by: M.A. Gertz and S.V. Rajkumar, DOI 10.1007/978-1-60761-631-3_14,
© Springer Science+Business Media, LLC 2010

Table 14-1. ATTR variants.

Mutation	Codon change	Clinical features	Geographic kindreds
Cys10Arg	TGT–CGT	Heart, eye, PN	USA (PA)
Leu12Pro	CTG–CCG	LM	UK
Asp18Glu	GAT–GAA	PN	South America, USA
Asp18Gly	– GGT	LM	Hungary
Asp18Asn	– AAT	Heart	USA
Val20Ile	GTC–ATC	Heart, CTS	Germany, USA
Ser23Asn	AGT–AAT	Heart, PN, eye	USA
Pro24Ser	CCT–TCT	Heart, CTS, PN	USA
Ala25Ser	GCC–TCC	Heart, CTS, PN	USA
Ala25Thr	– ACC	LM, PN	Japan
Val28Met	GTG–ATG	PN, AN	Portugal
Val30Met	GTG–ATG	PN, AN, eye, LM	Portugal, Japan, Sweden, USA (FAP I)
Val30Ala	– GCG	Heart, AN	USA
Val30Leu	– CTG	PN, heart	Japan
Val30Gly	– GGG	LM, eye	USA
Val32Ala	GTG–GCG	PN	Israel
Phe33Ile	TTC–ATC	PN, eye	Israel
Phe33Leu	– CTC	PN, heart	USA
Phe33Val	– GTC	PN	UK, Japan, China
Phe33Cys	– TGC	CTS, heart, eye, kidney	USA
Arg34Thr	AGA–ACA	PN, heart	Italy
Arg34Gly	AGA–GGA	Eye	UK
Lys35Asn	AAG–AAC	PN, AN, Heart	France
Lys35Thr	– ACG	Eye	USA
Ala36Pro	GCT–CCT	Eye, CTS	USA
Asp38Ala	GAT–GCT	PN, heart	Japan
Trp41Leu	TGG–TTG	Eye, PN	USA
Glu42Gly	GAG–GGG	PN, AN, heart	Japan, USA, Russia
Glu42Asp	– GAT	Heart	France
Phe44Ser	TTT–TCT	PN, AN, heart	USA
Ala45Thr	GCC–ACC	Heart	USA
Ala45Asp	– GAC	Heart, PN	USA
Ala45Ser	– TCC	Heart	Sweden
Gly47Arg	GGG–CGG/AGG	PN, AN	Japan
Gly47Ala	– GCG	Heart, AN	Italy, France
Gly47Val	– GTG	CTS, PN, AN, heart	Sri Lanka
Gly47Glu	– GAG	Heart, PN, AN	Turkey, USA, Germany
Thr49Ala	ACC–GCC	Heart, CTS	France, Italy
Thr49Ile	– ATC	PN, heart	Japan, Spain
Thr49Pro	– CCC	Heart, PN	USA
Ser50Arg	AGT–AGG	AN, PN	Japan, France/Italian, USA
Ser50Ile	– ATT	Heart, PN, AN	Japan
Glu51Gly	GAG–GGG	Heart	USA
Ser52Pro	TCT–CCT	PN, AN, heart, Kidney	UK
Gly53Glu	GGA–GAA	LM, heart	Basque, Sweden
Glu54Gly	GAG–GGG	PN, AN, eye	UK
Glu54Lys	– AAG	PN, AN, heart, eye	Japan
Glu54Leu	GAG–CTG	Heart, AN, eye	UK
Leu55Pro	CTG–CCG	LM	USA, Taiwan
Leu55Arg	– CGG	Eye, PN	Germany
Leu55Gln	– CAG	Heart, PN, AN	USA
Leu55Glu	CTG–CAG	Heart	Sweden
His56Arg	CAT–CGT	Heart	USA

(continued)

Table 14-1. (continued)

Mutation	Codon change	Clinical features	Geographic kindreds
Gly57Arg	GGG–AGG	CTS, heart	Sweden
Leu58His	CTC–CAC	CTS, AN, eye	USA (MD) (FAP II)
Leu58Arg	– CGC	Heart, PN, AN	Japan
Thr59Lys	ACA–AAA	Heart, CTS	Italy, USA (Chinese)
Thr60Ala	ACT–GCT	PN	USA (Appalachian)
Glu61Lys	GAG–AAG	Heart, PN	Japan
Glu61Gly	– GGG	PN, CTS, heart	USA
Phe64Leu	TTT–CTT/TTG	LM, PN, eye	USA, Italy
Phe64Ser	– TCT	Heart	Canada, UK
Ile68Leu	ATA–TTA	Eye, LM	Germany
Tyr69His	TAC–CAC	Heart, CTS, AN	Canada, USA
Tyr69Ile	– ATC[a]	Eye, CTS, PN	Japan
Lys70Asn	AAA–AAC	PN, eye, CTS	USA
Val71Ala	GTG–GCG	PN, AN	France, Spain
Ile73Val	ATA–GTA	Kidney	Bangladesh
Ser77Tyr	TCT–TAT	PN, AN, heart	USA (IL, TX), France
Ser77Phe	– TTT	PN, CTS, skin	France
Tyr78Phe	TAC–TTC	Heart	France
Ala81Thr	GCA–ACA	Heart	USA
Ala81Val	GCA–GTA	Heart, CTS, eye	UK
Ile84Ser	ATC–AGC	Heart, eye	USA (IN), Hungary (FAP II)
Ile84Asn	– AAC	Heart, PN	USA
Ile84Thr	– ACC	Heart	Germany, UK
His88Arg	CAT–CGT	PN, heart	Sweden
Glu89Gln	GAG–CAG	PN, heart	Italy
Glu89Lys	– AAG	Heart	USA
His90Asp	CAT–GAT	PN, CTS, heart	UK
Ala91Ser	GCA–TCA	Heart	France
Glu92Lys	GAG–AAG	Heart, PN, AN, Kidney	Japan
Val94Ala	GTA–GCA	Heart, PN	Germany, USA
Ala97Gly	GCC–GGC	PN, heart	Japan
Ala97Ser	– TCC	Heart, CTS, PN	Taiwan, USA
Ile107Val	ATT–GTT	PN, heart	USA
Ile107Met	– ATG	PN, AN	Germany
Ile107Phe	ATT–TTT	PN, AN	UK
Ala109Ser	GCC–TCC	Heart	Japan
Leu111Met	CTG–ATG	PN, heart	Denmark
Ser112Ile	AGC–ATC	PN, AN, eye, LM	Italy
Tyr114Cys	TAC–TGC	CTS, skin	Japan, USA
Tyy114His	– CAC	PN, CTS, AN	Japan
Tyr116Ser	TAT–TCT	Heart	France
Ala120Ser	GCT–TCT	Heart	Afro- Caribbean
Val122Ile	GTC–ATC	Heart, PN	USA
∆Val122	– ∆∆∆	Heart, eye, PN	USA (Ecuador), Spain
Val122Ala	– GCC	Heart, eye, PN	USA

AN, autonomic neuropathy; CTS, carpal tunnel syndrome; eye, vitreous deposits; LM, leptomeningeal; PN, peripheral neuropathy.

[a] Double nucleotide substitution.

the underlying cause. When the diagnosis is made late in the clinical course of the disease, treatment is either ineffective or impossible due to poor performance status. In a series of 52 North American patients with ATTR, the median time from onset of symptoms to diagnosis for patients presenting with peripheral neuropathy only was 30 months, while those with cardiomyopathy had a median time to diagnosis of 22 months [2]. Thus, the clinician must have a high degree of suspicion for the presence of amyloidosis in evaluating patients with progressive peripheral or autonomic neuropathy, congestive heart failure, nephrotic syndrome, or refractory diarrhea.

The diagnosis of systemic amyloidosis requires a pathologic demonstration of amyloid in some tissue. As with AL, the biopsy method of choice in ATTR is the subcutaneous fat aspirate, which is positive on Congo Red staining in about 75% of patients [2]. In patients with a negative fat aspirate in which a high clinical suspicion of amyloidosis remains, a biopsy of the organ suspected to be involved is indicated. The resulting Congo Red stain should be performed and interpreted at a center with experience in amyloidosis, as false-positive results are common. Thioflavin T staining and electron microscopy are used to confirm amyloid deposits in some cases of cardiac and renal amyloidosis, respectively.

Once the presence of amyloidosis has been confirmed by one of the above methods, care must be taken to identify the amyloid precursor protein correctly. It is not appropriate to rely solely on the presence of a monoclonal protein in the serum or urine to classify patients as having AL, as several studies have shown that a significant number of patients with hereditary amyloidosis have incidental monoclonal gammopathies [3, 4]. As patients with systemic amyloidosis are often quite ill at the time of diagnosis, it is crucial to obtain a definitive diagnosis with a high degree of sensitivity with a rapid turnaround time.

In an effort to identify patients with ATTR, we have been routinely screening the plasma of all newly diagnosed amyloid patients for variant forms of TTR by liquid chromatography-mass spectrometry [5, 6]. This methodology provides a relatively rapid and inexpensive means of detecting a high percentage of variant TTR proteins. Others have shown that screening by isoelectric focusing can also be used to detect circulating variants of TTR [7, 8]. Much like the finding of a monoclonal protein in the serum or urine, the presence of a variant form of TTR in the serum cannot be used as definitive evidence to establish the diagnosis of ATTR, but must be confirmed by direct sequencing of the TTR gene and examination of the amyloid deposits themselves. However, such a finding should prompt the clinician to exclude ATTR from the diagnosis and is recommended for all newly diagnosed systemic amyloidosis patients.

Immunohistochemical staining of the amyloid deposits with a battery of antibodies directed against the proteins known to cause amyloidosis has been the gold standard of identifying the amyloid-forming precursor. The results of immunostaining must be interpreted with caution, however, as most of the proteins implicated in systemic amyloidosis are abundant in the serum, resulting in high background levels [9]. Immunostaining remains highly sensitive for the detection of AA deposits, but equivocal staining for immunoglobulin light chains and TTR is not uncommon [10, 11].

The recent advances in proteomics using mass spectrometry to identify proteins present in minute quantities have led to the use of this technology in identifying amyloid precursor proteins. Chemical typing of amyloid deposits can be accomplished from formalin-fixed, paraffin-embedded biopsy specimens, as well as from subcutaneous fat aspirates [12]. We routinely perform mass spectrometry-based analysis on all positive fat aspirate samples to confirm the identity of the amyloid precursor protein. While this type of analysis is not widely available, it can be performed at our center as well as others on a send-in basis with reasonable turnaround time.

Prognosis

The prognosis of patients with ATTR varies considerably based on the predominant organ involvement. As in AL, amyloid deposition can occur in any organ system, but patients tend to present with symptomatic involvement of a single organ or system. Different TTR variants predispose patients to predominant cardiac, nerve, CNS, and other presentations, but there is considerable variation among individuals with the same mutation (Table 14-1).

Cardiac

Cardiac involvement is not uncommon, with a fourth of patients having evidence of cardiomyopathy at the time of diagnosis [2]. Symptomatic cardiac disease becomes more common as the disease progresses, with nearly two-thirds of all patients ultimately developing appreciable cardiac amyloid. The typical presentation of cardiac involvement in ATTR is congestive heart failure, with no history of ischemia. Deposition of amyloid within the myocardium is not always uniform, but symmetric thickening of the intraventricular septum (IVS) and posterior free wall are typically seen. The electrocardiogram may show low-voltage changes in the limb leads or the pseudoinfarction pattern due to loss of anterior forces.

The echocardiogram is the gold standard for diagnosing cardiac amyloid, with demonstration of concentric ventricular hypertrophy as the classic finding. A granular, sparkling pattern indicative of an infiltrative cardiomyopathy is pathognomonic. More rarely, thickening of the valves occurs. Preservation of systolic function is seen in earlier stages of the disease, when diastolic dysfunction is the predominant finding. The measurement of strain rate by Doppler echocardiography can be useful to detect early systolic dysfunction [13, 14]. Cardiac biomarkers, which have been found to be highly sensitive predictors of outcome in AL, have not been studied extensively in regard to prognosis in ATTR [15]. It appears that the heart is more tolerant of ATTR amyloid deposits than those of AL, as it is not uncommon for ATTR patients to have an IVS thickness in excess of 20 mm at diagnosis with minimal symptoms. Patients with AL are usually symptomatic with much earlier cardiac involvement. This finding is in keeping with a study of troponins and B-natriuretic peptide (BNP) in ATTR patients, in which the BNP correlated significantly with IVS thickness and strain rate abnormalities [16].

Other imaging modalities may be helpful, such as cardiac magnetic resonance imaging (MRI) to detect delayed gadolinium enhancement, which has been found to be informative in three-fourths of patients with cardiac amyloidosis [17]. The use of scintigraphy using 99^{m}Tc-labeled phosphonates has been reported to allow discrimination of cardiac involvement by AL from ATTR, but is not widely used for diagnostic purposes [18]. More commonly, retention of these compounds in the myocardium is incidentally noted on a routine bone scan, leading to the ultimate diagnosis of cardiac involvement by ATTR. Whole body amyloid load can be assessed using radioiodine-labeled SAP scintigraphy, but is not available in the USA [19].

In addition to the purely mechanical effects of amyloid deposition on cardiac function, advanced disease can result in conduction delays. This most commonly presents as asymptomatic bundle-branch block or atrial fibrillation; however, atrioventricular nodal block and even tachyarrhythmias can occur. Sudden death is a common cause of mortality among those with cardiac involvement. Rarely, classical angina symptoms may occur due to extensive vascular deposits, which result in diffuse subendocardial ischemia.

Of particular note in regard to cardiac involvement in ATTR is the V122I mutation found in a high percentage of African-Americans. Estimates of the allele frequency have shown that 3–4% of African-Americans carry the V122I mutation, which may account in part for the increased incidence of cardiovascular mortality in older blacks [20, 21]. Despite the relatively high frequency of the allele, recognition of the disease is poor, and therefore treatment is often inappropriate.

Overall survival in ATTR, as in AL, is directly related to the extent of cardiac involvement. In ATTR patients with symptomatic cardiomyopathy, the median survival is 3.4 years, which is considerably better than the median survival of less than 1 year for AL patients with cardiac involvement [2, 22]. As noted previously, this may reflect a less toxic effect of ATTR amyloid deposits compared to AL deposits. Alternatively, the pace of amyloid deposition may be slower in ATTR than in AL. While cardiac involvement in ATTR is directly related to prognosis, the clinical impact of ATTR deposits is less significant than those in AL patients.

Renal

Involvement of the kidneys is less frequent in ATTR than in AL, with up to one-third of ATTR patients showing evidence of proteinuria at some stage of the disease [23]. Renal deposits can occur in a glomerular, tubular, or vascular pattern, resulting in proteinuria and/or renal insufficiency. As with cardiac disease, the incidence of renal involvement varies between the different known TTR mutations, as well as among individuals with the same mutation. Up to 10% of patients may develop end-stage renal disease and eventually require hemodialysis [23].

A study of Japanese patients with the V30M mutation identified pre-transplant renal amyloid burden, as detected by the amount of affected glomeruli on renal biopsy, and extent of proteinuria as independent predictors of successful outcome with liver transplantation [24]. Progression to end-stage renal failure requiring hemodialysis confers an unfavorable prognosis, with survival rates of 54.5% at 1 year and 38.4% at 2 years [25].

GI

Gastrointestinal symptoms are quite common in ATTR patients, with over 50% exhibiting some form of GI disturbance at diagnosis [26]. The prevalence of GI tract involvement increases with disease duration, ultimately affecting nearly all patients with some mutations [27]. Patients may develop either malabsorption due to submucosal amyloid deposition or dysmotility as a result of autonomic neuropathy. Diarrhea is a common complaint in ATTR, and it can be difficult to differentiate between direct involvement of the GI tract and dumping due to denervation from the history alone. Autonomic dysfunction typically results in alternating diarrhea and constipation. In some cases, endoscopy with full thickness biopsy of the intestinal lumen can often be helpful in establishing the underlying cause. Steatorrhea can result from direct involvement of the GI tract or rapid transit secondary to autonomic dysfunction. Fecal fat measurement is the gold standard for quantifying malabsorption, but measurement of the serum beta-carotene level has been proposed as an easier and reliable alternative [28]. Malnutrition due to GI involvement is a strong predictor of poor outcome, and duration of GI symptoms correlates with survival in some studies [26].

Ocular

Vitreous opacities are common in ATTR, resulting in vision loss and often requiring vitrectomy to restore vision [29]. Increased intraocular pressure with resultant glaucoma can also be seen, requiring more aggressive surgery [30]. More rarely, direct involvement of the ciliary body can cause the scalloped pupil deformity seen in both Japanese and Swedish patients [1]. TTR is synthesized locally in the eye by the pigmented retinal epithelium [31]. As a result, case reports of progressive vitreous amyloidosis following curative liver transplantation have been reported, suggesting that continued local synthesis of variant TTR by the retina can lead to progressive intraocular deposits [32, 33].

Peripheral and Central Nervous System

One of the cardinal clinical features of ATTR is a progressive length-dependent, axonal sensorimotor neuropathy, seen in up to 90% of patients with ATTR [2]. Nearly half of the patients will develop bilateral carpal tunnel syndrome. The initial reports of ATTR by Andrade emphasized the peripheral neuropathy associated with the V30M mutation in Portuguese patients [34]. This predominant peripheral nerve involvement led to the use of the term familial amyloidotic polyneuropathy (FAP) to describe the clinical disease. Several distinct patterns of peripheral nerve involvement were characterized, with some patients exhibiting initial symptoms in the lower limbs. A second pattern was seen in the Indiana-Swiss form of the disease, with predominant upper limb symptoms [35]. This form was subsequently called type II FAP, to distinguish it from the earlier reported form of the disease, which became known as type I FAP. Eventually, with a growing number of cases identified without significant neuropathy and a change in the nomenclature of systemic amyloidosis to reflect the precursor protein, the term ATTR was proposed to replace FAP [36].

Considerable variability in the onset and pace of progression of peripheral neuropathy has been noted since the original descriptions of the disease. Portuguese patients tend to develop symptomatic disease in their twenties and thirties and show rapid progression of the disease with death resulting in 7–10 years, while Swedish patients with the same V30M mutation are frequently asymptomatic until the sixth or seventh decade [37]. Japanese patients with the V30M mutation can develop either early-onset or late-onset symptoms, with a milder disease course seen in older patients [38, 39]. While genetic and environmental effects have been postulated to explain this difference in phenotype, no specific factors have been identified.

Autonomic dysfunction can proceed peripheral nerve involvement in many cases, resulting in orthostatic hypotension, gastrointestinal dysmotility, sexual impotence, dyshidrosis, and urinary retention. In some cases, evidence of autonomic neuropathy can be clearly detected before other neurologic features are evident [40]. In severe cases of gastrointestinal involvement, pseudo-obstruction can occur with resulting intractable nausea, vomiting, and malnutrition.

More recent case reports have demonstrated direct involvement of the central nervous system (CNS) in some cases of ATTR [41–44]. Amyloid deposition in the leptomeninges has been shown in patients with cerebral infarction, hemorrhage, ataxia, seizures, and even dementia. Interestingly, TTR has also been implicated in the localized amyloid plaques characteristic of Alzheimer's disease, but no evidence of deposition within the brain parenchyma has been demonstrated in these patients [45, 46]. The mechanism by which the amyloid deposits lead to the above clinical symptoms is unclear, but it appears that local expression of variant TTR by the choroid plexus, rather than circulating plasma protein, contributes directly to the amyloid deposits in these cases [47]. This theory is supported by evidence of new leptomeningeal amyloidosis in patients following orthotopic liver transplantation, as only variant TTR produced by the choroid plexus could produce such deposits [32].

Overall Prognosis

Given the wide variation in clinical presentation in individual patients with ATTR, even those with the same underlying variant, it is difficult to predict overall survival at diagnosis. As a group, patients with ATTR tend to fare better than those with AL. The median survival in ATTR is between 5 and 15 years, compared to a median of only 20 months for AL [2, 22]. As in AL, the site of predominant organ involvement is crucial in determining survival. The presence of symptomatic cardiomyopathy in ATTR patients is associated with a median survival of only 3.4 years, compared to less than 1 year for AL patients with heart failure due to amyloid. This discrepancy suggests that the rate of amyloid deposition and/or toxic effects of the deposits themselves are different in the two diseases. Other factors that have been identified as prognostic are age at diagnosis, male sex, and the presence of peripheral or autonomic neuropathy. Death in ATTR can result from progressive cardiac impairment, leading to sudden death in some cases. Inanition due to progressive neuropathy has also been reported. End-stage renal disease is a significant cause of mortality in some kindreds [25].

Treatment of ATTR

No specific therapy currently exists to remove existing amyloid deposits of any source. Therefore treatment for all types of amyloid involves removing or reducing the supply of the precursor protein. In the case of ATTR, the liver is primarily responsible for the production of circulating TTR. As a result, orthotopic liver transplantation (OLT) has been used as potentially curative therapy beginning in 1990 in Sweden [48]. The excellent surgical outcome and reported symptomatic improvement in the original patients have led to widespread acceptance of the procedure. The Familial Amyloidotic Polyneuropathy World Transplant Registry (FAPWTR) reports over 1,450 transplants performed in 17 countries as of June 2008 [49].

Surgical outcomes are generally excellent, as ATTR patients are not in liver failure at the time of transplant, reducing the perioperative mortality and morbidity. Overall survival is also good with 77% alive at 5 years [50]. Death is primarily due to cardiac causes and sepsis. Factors prognostic of a better outcome are modified body mass index (mBMI) $\geq$ 600, disease duration $\leq$ 7 years, and V30M mutation (versus non V30M) [50]. Others have shown the presence of severe neuropathy or autonomic symptoms at the time of transplant confer a worse prognosis [51].

One of the main benefits of OLT in ATTR is a subjective improvement in neurologic symptoms. According to the latest FAPWTR report, 42% of patients reported improvement in their neurologic symptoms [50]. Motor deficits were noted to improve in 37%. In a report from Japan, seven of eight patients experienced an improvement in neurologic symptoms with associated improvement in EMG findings following OLT [52]. Similar improvement was noted in a more heterogeneous cohort of nine FAP patients in the USA, with all showing an improvement in symptomatic, autonomic, and sensorimotor neuropathy following OLT [53]. Other studies have failed to demonstrate such a benefit. In a report on 25 French FAP patients that underwent OLT, no improvement was noted in any patient and 40% showed progression of their neurologic deficit following OLT [51]. Similarly, stable peripheral neuropathy with no objective improvement has been reported from the UK [54]. Our experience has been similar, with only 35% of patients undergoing OLT showing stable or improved peripheral neuropathy [55]. It has been argued that the lack of improvement seen in the latter series may be associated with a longer duration of disease, more severe neurologic deficits at the time of transplant, and/or the presence of patients with a non-V30M mutation. In any case, it appears that OLT can be beneficial in halting the progression of peripheral neuropathy in some patients.

A second reported benefit of OLT is an improvement in nutritional status. In a long-term follow-up of the first 20 Swedish patients to undergo OLT, the nutritional status improved in a majority of patients [56]. Similarly, BMI improved in five of six (83%) patients with pre-operative evidence of malnutrition in a series from Boston University [57]. This has been attributed in large part to improved gastrointestinal motility. In fact, autonomic symptoms were among the first signs of improvement following OLT in some cases.

The benefit of OLT for patients with significant cardiac involvement is less clear. Cardiac complications are a significant cause of mortality following OLT [50, 57]. Early reports suggested stable or improved cardiac status following OLT, but subsequent studies have shown that progression of cardiac involvement based on echocardiographic findings is not uncommon [55, 57–59]. Conduction defects have also been demonstrated to worsen following OLT, even leading to potentially fatal arrhythmias [60]. Progressive cardiac disease can occur in patients with no known pre-operative cardiac involvement and is not limited to specific TTR mutations.

Of greater concern is the more recent suggestion of a paradoxical increase in the rate of amyloid deposition in the myocardium following OLT [59]. The rationale for the use of OLT in FAP assumes that removal of the circulating amyloid precursor should halt the formation of additional amyloid deposits. Analysis of the composition of amyloid deposits from patients noted to have progressive disease after OLT has shown that the proportion of wild-type TTR increases after transplant [61, 62]. Thus, it appears that pre-existing amyloid fibrils can induce the formation of rapidly progressive deposits composed primarily of wild-type TTR after OLT.

A similar situation occurs in the eye, in which progressive vitreous deposits have been documented in patients following OLT [33]. Presumably localized production of variant TTR by the pigmented retinal epithelium is responsible in this scenario, as opposed to circulating wild-type TTR as seen in the heart. More disturbingly, progressive amyloid deposits in the leptomeninges after OLT have also been shown to result in fatal intracranial hemorrhage, presumably due to de novo deposition of variant TTR produced by the choroid plexus [63, 64]. The concern of unmasking silent leptomeningeal deposits or accelerating clinically insignificant cardiac deposition with potentially fatal consequences has resulted in confusion regarding the utility of OLT in ATTR patients, particularly those with non-V30M variants. Further longitudinal studies must be performed to document and quantify the risks and benefits of liver transplantation in these patients.

Of interest, since the synthetic function of the liver is intact in patients with ATTR, the explanted liver can be transplanted into another individual through a procedure known as a domino transplant [65–67]. The result is a net increase in the number of available organs. It is assumed that the long latency before symptoms develop in ATTR patients will reduce the risk of symptomatic amyloid developing in recipients of the variant-producing liver. The FAPWTR reports that a total of 655 domino transplants have been performed in 17 countries as of June 2008 [49]. Recipients most often had end-stage liver disease secondary to malignancy or viral hepatitis. Tumor recurrence is the leading cause of mortality among domino recipients. The first reports of amyloid deposits in the peripheral nervous system and gastric mucosa in recipients of ATTR livers have now appeared [68, 69]. At least one of these cases has necessitated a second liver transplant [68].

In areas where ATTR is endemic, such as Sweden, Portugal, and Japan, it is possible to recognize affected individuals at a point in the disease at which a liver transplantation is apparently beneficial. Unfortunately, patients in most other countries may have a prolonged period of symptoms before the underlying disease is correctly identified. As a result, many patients are either too old or have advanced symptoms at the time of diagnosis and are therefore not considered candidates for such an aggressive surgical approach. This has prompted the search for alternative forms of treatment.

It was initially noted in some Portuguese V30M patients that a more benign clinical course occurred when a second mutation, T119M, was present [70]. The T119M variant was not found in patients with ATTR by itself, suggesting it was a non-amyloidogenic polymorphism. Further studies showed that hybrid TTR tetramers containing both the T119M and the V30M variants had a reduced amyloid-forming potential compared to those composed solely of V30M [71]. The reduced amyloidogenic potential was attributed to an increase in the stability of the tetramer when both variants were present, thereby resulting in a decrease in the availability of the V30M monomer.

Additional studies showed that small molecules could bind to the TTR tetramer and confer a similar increase in stability [72]. One of the compounds shown to have a stabilizing effect is the non-steroidal anti-inflammatory diflunisal. While not the most potent in terms of stabilization, the safety profile of diflunisal makes it an ideal choice for use in clinical trials in humans. Orally administered diflunisal has been shown to provide sufficient serum levels to stabilize TTR tetramers and prevent dissociation [73]. These findings have prompted a randomized, placebo-controlled, double-blind international phase III clinical trial evaluating the efficacy of diflunisal in ATTR patients with neuropathy as the major endpoint. An even more potent stabilizer of the TTR tetramer has been designed and is currently being tested in patients with ATTR in a phase II/III clinical trial [74]. The results of these trials are eagerly awaited as proof of the concept that stabilization of the TTR tetramer will slow or halt the development of amyloid deposits and result in clinical benefit.

Alternative approaches have sought to block production of TTR altogether, based on the finding that mice in which the TTR gene was knocked out show no phenotypic effects attributable to the loss of the TTR protein [75]. The use of antisense oligonucleotides in mice transgenic for the I84S human TTR gene has shown the feasibility of using this approach to suppress TTR expression for substantial periods [76]. Others have shown that ribozymes can be used to similarly suppress TTR synthesis [77]. Gene therapy via targeted conversion of the mutant allele has also been reported to be possible both in vitro and in vivo [78]. Doxycycline has been shown to disrupt existing TTR amyloid fibrils in vitro [79]. When tested in vivo in a mouse model of ATTR, administration of doxycycline to transgenic mice resulted in a lack of congophilic amyloid deposits. These approaches hold promise for the development of effective therapy for patients unable to undergo liver transplantation. In summary, ATTR remains a devastating disease despite the significant gains in understanding the pathogenesis of the disease. However, for the first time since the advent of liver transplantation nearly 20 years ago, there is new hope for patients that effective treatment may soon be available.

References

1. Benson MD, Kincaid JC. The molecular biology and clinical features of amyloid neuropathy. Muscle Nerve. 2007;36(4):411–23.
2. Gertz MA, Kyle RA, Thibodeau SN. Familial amyloidosis: a study of 52 North American-born patients examined during a 30-year period. Mayo Clin Proc. 1992;67(5): 428–40.
3. Comenzo RL, et al. Seeking confidence in the diagnosis of systemic AL (Ig light-chain) amyloidosis: patients can have both monoclonal gammopathies and hereditary amyloid proteins[see comment]. Blood. 2006;107(9):3489–91.
4. Lachmann HJ, et al. Misdiagnosis of hereditary amyloidosis as AL (primary) amyloidosis[see comment]. N Engl J Med. 2002;346(23):1786–91.
5. Bergen HR 3rd, et al. Identification of transthyretin variants by sequential proteomic and genomic analysis [see comment]. Clin Chem. 2004;50(9):1544–52.
6. Nepomuceno AI, et al. Detection of genetic variants of transthyretin by liquid chromatography-dual electrospray ionization fourier-transform ion-cyclotron-resonance mass spectrometry [see comment]. Clin Chem. 2004;50(9):1535–43.
7. Altland K, et al. Genetic microheterogeneity of human transthyretin detected by IEF. Electrophoresis. 2007;28(12):2053–64.
8. Rosenzweig M, et al. A new transthyretin variant (Glu61Gly) associated with cardiomyopathy. Amyloid. 2007;14(1):65–71.
9. Picken MM, Herrera GA. The burden of "sticky" amyloid: typing challenges [see comment]. Arch Pathol Lab Med. 2007;131(6):850–1.
10. Kebbel A, Rocken C. Immunohistochemical classification of amyloid in surgical pathology revisited. Am J Surg Pathol. 2006;30(6):673–83.
11. Satoskar AA, et al. Typing of amyloidosis in renal biopsies: diagnostic pitfalls.[see comment]. Arch Pathol Lab Med. 2007;131(6):917–22.
12. Murphy CL, et al. Characterization of systemic amyloid deposits by mass spectrometry. Methods Enzymol. 2006;412:48–62.
13. Bellavia D, et al. Evidence of impaired left ventricular systolic function by Doppler myocardial imaging in patients with systemic amyloidosis and no evidence of cardiac involvement by standard two-dimensional and Doppler echocardiography. Am J Cardiol. 2008;101(7):1039–45.
14. Bellavia D, et al. Detection of left ventricular systolic dysfunction in cardiac amyloidosis with strain rate echocardiography. J Am Soc Echocardiogr. 2007;20(10):1194–202.
15. Dispenzieri A, et al. Serum cardiac troponins and N-terminal pro-brain natriuretic peptide: a staging system for primary systemic amyloidosis. J Clin Oncol. 2004;22(18):3751–7.
16. Suhr OB, et al. Do troponin and B-natriuretic peptide detect cardiomyopathy in transthyretin amyloidosis? J Intern Med. 2008;263(3):294–301.
17. Perugini E, et al. Non-invasive evaluation of the myocardial substrate of cardiac amyloidosis by gadolinium cardiac magnetic resonance. Heart. 2006;92(3):343–9.
18. Perugini E, et al. Noninvasive etiologic diagnosis of cardiac amyloidosis using 99mTc-3,3-diphosphono-1,2-propanoldicarboxylic acid scintigraphy. J Am Coll Cardiol. 2005;46(6):1076–84.
19. Hazenberg BPC, et al. Diagnostic performance of 123I-labeled serum amyloid P component scintigraphy in patients with amyloidosis. Am J Med. 2006;119(4):355.e15–24.
20. Afolabi I, et al. Transthyretin isoleucine-122 mutation in African and American blacks. Amyloid. 2000;7(2):121–25.
21. Jacobson DR, et al. Variant-sequence transthyretin (isoleucine 122) in late-onset cardiac amyloidosis in black Americans.[see comment]. N Engl J Med. 1997;336(7):466–73.
22. Ando Y, Nakamura M, Araki S. Transthyretin-related familial amyloidotic polyneuropathy. Arch Neurol. 2005;62(7):1057–62.
23. Lobato L. Portuguese-type amyloidosis (transthyretin amyloidosis, ATTR V30M). J Nephrol. 2003;16(3):438–42.
24. Oguchi K, Takei Y-I, Ikeda S-I. Value of renal biopsy in the prognosis of liver transplantation in familial amyloid polyneuropathy ATTR Val30Met patients. Amyloid. 2006;13(2):99–107.

25. Lobato L, et al. End-stage renal disease and dialysis in hereditary amyloidosis TTR V30M: presentation, survival and prognostic factors. Amyloid. 2004;11(1):27–37.

26. Tashima K, et al. Gastrointestinal dysfunction in familial amyloidotic polyneuropathy (ATTR Val30Met)–comparison of Swedish and Japanese patients. Amyloid. 1999;6(2):124–9.

27. Steen L, Ek B. Familial amyloidosis with polyneuropathy. A long-term follow-up of 21 patients with special reference to gastrointestinal symptoms. Acta Medica Scandinavica. 1983;214(5):387–97.

28. Galvan-Guerra E, et al. Diagnostic utility of serum beta-carotenes in intestinal malabsorption syndrome. Revista de Investigacion Clinica. 1994;46(2):99–104.

29. Falls HF, et al. Ocular manifestations of hereditary primary systemic amyloidosis. AMA. Arch Ophthalmol. 1955;54(5):660–64.

30. Tsukahara S, Matsuo T. Secondary glaucoma accompanied with primary familial amyloidosis. Ophthalmologica. 1977;175(5):250–62.

31. Ong DE, et al. Synthesis and secretion of retinol-binding protein and transthyretin by cultured retinal pigment epithelium. Biochemistry. 1994;33(7):1835–42.

32. Ando Y, et al. A different amyloid formation mechanism: de novo oculoleptomeningeal amyloid deposits after liver transplantation. Transplantation. 2004;77(3):345–49.

33. Munar-Ques M, et al. Vitreous amyloidosis after liver transplantation in patients with familial amyloid polyneuropathy: ocular synthesis of mutant transthyretin. Amyloid. 2000;7(4):266–9.

34. Andrade C. A peculiar form of peripheral neuropathy; familiar atypical generalized amyloidosis with special involvement of the peripheral nerves. Brain. 1952;75(3):408–27.

35. Block WD, Curtis AC, Rukavina JG. Familial primary systemic amyloidosis: an experimental, genetic and clinical study. J Invest Dermatol. 1956;27(3):111–31.

36. Husby G. Nomenclature and classification of amyloid and amyloidoses. J Intern Med. 1992;232(6):511–2.

37. Andersson R. Hereditary amyloidosis with polyneuropathy. Acta Medica Scandinavica. 1970;1–2(1):85–94.

38. Misu KI, et al. Late-onset familial amyloid polyneuropathy type I (transthyretin Met30-associated familial amyloid polyneuropathy) unrelated to endemic focus in Japan. Clinicopathological and genetic features. Brain. 1999;122(Pt 10):1951–62.

39. Sobue G, et al. Clinicopathologic and genetic features of early- and late-onset FAP type I (FAP ATTR Val30Met) in Japan. Amyloid. 2003;10(Suppl 1):32–8.

40. Ducla-Soares J, et al. Correlation between clinical, electromyographic and dysautonomic evolution of familial amyloidotic polyneuropathy of the Portuguese type. Acta Neurol Scand. 1994;90(4):266–9.

41. Ellie E, et al. Recurrent subarachnoid hemorrhage associated with a new transthyretin variant (Gly53Glu). Neurology. 2001;57(1):135–37.

42. Goren H, Steinberg MC, Farboody GH. Familial oculoleptomeningeal amyloidosis. Brain. 1980;103(3):473–95.

43. Petersen RB, et al. Transthyretin amyloidosis: a new mutation associated with dementia. Ann Neurol. 1997;41(3):307–13.

44. Ushiyama M, Ikeda S, Yanagisawa N. Transthyretin-type cerebral amyloid angiopathy in type I familial amyloid polyneuropathy. Acta Neuropathol. 1991;81(5):524–8.

45. Riisoen H. Reduced prealbumin (transthyretin) in CSF of severely demented patients with Alzheimer's disease. Acta Neurol Scand. 1988;78(6):455–9.

46. Serot JM, et al. Cerebrospinal fluid transthyretin: aging and late onset Alzheimer's disease. J Neurol Neurosurg Psychiatr. 1997;63(4):506–8.

47. Hammarstrom P, et al. D18G transthyretin is monomeric, aggregation prone, and not detectable in plasma and cerebrospinal fluid: a prescription for central nervous system amyloidosis? Biochemistry. 2003;42(22):6656–63.

48. Holmgren G, et al. Biochemical effect of liver transplantation in two Swedish patients with familial amyloidotic polyneuropathy (FAP-met30). Clinical Genetics. 1991;40(3):242–6.

49. Results from the Familial World Transplant Registry. Available from: http://www.fapwtr.org/ram_fap.htm. Accessed 30 June 2008 [cited 2009 June 1]

50. Herlenius G, et al. Ten years of international experience with liver transplantation for familial amyloidotic polyneuropathy: results from the Familial Amyloidotic Polyneuropathy World Transplant Registry. Transplantation. 2004;77(1):64–71.

51. Adams D, et al. The course and prognostic factors of familial amyloid polyneuropathy after liver transplantation. Brain. 2000;123(Pt 7):1495–504.

52. Shimojima Y, et al. Ten-year follow-up of peripheral nerve function in patients with familial amyloid polyneuropathy after liver transplantation. J Neurol. 2008;255(8):1220–5.

53. Bergethon PR, et al. Improvement in the polyneuropathy associated with familial amyloid polyneuropathy after liver transplantation. Neurology. 1996;47(4):944–51.

54. Stangou AJ, Hawkins PN. Liver transplantation in transthyretin-related familial amyloid polyneuropathy. Curr Opin Neurol. 2004;17(5):615–20.

55. Sharma P, et al. Outcome of liver transplantation for familial amyloidotic polyneuropathy. Liver Transpl. 2003;9(12):1273–80.

56. Suhr OB, et al. Liver transplantation in familial amyloidotic polyneuropathy. Follow-up of the first 20 Swedish patients. Transplantation. 1995;60(9):933–38.

57. Pomfret EA, et al. Effect of orthotopic liver transplantation on the progression of familial amyloidotic polyneuropathy. Transplantation. 1998;65(7):918–25.

58. Olofsson B-O, et al. Progression of cardiomyopathy after liver transplantation in patients with familial amyloidotic polyneuropathy, Portuguese type. Transplantation. 2002;73(5):745–51.

59. Stangou AJ, et al. Progressive cardiac amyloidosis following liver transplantation for familial amyloid polyneuropathy: implications for amyloid fibrillogenesis. Transplantation. 1998;66(2):229–33.

60. Hornsten R, et al. Liver transplantation does not prevent the development of life-threatening arrhythmia in familial amyloidotic polyneuropathy, Portuguese-type (ATTR Val30Met) patients. Transplantation. 2004;78(1):112–16.

61. Liepnieks JJ, Benson MD. Progression of cardiac amyloid deposition in hereditary transthyretin amyloidosis patients after liver transplantation. Amyloid. 2007;14(4):277–82.

62. Yazaki M, et al. Progressive wild-type transthyretin deposition after liver transplantation preferentially occurs onto myocardium in FAP patients. Am J Transplant. 2007;7(1):235–42.

63. De Carolis P, et al. Fatal cerebral haemorrhage after liver transplantation in a patient with transthyretin variant (gly53glu) amyloidosis. Neurol Sci. 2006;27(5):352–4.

64. Mascalchi M, et al. Transthyretin amyloidosis and superficial siderosis of the CNS. Neurology. 1999;53(7):1498–503.

65. Azoulay D, et al. Domino liver transplants for metabolic disorders: experience with familial amyloidotic polyneuropathy. J Am Coll Surg. 1999;189(6):584–93.

66. Furtado A, et al. Sequential liver transplantation. Transplant Proc. 1997;29(1–2):467–8.

67. Schmidt HH, et al. Familial Amyloidotic Polyneuropathy: domino liver transplantation. J Hepatol. 1999;30(2):293–8.

68. Stangou AJ, Heaton ND, Hawkins PN. Transmission of systemic transthyretin amyloidosis by means of domino liver transplantation. N Engl J Med. 2005;352(22):2356.

69. Takei Y-I, et al. Transthyretin-derived amyloid deposition on the gastric mucosa in domino recipients of familial amyloid polyneuropathy liver.[see comment]. Liver Transpl. 2007;13(2):215–18.

70. Coelho T, et al. A strikingly benign evolution of FAP in an individual compound heterozygote for two TTR mutations: TTR Met30 and TTR Met119. J Rheumatol. 1993;20:179.

71. Hammarstrom P, Schneider F, Kelly JW. Trans-suppression of misfolding in an amyloid disease. Science. 2001;293(5539):2459–62.

72. Hammarstrom P, et al. Prevention of transthyretin amyloid disease by changing protein misfolding energetics. Science. 2003;299(5607):713–6.

73. Sekijima Y, Dendle MA, Kelly JW. Orally administered diflunisal stabilizes transthyretin against dissociation required for amyloidogenesis. Amyloid. 2006;13(4):236–49.

74. Waddington-Cruz M, et al. A landmark clinical trial of a novel small molecule transthyretin (TTR) stabiliser, Fx-1006A, in patients with TTR amyloid polyneuropathy: a phase II/III, randomised, double-blind, placebo-controlled study. J Neurol. 2008;255(Suppl 2):107.

75. Wolf G. Retinol transport and metabolism in transthyretin-"knockout" mice. Nutr Rev. 1995;53(4 Pt 1):98–9.

76. Benson MD, et al. Targeted suppression of an amyloidogenic transthyretin with antisense oligonucleotides. Muscle Nerve. 2006;33(5):609–18.

77. Tanaka K, et al. Suppression of transthyretin expression by ribozymes: a possible therapy for familial amyloidotic polyneuropathy. J Neurol Sci. 2001;183(1):79–84.

78. Nakamura M, et al. Targeted conversion of the transthyretin gene in vitro and in vivo. Gene Therpy. 2004;11(10):838–46.

79. Cardoso I, Merlini G, Saraiva MJ. 4′-iodo-4′-deoxydoxorubicin and tetracyclines disrupt transthyretin amyloid fibrils in vitro producing noncytotoxic species: screening for TTR fibril disrupters. FASEB J. 2003;17(8):803–09.

Chapter 15

Other Systemic Forms of Amyloidosis

Merrill D. Benson

Abstract While the transthyretin amyloidoses are the most common form of hereditary amyloidosis, mutations in a number of other proteins are associated with systemic amyloidosis. Some give clinical features similar to TTR amyloidosis but others have unique phenotypes. Proteins that we now know cause familial forms of systemic amyloidosis include apolipoprotein-AI (ApoAI), fibrinogen Aα-chain, lysozyme, apolipoprotein-AII (ApoAII), gelsolin, and cystatin C. The diseases associated with these proteins are all inherited in an autosomal dominant Mendelian fashion with varying degrees of penetrance. In addition, the newly characterized systemic amyloidosis associated with leukocyte chemotactic factor 2 (LECT 2) is also included in the non-TTR forms of systemic amyloidosis, although no inheritance pattern has been noted. Several of these mutant proteins (fibrinogen, lysozyme, apolipoprotein-AI, apolipoprotein-AII) are characterized particularly by renal failure. Gelsolin has a unique phenotype of lattice corneal dystrophy, cranial nerve palsy, and cutis laxa. Cystatin C amyloidosis is characterized by cerebral vascular angiopathy and death from intracranial hemorrhage. While the numbers of patients with these various forms of amyloidosis are unknown they must be considered when evaluating any patient suspected of having familial amyloidosis.

Keywords Fibrinogen, Lysozyme, Apolipoprotein-AI, Apolipoprotein-AII, Gelsolin, Cystatin C, LECT 2

A number of human proteins can participate in amyloid fibril formation and produce systemic amyloidosis. While immunoglobulin light chain (AL) is the most common and amyloid A (AA) the longest recognized, the proteins that cause familial forms of systemic amyloidosis have a fascination of their own. Similar to Ig light chains and SAA, these proteins that give systemic amyloidosis are plasma proteins, unlike proteins that are associated with only localized deposition of amyloid fibrils [islet amyloid polypeptide (IAPP), procalcitonin, semenogelin I, keratoepithelin, atrial natriuretic factor (ANF), Aβ-protein precursor (AβPP)]. Unlike Ig light chains and SAA the plasma amyloid precursor proteins in general do not cause amyloidosis as a result of overproduction, but instead, most are mutant forms of their naturally occurring counterpart. While most familial amyloidosis patients are heterozygous for a causative mutant protein, only in transthyretin (TTR) amyloidosis are both the variant and the normal versions of the precursor protein found in the amyloid fibrils. Since TTR amyloidosis is discussed elsewhere (Chapter 14) we leave the reasoning for that phenomenon to others. The forms of systemic amyloidosis to be considered here are listed in Table 15-1. All are familial forms of amyloidosis with autosomal

From: *Amyloidosis*, Contemporary Hematology,
Edited by: M.A. Gertz and S.V. Rajkumar, DOI 10.1007/978-1-60761-631-3_15,
© Springer Science+Business Media, LLC 2010

Table 15-1. Other systemic forms of amyloidosis.

Type of amyloid	First clinical description	First characterized biochemically	Where first discovered
ApoAI	1969 [1]	1988 [2]	United States
Fibrinogen Aα-chain	1975 [27]	1993 [22]	United States
Lysozyme	1982 [39]	1993 [37]	United Kingdom
ApoAII	1973 [44]	2001 [46]	United States
Gelsolin	1969 [52]	1990 [53, 54]	Finland
Cystatin C	1972 [61]	1986 [62]	Iceland
LECT2	2008 [64]	2008 [64]	United States

dominant inheritance except for leukocyte chemotactic factor 2 (LECT 2) which is the most recent to be characterized, and there are insufficient data to speculate on the mechanism of pathogenesis.

Before we start a few words on pathogenesis...

Like TTR amyloidosis the other forms of familial amyloidosis are caused by mutations in the fibril precursor protein. Unlike TTR there is no evidence for incorporation of the normal allele product into the fibril, and most of the proteins are partially proteolyzed to give the fibril subunit. This suggests that metabolic processing of the precursor protein is a required step in the pathway to β configuration and fibril formation. In apolipoprotein-AII (ApoAII), reduction of a disulfide bond present in the plasma dimeric protein is required since only the variant allele product is incorporated into the amyloid fibrils. Certainly this is not a post-fibril formation event. In apolipoprotein-AI (ApoAI) amyloidosis caused by amino acid substitutions in the C-terminal region of the protein, the amyloid fibrils contain only the N-terminal approximately 93 amino acid residues. It has not been determined whether the amyloid fibril subunit is all from the variant precursor protein, but this does suggest that the causative mutation, which is remote from the fibril product, exerts its effect somewhere in the cellular degradative machinery. Also in favor of an important role for proteolytic processing in amyloid formation is the fact that many of the amyloid proteins, unlike Ig light chains and TTR, do not have significant β-structure in their native state. In fact ApoAI and ApoAII are more like SAA which has amphipathic structure and is part of HDL. Only lysozyme has been shown to have significant β-structure.

Table 15-1 lists the types of systemic amyloidoses that are discussed in this chapter. When possible the year of the first clinical description of each type, which has subsequently been verified by biochemical analysis, and the first year of the biochemical verification are noted. Otherwise the order of tabulation is at the author's discretion. Apolipoprotein-AI (ApoAI) which has the greatest number of recognized amyloidogenic mutations and fibrinogen Aα-chain amyloidosis are the most prevalent of these types of hereditary amyloidosis and deserve a working knowledge by the practicing internist. Lysozyme and apolipoprotein-AII (ApoAII) amyloidoses are relatively uncommon and are usually considered only when the more common forms have been excluded. Gelsolin and cystatin C amyloidoses are mostly restricted to their countries of origin (gelsolin in Finland; cystatin C in Iceland). While affected individuals and/or families may be seen in other countries, a high degree of penetrance makes family history a significant factor in bringing this diagnosis to attention. Leukocyte chemotactic factor 2 (LECT2) is only recently discovered and, while a systemic disease, a genetic predisposition has not been determined.

Apolipoprotein-AI (ApoAI) Amyloidosis

The first clinical description of ApoAI amyloidosis which was subsequently veri-fied by biochemical analysis was by Van Allen et al. in 1969 [1]. A family with ApoAI amyloidosis came to attention because of peripheral neuropathy, although most affected members died from renal insufficiency. It was not until 1988 that tissue became available for isolation of amyloid fibrils. Characterization of the amyloid fib-ril protein revealed that it contained an amino terminal portion of apolipoprotein-AI with a substitution of arginine for glycine at position 26 from the amino terminus [2]. Since that time, 14 other mutations in ApoAI associated with systemic amyloido-sis have been described. Table 15-2 lists these mutations and the clinical features of the various syndromes that they cause. While most of the ApoAI amyloidoses show typical autosomal dominant inheritance, inheritability has not been verified for all of them. The ApoAI amyloidoses show considerable degree of clinical variation. Muta-tions within the amino terminal 75 amino acid sequence usually cause nephropathy with interstitial and medullary renal amyloid deposition. In some instances hepatic amyloid may be a more prominent feature. Only the Gly26Arg mutation has been shown to be associated with peripheral neuropathy. An interesting observation is the difference between the clinical manifestations of ApoAI mutations in the amino ter-minal compared to the carboxyl terminal portion of the molecule. Mutations in the first 75 amino acid portion of ApoAI cause renal, hepatic, and occasionally cardiac amyloid deposition. Mutations in the carboxyl terminal portion of the protein from residue 90 and including residues 170–178 cause dermal and laryngeal amyloid depo-sition and patients die with amyloid cardiomyopathy. In all types of ApoAI, however, it is the amino terminal 80–96 amino acid residues that are found in the amyloid fibrils.

Gly26Arg: This first amyloid-associated mutation in ApoAI was discovered in the Midwestern United States [1]. The original report gives an in-depth clinical descrip-tion of the manifestations of the systemic disease and deserves review. Subsequent reports of amyloid-associated ApoAI mutations have concentrated on the biochemical and molecular biology aspects of the disease and have been relatively short on clinical description. While renal failure was the major cause of death peripheral neuropathy was the uniform factor that brought the Iowa kindred to medical attention. Clinically, the neuropathy is similar to that described for TTR amyloidosis beginning in the lower extremities with shooting pains, dysesthesias, and weakness. The neuropathy is steadily progressive and subsequently involves the upper extremities. In severe cases muscle atrophy and diminished stretch reflexes are noted. The average age of onset of disease in the original report was 35 years and the average life span after onset was 16 years. Amyloid deposition in surgical biopsies was demonstrated in liver, stomach, testis, duodenum, and vagus nerve. At autopsy, generalized amyloid deposition with significant deposits in spleen, liver, adrenals, meninges, choroid plexus, nerve trunks, and ganglia was found. In particular, large deposits were found in testis and kidneys. The renal amyloid was described as mainly interstitial with little glomerular involve-ment, and this has been the finding with other forms of ApoAI amyloidosis where nephrotic syndrome, or even significant proteinuria, is rare. Another observation in this family was elevation of cerebral spinal fluid protein concentration, a finding that has not been appreciated or investigated with other families. A high incidence of gastric ulcer disease was found in members of this family, but its relationship to the amyloid syndrome is still not known. This has not been a reported finding with other families with ApoAI amyloidosis, even those with the Gly26Arg variety. One clinical

Table 15-2. Mutant proteins other than transthyretin associated with autosomal dominant systemic amyloidosis.

Protein	cDNA change[a]	Amino acid change[b]	Codon change	Clinical features	Geographic kindreds
Apolipoprotein-AI	148G→C	Gly26Arg	GGC26CGC	PN[c], nephropathy	United States
	251T→G	Leu60Arg	CTG60CGG	Nephropathy	United Kingdom
	220T→C	Trp50Arg	TGG50CGG	Nephropathy	United Kingdom
	del250-284insGTCAC	del60-71insVal/Thr	del60-71ins GTCAC	Hepatic	Spain
	263T→C	Leu64Pro	CTC64CCC	Nephropathy	United States
	del1280-288	del70-72	del70-72	Nephropathy	South Africa
	294insA(fs)[d]	Asn74Lys(fs)[d]	AAC74AAAC(fs)[d]	Nephropathy	Germany
	296T→C	Leu75Pro	CTG75CCG	Hepatic	Italy, United States
	341T→C	Leu90Pro	CTG90CCG	Cardiomyopathy, cutaneous, laryngeal	France
	532insGC(fs)[d]	Ala154(fs)[d]	GCC154GGC(fs)[d]	Nephropathy	Germany
	581T→C	Leu170Pro	CTG170CCG	Laryngeal	Germany
	590G→C	Arg173Pro	CGC173CCC	Cardiomyopathy, cutaneous, laryngeal	United States
	593T→C	Leu174Ser	TTG174TCG	Cardiomyopathy	Italy
	595G→C	Ala175Pro	GCX175CCX[e]	Laryngeal	United Kingdom
	604T→A	Leu178His	TTG178CAT	Cardiomyopathy, laryngeal	France
Gelsolin	640G→A	Asp187Asn	GAC187AAC	PN[c], lattice corneal dystrophy	Finland, United States, Japan
	640G→T	Asp187Tyr	GAC187TAC	PN[c]	Denmark, Czech

Table 15-2. (continued)

Protein	cDNA change[a]	Amino acid change[b]	Codon change	Clinical features	Geographic kindreds
Cystatin C	280T→A	Leu68Gln	CTG68CAG	Cerebral hemorrhage	Iceland
Fibrinogen A	1718G→T	Arg554Leu	CGT554CTT	Nephropathy	Mexico, United States, France
	1634A→T	Glu526Val	GAG526GTG	Nephropathy	United States
	1629delG	Glu524Glu(fs)[d]	GAG524GA_	Nephropathy	United States
	1622delT	Val522Ala(fs)[d]	GTC522G_C	Nephropathy	France
	1676A→T	Glu540Val	GAA540GTA	Nephropathy	Germany
	del1636-1650insCA 1649-1650			Nephropathy	Korea
	1712C→A	Pro552His	CCT552CAT	Nephropathy	Afro-Caribbean
	1670C→A	Thr538Lys	ACA538AAA	Nephropathy, neuropathy	Chinese
Lysozyme	1632delT	Thr525fs	ACT525AC_	Nephropathy	Chinese
	221T→C	Ile56Thr	ATA56ACA	Nephropathy, petechiae	United Kingdom
	253G→C	Asp67His	GAT67CAT	Nephropathy	United Kingdom
	244T→C	Trp64Arg	TGG64CGG	Nephropathy	France
	223T→A	Phe57Ile	TTT57ATT	Nephropathy	Canada
	413T→A	Trp112Arg	TGG112AGG	Nephropathy, GI	Germany
Apolipoprotein-AII	301T→G	Stop78Gly	TGA78GGA	Nephropathy	United States
	302G→C	Stop78Ser	TGA78TCA	Nephropathy	United States
	301T→C	Stop78Arg	TGA78CGA	Nephropathy	United States, Russia
	301T→A	Stop78Arg	TGA78AGA	Nephropathy	Spain
	302G→T	Stop78Leu	TGA78TTA	Nephropathy	United States

[a] cDNA numbering is from initiation codon (ATG)
[b] Amino acids numbered for N-terminus of mature protein
[c] PN, peripheral neuropathy
[d] fs, frameshift
[e] Deduced

finding that is relatively consistent among the Gly26Arg patients is the early onset of hypertension which is probably related to the renal amyloid.

Other families with this mutation have been described and most have not shown evidence of neuropathy, even when followed for long periods of time [3]. A revisit to the Iowa kindred, however, has shown that the first sign of disease in several family members has been elevated serum creatinine, and renal biopsies have shown interstitial amyloid deposition. In one case testicular biopsy has also been positive for amyloid. Neuropathy has developed later. Metabolic studies of members of this family using radiolabeled ApoAI demonstrated a reduced plasma residence time of the variant AI supporting the hypothesis that increased catabolic processing of the amyloid precursor protein is an important factor in amyloidogenesis [4]. A G→C transition in codon 26 (exon 3) is the causative mutation [5].

Trp50Arg: This mutation was first reported in the amyloid of a 45-year-old Polish man who developed hematuria by age 34 and died shortly after kidney transplantation [6]. His clinical course was characterized by a moderate degree of proteinuria, hepatomegaly, splenomegaly, and subsequent renal failure. His father had hepatic and renal amyloidosis and died at age 45. This mutation has also been discovered in patients from Israel. The mutation is the result of a T→C transition in codon 50 of ApoAI causing a substitution of normal tryptophan by arginine. Biochemical analysis of isolated amyloid revealed amino terminal fragments of ApoAI extending as far as residue 93. Diagnosis is usually made by restriction fragment length polymorphism (RFLP) analysis using the restriction enzyme *Msp* 1 which cuts the variant allele PCR product. The mutation can also be identified by direct nucleotide sequencing of ApoAI exon 4.

Leu60Arg: This mutation, the result of a T→G transversion at the second neucleotide position of codon 60, causes relatively early-onset renal amyloidosis with members of the kindred affected by age 25 [7]. Hypertension and heart failure have been reported and, as with the Trp50Arg mutation, N-terminal ApoAI peptides of residue 1–93 were found biochemically.

Leu64Pro: This mutation causes renal amyloid, but unlike other ApoAI mutations in the N-terminal region it is associated with nephrotic range proteinuria [8]. Renal biopsy showed extensive glomerular as well as interstitial amyloid deposition. Biochemical analysis of fibril subunit protein showed the N-terminal ApoAI fragment to span from 1 to approximately 96 residues. As with other ApoAI amyloid proteins only the variant was found in the fibril deposits.

Δ60–71 *ins Val/Thr*: This mutation was reported in a Spanish family with slowly progressive and fatal liver amyloidosis which was clinically diagnosed by age 40 [9]. DNA sequencing revealed a deletion of 35 nucleotides (codons 60–71) with a five nucleotide insertion which maintained the wild-type reading frame. Diagnosis can be made by direct nucleotide sequencing of ApoAI exon 4 and the variant protein can be detected by gel electrophoresis because of the ten amino acid difference from the wild-type protein.

Δ70–72: This mutation was found in a South African family with renal amyloidosis [10]. It is the result of a 9-base pair deletion in exon 4 of ApoAI which gives loss of residues Glu70Phe71Trp72. Disease onset is in the mid-twenties and death is from renal failure. DNA diagnosis is made by direct nucleotide sequencing.

Asn74 Frameshift: This mutation was discovered in a 48-year-old woman with renal failure who had massive vascular and interstitial amyloid deposits in the uterus, ovaries, and pelvic lymph nodes [11]. A 67-year-old woman relative also had amyloid deposits in biopsies of the large intestine. The mutation is an insertion of an adenine in the third base position of codon 74 causing a change of asparagine to lysine and a frameshift theoretically coding a new carboxyl peptide of 105 amino acids.

Leu75Pro: This mutation was found in several families in Northern Italy. It has also been discovered in at least three unrelated families in the United States [12, 13]. The amyloid is mainly hepatic, although some individuals have decreased renal function with hypertension and modest increase of serum creatinine. Renal amyloid has not been documented in most of the individuals who were diagnosed by liver biopsy. The amyloid is deposited mainly in the portal tracts of the liver and appears not to shorten life span. Most individuals are over 50 years of age. The mutation is a T→C transition in the second position of codon 75 and can be detected by RFLP using the restriction enzyme *Hpa*II.

Leu90Pro: This mutation was first identified in a family from France in which affected individuals had skin infiltration of amyloid in the face and upper torso [14]. They also had laryngeal amyloid deposits causing hoarseness. Affected individuals died from cardiac amyloidosis in sixth decade of life. Individuals in this family did not have evidence of renal amyloidosis, and it would appear that residue 90 of ApoAI is the dividing point between the renal phenotype and the cardiac phenotype of ApoAI amyloidosis. The mutation is the result of thymine to cytosine point mutation in the second position of codon 90 [15].

Ala154 Frameshift: This mutation was reported in a woman who presented with nephrotic syndrome at age 58 [11]. Renal biopsy showed glomerular amyloid deposits. The only other clinical information was that the patient did not have hypertension. The mutation is a duplication of GC in codon 154 of the cDNA which would still code for Ala154 but causes a frameshift which theoretically would give a total protein length of 200 amino acid residues. The presence of nephrotic syndrome in a patient with an ApoAI mutation is unusual. So far only one affected subject has been described.

Leu170Pro: This mutation was reported in a 52-year-old man who had swallowing difficulties [11]. Amyloid was demonstrated on biopsy of vocal chords but the patient did not have evidence of systemic disease. This is included in the list of systemic ApoAI amyloidosis because of the laryngeal involvement and similarity to the phenotype of other mutations in this region of the ApoAI protein. The original description said there was no family history of amyloidosis, so there is a possibility that this is the result of a somatic mutation.

Arg173Pro: This mutation is associated with cutaneous, laryngeal, and cardiac amyloid deposition very similar to Leu90Pro [16]. The original diagnosis was from skin biopsy. Affected subjects develop thickened skin with nodularity often by age 20 and have hoarseness from laryngeal deposits at an early age (Fig. 15-1). Cardiac amyloid is slowly progressive but is eventually the cause of death. The disease is the result of a G→C transversion in the second base position of codon 173 (CGC→CCC) resulting in an Arg to Pro substitution. The mutation can be detected by direct nucleotide sequencing of ApoAI exon 4 or by an *Nco*1 restriction enzyme recognition site when PCR products are produced with an induced mutation restriction analysis (IMRA) primer [16]. The mutation was originally discovered in related families on the west coast of the United States. Affected individuals have also been evaluated in the Netherlands and in England. Individuals with this mutation have had heart transplantation and some have survived at least 10 years after transplantation.

Leu174Ser: This mutation in the carboxyl terminal region of ApoAI was found in an Italian family in which affected individuals had severe restrictive cardiomyopathy [17]. The mutation is a T→C transition in the second position of codon 174 giving a Leu to Ser substitution. Amyloid protein from the heart of one affected individual

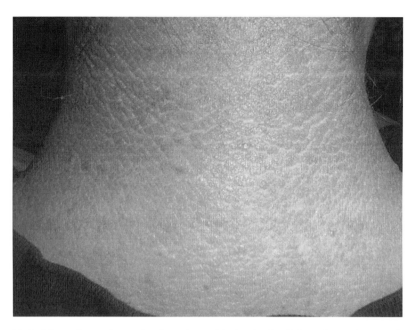

Fig. 15-1. View of posterior neck of a patient with ApoAI Arg173Pro Systemic amyloidosis. Amyloid deposits beneath the epidermal basement cell layer cause a macular appearance and darkened pigmentation.

revealed the amino terminal ApoAI subunit to end at position 93. Affected individuals have low plasma levels of ApoAI similar to those with the Gly26Arg mutation [4]. At least one individual in the family had good results from heart transplantation at age 56. The mutation can be identified by direct nucleotide sequencing of exon 4 or by use of RFLP with Eag I.

Ala175Pro: This mutation was found associated with laryngeal amyloid in a young British man. No cardiac involvement was reported but, as with Leu170Pro, the similarity to other amyloidosis mutations in this region deserves consideration as a systemic form of the disease [18].

Leu178His: This mutation was reported in a French family with cardiac, laryngeal, and dermal amyloidosis with onset in the fourth decade of life [19]. It is due to a thymine to adenine transversion in the second base position of codon 178.

Diagnosis and Treatment

As mentioned previously, diagnosis of many of the ApoAI mutations can be made by RFLP using specific endonucleases. This is appropriate for members of a kindred with a known mutation; however, with the increased availability of direct nucleotide sequencing, this is probably the best approach to making DNA diagnosis in individuals suspected of having this type of amyloidosis. Only the Gly26Arg mutation is in exon 3, the rest in exon 4 which, while a fairly large exon, is now amenable to PCR amplification and direct nucleotide sequencing. As for treatment, there is no specific medical therapy. Renal and/or cardiac transplantations, however, have been quite successful for many individuals. Survival with renal transplantation has been as long as 27 years and with heart transplantation as long as 13 years [20]. In one patient with Gly26Arg mutation who was studied in detail it was demonstrated that liver transplantation reduced the serum concentration of the variant ApoAI to a degree commensurate with previous studies that indicated 50% of ApoAI is synthesized by the liver and the remaining by the gastrointestinal tract [21]. That patient was reported as alive at 7.8 years with a combined liver/kidney transplant and no recurrence of amyloid. Transplantation of only the affected organ (kidney, heart) without liver transplantation may also be associated with prolonged survival [20]. Heart transplantation has been performed for patients with Gly26Arg, Arg173Pro, and Leu174Ser with good results. While it is hypothesized that early liver transplantation may prevent the renal amyloid disease, the picture is not clear. In light of the variable penetrance of these syndromes, preemptive liver transplantation is not indicated before vital organ involvement has been demonstrated. However, once an organ such as the kidney has been seeded with amyloid fibrils, it is not clear whether liver transplantation would stop the amyloid process even though serum levels of the mutant protein have been halved. Obviously development of a medical therapy would be advantageous.

Fibrinogen Aα-Chain Amyloidosis (A Fib)

Hereditary renal amyloidosis has been associated with nine different mutations in the fibrinogen Aα-chain protein. The first was described in 1993 in a patient who had a syndrome characteristic of this disease (hypertension, proteinuria, and progressive azotemia) [22]. Glomerular amyloid deposition without significant medium-sized vessel involvement is characteristic of this disease (Fig. 15-2). Other organ systems may be involved including the liver and spleen, especially in patients who have been maintained on dialysis for renal failure. Recently peripheral vascular and cardiac amyloid deposition has been appreciated in some patients. For those cases that have been studied biochemically, the amyloid fibrils are composed of a fragment of the protease-sensitive carboxyl terminal region of the fibrinogen Aα-chain [23]. In

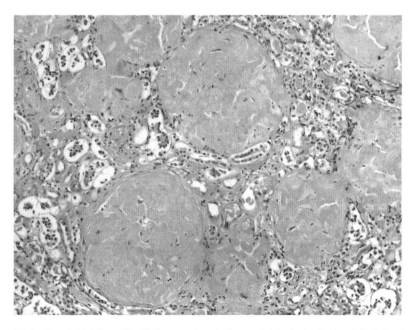

Fig. 15-2. Renal histology in fibrinogen Aα-chain amyloidosis is distinguished by dense glomerular amyloid deposition and loss of renal tubules giving an appearance of glomeruli collapsing on one another.

all cases the patients have been heterozygous for the disease mutation, but only the variant peptide has been found in fibril deposits. While the first mutation described with A Fib was a substitution of leucine for arginine at position 554 of the fibrinogen Aα-chain, the most prevalent form is the glutamic acid to valine substitution at position 526. Thus far all amyloid-associated mutations in the fibrinogen Aα-chain gene have been found to be associated with nephropathy and they all give a similar clinical picture.

Arg554Leu: This mutation was first discovered in a family of Mexican and Peruvian descent in which the propositus had hypertension and proteinuria in the third and fourth decade of life [22]. He had renal transplantation at age 40 but died 10 years later with recurrent amyloid nephropathy. Members of his family were affected with nephrotic syndrome by as early as age 24 with rapid progression of azotemia. This mutation has also been found in an African-American kindred in the United States with a later age of onset and a French kindred with proteinuria and renal failure occurring at approximately age 50 [24, 25]. The mutation, a G→T transversion in the second position of codon 554, can be detected by RFLP with the restriction endonuclease *Sty*I.

Glu526Val: The most common type of fibrinogen Aα-chain amyloidosis was originally discovered in the United States in families of Irish origin but affected individuals have been identified in the United Kingdom and Europe [26]. The clinical syndrome is typical of fibrinogen Aα-chain amyloidosis with hypertension, proteinuria, and subsequent renal failure. Clinical onset of proteinuria may occur by age 40, but later onset has been documented and penetrance would not appear to be 100%. The clinical course from onset of proteinuria to dialysis or death is approximately 10 years. The diagnosis can be made by DNA sequencing or by RFLP to detect the *Mae*III restriction endonuclease site created by the A→T transversion in the second position of codon 526. The first clinical description of a family that was subsequently proven to have this mutation was by Alexander and Atkins in 1975 [27]. A family described by Mornaghi et al. in 1982 also had this mutation [28, 29].

1629delG: This fibrinogen Aα-chain mutation was discovered in an American family with affected individuals presenting with proteinuria and azotemia by approximately age 40. Deletion of guanine in the third position of codon 524 gives a reading frameshift which results in a novel 23 residue peptide and a premature stop codon [30]. In this family, decreased plasma fibrinogen levels were found. DNA diagnosis can be made by direct nucleotide sequencing.

1622delT: This fibrinogen Aα-chain gene mutation (deletion of a thymine in the second position of codon 522) causes a clinical syndrome which is similar to the 1629delG [31]. In the only family studied, nephrotic syndrome occurred as early as age 12 and amyloid recurred in a transplanted kidney within 1 year. Direct DNA sequencing was used to detect this mutation which gives a reading frameshift.

Glu540Val: This mutation was discovered in a German family with a clinical syndrome typical of the other fibrinogen Aα-chain renal amyloidoses [32]. Affected subjects presented with proteinuria in the fifth decade of life and progressive azotemia within 10 years.

Del1636-1650, InsCA1649-1650: This mutation was discovered in a 7-year-old Korean girl who presented with proteinuria and renal failure [33]. She also had hepatomegaly. The renal pathology was similar to the other forms of fibrinogen Aα-chain amyloidosis. This single case probably represents a somatic or novel germline mutation since analysis of DNA from the propositus' parents failed to detect the mutation. Since the amyloid was not biochemically analyzed, it is not certain that it represents the same fibrinogen Aα-chain fragment as the other types.

1632*delT*: Recently three additional mutations in fibrinogen Aα-chain have been found in patients with renal amyloidosis [34]. One was discovered in a Chinese patient with a deletion of a thymine in the third base position of codon 525. This would leave the coding for threonine at 525 followed by a 22 residue novel peptide. This patient was reported to have a family history of amyloidosis with proteinuria presenting in the fourth decade

*Thr*538*Lys*: This mutation is the result of a cytosine to adenine transversion in the second position of codon 538 [34]. It was discovered in a Chinese patient who presented with proteinuria in the fourth decade and also had biopsy-proven amyloid neuropathy.

*Pro*552*His*: This mutation was found in an Afro-Caribbean patient with nephrotic syndrome. It is the result of a cytosine to adenine transversion in the second position of codon 552 which gives a substitution of histidine for the normal proline [34].

As with many of the TTR ApoAI mutations some of the fibrinogen Aα-chain mutations have been described in only single individuals and there are very limited clinical data available. However, unlike ApoAI and TTR, all fibrinogen Aα-chain mutations thus far described have been associated with glomerular amyloidosis causing significant proteinuria as a presenting clinical feature. Only the one patient with Thr538Lys has been proven to have amyloid neuropathy by biopsy.

Treatment

There is no specific medical treatment for fibrinogen Aα-chain amyloidosis. A number of renal transplants have been done, but practically all have resulted in amyloid deposition in the graphs within 10 years. In patients who are maintained on renal dialysis, amyloid involvement of liver and spleen may become massive. Of great significance is the fact that hepatic transplantation would appear to be curative for this condition [35, 36]. Fibrinogen is synthesized strictly by the liver, and hepatic transplantation removes the variant protein. The question arises, of course, after DNA diagnosis when should a DNA-positive subject receive liver transplantation? If the liver transplant is done early enough, then no kidney transplantation would be needed. On the other hand, the lack of complete penetrance of the mutation would suggest that liver transplantation should not be done until renal amyloid deposition is documented. It would appear that there should be a window of opportunity between time of development of proteinuria or elevated serum creatinine with proof of diagnosis by renal biopsy when hepatic transplantation can be accomplished and native kidney function maintained. One problem may be the association of hypertension with this syndrome, but this may respond to conventional medical therapy.

Lysozyme Amyloidosis (A Lys)

Lysozyme amyloidosis was first characterized biochemically in 1993 when tissues from a member of a family described by Zalin et al. in 1991 became available [37, 38]. Characterization of lysozyme as an amyloid subunit protein led to identification of a second mutation which was in a family originally described by Lanham et al. in 1982 [39]. These clinical descriptions of lysozyme amyloidosis note predominantly renal involvement with both glomerular and interstitial amyloid deposition. Spleen, liver, and lung amyloid was also noted, but evidence of peripheral nerve involvement was lacking. Three other mutations in lysozyme associated with amyloidosis have now been described and are characterized by renal amyloidosis.

Lysozyme is a bacteriolytic enzyme synthesized by polymorphonuclear leukocytes and macrophages. Its molecular size is approximately 14,000 daltons and the tertiary structure has been characterized by X-ray diffraction. Lysozyme has considerable beta sheet configuration, and it is suggested that the amyloid-associated mutations result in partly folded intermediates which allow aggregation of full-length lysozyme protein as β-fibrils [40].

Ile56Thr: This mutation was identified in amyloid protein isolated from renal tissue of a 50-year-old man who died from staphylococcal septicemia [37]. He also had amyloid in the ileum, liver, lymph nodes, peripheral nervous system, rectum, thyroid, and spleen. Death in the family was usually associated with renal failure. An interesting observation was the tendency to develop petechiae or purpura. A T→C transition in second position of codon 56 of exon 2 of the lysozyme gene can be identified by direct nucleotide sequencing. All affected individuals have been heterozygous for the mutant allele.

Asp67His: This mutation was discovered in a family originally described clinically in 1982 [39]. Renal amyloidosis was associated with hypertension and death in the late thirties or forties. Amyloid was also present in the adrenals and spleen and only vascular amyloid in the liver. A G→C transversion in the first base of codon 67 produces an Asp to His substitution [37]. Direct DNA sequencing is used to identify this exon 2 mutation.

Trp64Arg: This mutation was first described in a French family with hereditary amyloidosis characterized by renal failure [41]. Affected individuals demonstrated nephrotic syndrome by age 30 with subsequent azotemia within approximately 10 years and also had Sicca syndrome due to salivary gland amyloid. The mutation is a T→C transition at the first nucleotide position of codon 64 in exon 2. This results in an arginine replacement of tryptophan. Affected individuals have received renal transplantation with greater than 15 years of survival despite evidence of amyloid deposition in the transplanted kidney.

Phe57Ile: This mutation was discovered in a Canadian family of Italian origin with amyloidosis characterized by hypertension by age 20, renal insufficiency by age 30, and death or need for dialysis by approximately age 40 [42]. As with other lysozyme amyloidoses, renal involvement is glomerular with some interstitial deposition, but vascular amyloid also may be a prominent feature. One affected individual had kidney transplantation at age 23 and has survived greater than 15 years. The mutation is a T→A transversion at the first position of codon 57 resulting in the replacement of Phe by Ile and can be detected by direct nucleotide sequencing or by RFLP analysis using a restriction enzyme *Tsp*509I. Members of this family also had a DNA polymorphism C→A transversion at the second position of codon 70 giving replacement of threonine by asparagine, but this polymorphism did not segregate with the amyloidosis.

Trp112Arg: This mutation was discovered in a 36-year-old German patient with renal and gastrointestinal amyloid deposition [43]. The mutation is a T→A transversion at the first position of codon 112 giving replacement of tryptophan by arginine and can be detected by direct DNA sequencing.

Diagnosis and Treatment

Lysozyme amyloidosis does not give quite as clear a clinical picture as the fibrinogen Aα-chain amyloidoses. Gastrointestinal, liver, and spleen deposition may lead to medical attention before end-stage renal disease. Some patients with nephrotic syndrome come to clinical attention due to this manifestation. Also, not all affected patients have hypertension. The presence of Sicca syndrome (associated with the salivary gland amyloid deposition) may be a clue in a patient who also has either gastrointestinal or renal manifestations. There is no specific medical treatment; however, lysozyme amyloid usually occurs quite early in adult life and appears to be relatively slow to progress. A number of individuals have had satisfactory renal transplantation with graft function for greater than 15 years.

Apolipoprotein-AII (Apo AII) Amyloidosis

Weiss and Page in 1973 described a family with non-neuropathic amyloidosis in which renal failure was the cause of death [44]. For this reason it was dubbed the Ostertag type of amyloidosis, although obviously we have never been able to document the type of amyloidosis described by Ostertag first in 1932 and later in 1950 [45]. In the family of Weiss and Page two sisters died at ages 47 and 52 after demonstrating hypertension, edema, and subsequent azotemia. Involvement of adrenals and blood vessels of many organs was described. When one of the members of the next generation died 25 years later, amyloid fibrils were extracted from renal tissue and found to have ApoAII as the fibril subunit protein [46]. The amyloid protein was found to be the entire ApoAII molecule plus a 21 amino acid residue extension which was coded by the 3′ untranslated region of the gene. The causative mutation was a T→G transversion in the first position of the stop codon of ApoAII. This resulted in a replacement of the stop codon by glycine which was then followed by 20 additional residues before a new stop codon was encountered. ApoAII, normally part of the HDL fraction of plasma, and the 21 amino acid extension of the amyloid precursor protein are predicted to have amphipathic helix structure, a finding that is characteristic of serum amyloid A and apolipoprotein-AI. The finding of full-length ApoAII in the amyloid fibril is against proteolysis of the precursor protein being an important factor in amyloidogenesis as is suspected for SAA and ApoAI where only portions of the molecules are incorporated into the fibrils.

*Stop*78*Gly*: This mutation causes amyloidosis at a relatively early adult age. The amyloid deposition is prominent not only in kidney glomeruli but also in the walls of blood vessels. The causative mutation, a T→G transversion in the first position of the stop codon, can be detected by direct nucleotide sequencing or use of Bst 1 restriction endonuclease which recognizes the site caused by the mutation [46]. Identification of carriers, however, is easily accomplished with Western analysis since the protein product of the variant allele has a significantly larger molecular mass and can be identified by electrophoresis of non-reduced plasma which shows both normal and variant forms of ApoAII, plus their hetero-dimers since Apo AII is covalently linked through its one cysteine residue by a disulfide bond. While proteolytic processing is not suspected as a culprit in amyloid pathogenesis, it is obvious that the disulfide bond must be reduced before incorporation into amyloid since only the variant ApoAII is found in fibril isolates.

*Stop*78*Ser*: This mutation was identified in a Caucasian male at age 42 [47]. A renal biopsy showed glomerular and vascular wall amyloid deposition. The patient had very slowly progressive deterioration in renal function over at least 10 years. The mutation, a G→C transversion in the second position of the stop codon, results in coding for a serine residue followed by the same 20 amino acid elongation at the carboxyl terminus as with the stop 78 glycine mutation. Western blot analysis can be used for testing carriers or an RFLP with Nla3 restriction endonuclease can be used.

*Stop*78*Arg*: This mutation was discovered in a Russian gentleman who had immigrated to the United States [48]. Proteinuria and hypertension were noted by age 34 and slowly progressive renal insufficiency led to dialysis by age 60. He gave a history that his father had died from kidney failure. The mutation is a T→C transition in the first position of the stop codon resulting in an arginine residue followed by the same 20 amino acid extension as with the other stop codon mutations. A Spanish family with a stop to Arg ApoAII mutation has also been described, but the mutation was found to be a TGA to AGA instead of TGA to CGA [49].

*Stop*78*Leu*: This mutation, a G→T transition in the second position of the stop codon, has been reported in a patient with renal amyloidosis with glomerular, interstitial, and vascular amyloid deposits associated with slowly progressive renal failure [50].

Diagnosis and Treatment

ApoAII amyloidosis is one of the rarer forms of renal amyloidosis and is not likely to be the subject of initial laboratory testing for a patient who presents with unknown type of familial amyloidosis. Even so, since all of the mutations have been in the stop codon and the amyloid precursor protein is significantly larger than the normal allele product, Western analysis using ApoAII-specific antibodies easily detects carriers of the causative mutations. The disease does tend to occur at a relatively early age (30–40 years) and should be suspected in patients with renal insufficiency without evidence of neuropathy. Cardiac amyloidosis is associated with this form of amyloid in some individuals, but would not appear to be a defining factor in the life span unless the patient has renal transplantation or is maintained on dialysis for a number of years. One individual with the stop to Gly mutation has recently had a second renal transplant after his first graft failed at 14 years [51].

Gelsolin Amyloidosis (AGel)

Meritoya described the syndrome of lattice corneal dystrophy, cranial neuropathy, and cutis laxa of facial skin in 1969 [52]. It is a systemic form of amyloidosis with deposits in the heart, kidney, and other internal organs. The largest focus of this disease is in Finland where it is appreciated with autosomal dominant inheritance. The causative mutation is substitution of aspartic acid by asparagine at position 187 of plasma gelsolin [53, 54]. Affected individuals often have lattice corneal dystrophy by the third decade of life. Some patients need corneal transplantation, but this condition is not life threatening. Facial palsy particularly with blepharoptosis can become very distressing and often requires intervention by plastic surgery. Families with this mutation have been found in the United States, Holland, and Japan [55, 56]. Haplotype analysis suggests that the mutation in Japanese patients represents a second mutation event.

Another mutation in gelsolin Asp187Tyr was found in kindreds in Denmark and Czechoslovakia [57]. Clinically the syndrome is similar to the Finnish disease. Normally, gelsolin amyloidosis is not associated with shortened life span, although individuals who are homozygous for the Asp187Asn mutation have been shown to have accelerated renal disease. The amyloid fibril protein represents a 71 amino acid residue internal fragment of gelsolin which contains the mutated residue. No evidence of incorporation of the normal allele product has been found in the few cases that have been studied biochemically. Gelsolin is synthesized by both skeletal muscle and macrophages and is encoded by a single gene on chromosome 9 [58–60]. It is essential for cytoskeletal reorganization through its actin cleaving property; however, the amyloid precursor is probably plasma gelsolin which has a higher molecular weight than cellular gelsolin due to an alternative splicing site. The genetic mutation is caused by a G→A transition in the Asp187Asn disease and a G→T transversion in the Asp187Tyr families. There is no treatment other than plastic surgery to alleviate disturbing features of facial palsy (drooling) and blepharoplasty to aid with vision (Fig. 15-3). Corneal transplantation is occasionally needed for the lattice corneal dystrophy.

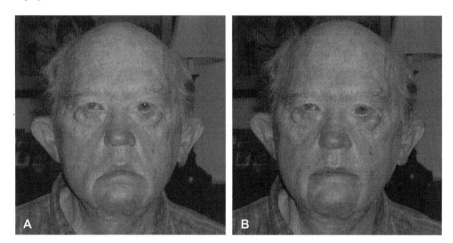

Fig. 15-3. This gentleman with gelsolin amyloidosis has had blepharoplasty to aid vision and plastic surgery to decrease drooling caused by the facial palsy. The neuropathy is exemplified by the two photos: (**a**) facial view, and (**b**) attempt to smile.

Cystatin C

Hereditary cerebral hemorrhage with amyloidosis (HCHWA) was first described in families in Iceland who were affected with leptomeningeal amyloidosis [61]. It is an autosomal dominant disease which presents in the third or fourth decade of life and causes death by repeated intracranial hemorrhage. This is a systemic disease with deposits of amyloid in internal organs which have been demonstrated at autopsy. The causative mutation is a T→A transversion in the second nucleotide of codon 68 which results in substitution of leucine by glutamine (Leu68Gln) in cystatin C, and biochemical analysis reported only the mutant peptide in fibril isolates [62]. This disease can be confused with leptomeningeal forms of TTR amyloidosis or hereditary cerebral hemorrhage with mutations in the Alzheimer βPP gene; however, family history and ethnic origin help to differentiate these syndromes. Cystatin C, originally named gamma trace protein when isolated from urine, is a serine protease inhibitor. The amyloid subunit protein lacks the first ten residues of mature cystatin C. While there is no specific treatment for this disease it has been shown that increased temperature causes aggregation of the variant cystatin C protein in vitro and it has been hypothesized that fever may promote amyloid formation in carriers of the mutant gene [63].

Leukocyte Chemotactic Factor 2 (LECT2)

LECT2 was first described as an amyloid fibril subunit protein in 2008 [64]. It was isolated from the kidney tissue of a patient who presented at 54 years with nephrotic syndrome and subsequently had progressive renal insufficiency requiring hemodialysis by age 61. While this type of amyloidosis would appear to be primarily nephropathic it fits the pattern of other types of systemic amyloidosis. LECT2 is synthesized by the liver, and previous studies suggest that it is a possible chemotactic and growth factor [65–68]. So far other patients with this type of amyloidosis have presented with kidney disease, but to date there have been too few patients identified to expand on the clinical picture of this disease. The renal biopsies show a fairly unique pattern of glomerular and interstitial amyloid and medium-sized blood vessels also have amyloid deposition. There is no evidence that this is a hereditary type of amyloidosis and, therefore, no DNA testing is available. At present diagnosis depends on immunohistochemistry using specific anti-LECT2 antibody or biochemical analysis of fibril protein. The standard approach to this disease from the renal pathology viewpoint is to examine those cases of kidney biopsies in which evaluation for other forms of nephropathic amyloidosis has been nonrevealing. Discovery of LECT2 renal amyloidosis has extended the list of proteins that can cause amyloidosis and suggests that there are probably more to come.

Differential Diagnosis of Systemic Amyloidosis

In this chapter we have been mainly interested in reviewing aspects of the systemic amyloidoses other than immunoglobulin light chain (AL), reactive (AA), and transthyretin (hereditary or senile systemic). In evaluating the patient with systemic amyloidosis, however, we must keep all types of amyloidosis in mind since there is often considerable overlap in the clinical features of these diseases. A precise diagnosis is essential if we are to offer the best counseling as to prognosis and recommendations for appropriate treatment if available. With hereditary amyloidosis, genetic counseling is of great importance. Patients want to know whether their children will develop the disease and whether testing positive for the gene mutation means the subject will inevitably develop amyloidosis. Many of the hereditary amyloidoses appear sporadic due to lack of diagnostic expertise in evaluation of their ancestors or incomplete penetrance of the gene mutation. The diagnosis of a hereditary form of amyloidosis with its implications for future generations can be devastating news to the patient. We have seen from the previous pages that essentially all of the hereditary forms of amyloidosis can be detected by DNA or protein analysis. As the numbers of proteins and their mutations have expanded a strict laboratory approach to diagnosis is neither cost-effective nor prudent. As clinicians we must recognize distinguishing features of these diseases so that we can formulate a rational differential diagnosis. Confirmation can then be made by specific laboratory tests. Two things must be kept in mind in this exercise: First, incomplete penetrance of many of the hereditary mutations makes the taking of a thorough family history, while very important, not as useful as one would hope. We must always remain suspicious. Second, the patient with systemic amyloidosis may present with diagnostic features that are misleading. Many patients with late-onset disease have monoclonal immunoglobulin proteins in the serum or urine and these may be only incidental findings [69]. Patients with hereditary forms of amyloidosis can also have one of the common inflammatory conditions such as Crohn's disease, rheumatoid arthritis, or ankyloisng spondylitis which are unrelated to the systemic amyloidosis. An increasing problem is presented by the elderly individual who has cardiomyopathy which may be a manifestation of AL amyloidosis, senile cardiac amyloidosis, or a hereditary form of transthyretin amyloidosis associated with TTR mutations which give amyloidosis in the later stages of life.

Where to Start with Laboratory Testing

There are actually a few clues which point in some direction: Peripheral neuropathy in a patient with a family history of amyloidosis is in favor of transthyretin amyloidosis; however, neuropathy associated with strong family history of kidney failure is suggestive of the ApoAI Gly26Arg amyloidosis. Cutaneous amyloidosis with a history of vocal hoarseness is consistent with ApoAI amyloidosis. Slowly progressive renal insufficiency is more consistent with lysozyme or ApoAII amyloidosis. Proteinuria and hypertension with subsequent azotemia suggest fibrinogen Aα-chain amyloidosis. For many patients with diagnosis of amyloidosis made by kidney biopsy, there are histologic features which suggest one form of systemic amyloidosis versus the others. ApoAI amyloidosis almost always gives interstitial renal amyloid deposition. Fibrinogen Aα-chain amyloid gives extensive glomerular deposits (Fig. 15-2). Lysozyme amyloidosis and ApoAII amyloidosis usually show glomerular, blood vessel, and interstitial deposits. These clues should be considered before proceeding with either DNA analysis or biochemical characterization of amyloid fibrils. Recently, mass spectroscopy or amino acid sequencing of isolated fibril proteins has added to our ability to precisely identify the form of amyloidosis involved [70]. Immunohistochemistry has been and continues to be a valuable tool in differential diagnosis, but unfortunately it may be noninformative or misleading when not performed in laboratories with extensive experience.

When Is the Time to Proceed to DNA Testing?

For the patient who is a member of a family with a known amyloid-associated gene mutation, this is easy. Genetic testing should be done, however, if only to confirm that the patient's symptoms are not expression of some other disease which warrants different treatment. Unlike TTR, for which a number of commercial DNA diagnostic laboratories are available, DNA analysis for other types of hereditary amyloidosis is quite limited. Consultation with a medical center that specializes in the evaluation and treatment of patients with amyloidosis is advised.

Treatments

Specific treatments for the types of systemic amyloidosis discussed in this chapter have not advanced any further than the treatment for TTR amyloidosis. Transplantation of affected organs in ApoAI, including either kidney or heart, has shown varying results. Whether liver transplantation to reduce the amount of circulating precursor protein adds to the survival outcome is not clear. Some patients have obviously benefitted, but variation in natural progression of disease has obscured a definitive assessment. Both lysozyme and ApoAII amyloidoses appear to be relatively slowly progressive, and renal transplantation has met with good results for many patients. In the case of fibrinogen Aα-chain amyloidosis, however, most of the mutations are associated with relatively rapid progressive loss of renal function and kidney transplantation is usually met with recurrence of amyloid in the graft. This form of hereditary amyloidosis, however, appears to be the only one that can be cured by liver transplantation. Biochemical analysis has shown that only the variant form of fibrinogen Aα-chain is incorporated into the fibrils. Therefore, liver transplantation stops the supply of the necessary ingredient for advancement of disease. Obviously, continued research is needed to develop specific medical treatments for each of these conditions either by modulating the production of mutant proteins or by interfering with their transition to β-fibrils.

References

1. Van Allen MW, Frohlich JA, Davis JR. Inherited predisposition to generalized amyloidosis. Neurology. 1969;19:10–25.
2. Nichols WC, Dwulet FE, Liepnieks J, Benson MD. Variant apolipoprotein AI as a major constituent of a human hereditary amyloid. Biochem Biophys Res Commun. 1988;156:762–68.
3. Vigushin DM, Gough J, Allan D, Alguacil A, Penner B, Pettigrew NM, et al. Familial nephropathic systemic amyloidosis caused by apolipoprotein AI variant Arg26. Q J Med. 1994;87:149–54.
4. Rader DJ, Gregg RE, Meng MS, Schaefer Jr, Kindt MR, Zech LA. In vivo metabolism of a mutant apolipoprotein, apoAI Iowa, associated with hypoalphalipoproteinemia and hereditary systemic amyloidosis. J Lipid Res. 1992;33:755–63.
5. Nichols WC, Gregg RE, Brewer HB Jr, Benson MD. A mutation in apolipoprotein A-I in the Iowa type of familial amyloidotic polyneuropathy. Genomics. 1990;8:318–23.
6. Booth DR, Tan SY, Booth SE, Hsuan JJ, Totty NF, Nguyen O, et al. A new apolipoprotein AI variant, Trp 50 Arg, causes hereditary amyloidosis. Q J Med. 1995;88:695–702.
7. Soutar AK, Hawkins PN, Vigushin DM, Tennent GA, Booth SE, Hutton T, et al. Apolipoprotein AI mutation Arg-60 causes autosomal dominant amyloidosis. Proc Natl Acad Sci USA. 1992;89:7389–93.
8. Murphy CL, Wang S, Weaver K, Gerta MA, Weiss DT, Solomon A. Renal apolipoprotein A-I amyloidosis associated with a novel mutant Leu64Pro. Am J Kidney Dis. 2004;44:1103–9.
9. Booth DR, Tan SY, Booth SE, Tennent GA, Hutchinson WL, Hsuan JJ, et al. Hereditary hepatic and systemic amyloidosis caused by a new deletion/insertion mutation in the apolipoprotein AI gene. J Clin Invest. 1996;97:2714–21.
10. Persey MR, Booth DR, Booth SE, Van Zyl-Smit R, Adams BK, Fattaar AB, et al. Hereditary nephropathic systemic amyloidosis caused by a novel variant apolipoprotein A-I. Kidney Int. 1998;53:276–81.
11. Eriksson M, Schönland S, Yumlu S, Hegenbart U, von Hutten H, Gioeva Z, Lohse P, Büttner J, Schmidt H, Röcken C. Hereditary apolipoprotein AI-associated amyloidosis in surgical pathology specimens: identification of three novel mutations in the APOA1 gene. J Mol Diagn. 2009;11:257–62.
12. Obici L, Palladini G, Giorgetti S, Bellotti V, Gregorini G, Arbustini E, et al. Liver biopsy discloses a new apolipoprotein A-I hereditary amyloidosis in several unrelated Italian families. Gastroenterology. 2004;126:1416–22.
13. Coriu D, Dispenzieri A, Stevens FJ, Murphy CL, Shuching W, Weiss DT, et al. Hepatic amyloidosis resulting from deposition of the apolipoprotein A-I variant Leu75Pro. Amyloid J Protein Folding Disord. 2003;10:215–33.
14. Moulin G, Cognat T, Delaye J, Ferrier E, Wagschal D. Amylose disséminée primitive familiale (nouvelle forme clinique?). Ann Dermatol Venereal. 1988;115:565–70.
15. Hamidi Asl L, Liepnieks JJ, Hamidi Asl K, Uemichi T, Moulin G, Desjoyaux E, et al. Hereditary amyloid cardiomyopathy caused by a variant apolipoprotein AI. Am J Pathol. 1999;154:221–27.
16. Hamidi Asl K, Liepnieks JJ, Nakamura M, Parker F, Benson MD. A novel apolipoprotein A-I variant, Arg173Pro, associated with cardiac and cutaneous amyloidosis. Biochem Biophys Res Commun. 1999;257:584–88.
17. Obici L, Bellotti V, Mangione P, Stoppini M, Arbustini E, Verga L, et al. The new apolipoprotein A-I variant Leu174→Ser causes hereditary cardiac amyloidosis, and the amyloid fibrils are constituted by the 93-residue N-terminal polypeptide. Am J Pathol. 1999;155:695–702.

18. Hawkins PN, Bybee A, Goodman HJB, Lachmann HJ, Rowczenio D, Gilbertson JA, et al. Phenotype, genotype and outcome in hereditary apoAI amyloidosis. In: Grateau G, Kyle RA, Skinner M, editors. Amyloid and amyloidosis. Boca Raton, FL: CRC Press; 2005. p. 316.

19. de Sousa MM, Vital C, Ostler D, Fernandes R, Pouget-Abadie J, Carles D, Saraiva MJ. Apolipoprotein AI and transthyretin as components of amyloid fibrils in a kindred with apoAI Leu178His amyloidosis. Am J Pathol. 2000;156:1911–17.

20. Gillmore JD, Stangou AJ, Lachmann HJ, Goodman HJ, Wechalekar AD, Acheson J, Tennent GA, Bybee A, Gilbertson J, Rowczenio D, O'Grady J, Heaton ND, Pepys MB, Hawkins PN. Organ transplantation in hereditary apolipoprotein AI amyloidosis. Am J Transplant. 2006;6:2342–47.

21. Gillmore JD, Stangou AJ, Tennent GA, Booth DR, O'Grady J, Rela M, Heaton ND, Wall CA, Keogh JAB, Hawkins PN. Clinical and biochemical outcome of hepatorenal transplantation for hereditary systemic amyloidosis associated with apolipoprotein AI Gly26Arg. Transplantation. 2000;71:986–92.

22. Benson MD, Liepnieks J, Uemichi T, Wheeler G, Correa R. Hereditary renal amyloidosis associated with a mutant fibrinogen α-chain. Nature Genet. 1993;3:252–55.

23. Doolittle RF, Watt KWK, Cottrell BA, Strong DD, Riley M. The amino acid sequence of the α-chain of human fibrinogen. Nature. 1979;280:464–68.

24. Uemichi T, Liepnieks JJ, Gertz MA, Benson MD. Fibrinogen Aa chain Leu554: an African-American kindred with late onset renal amyloidosis. Amyloid Int J Exp Clin Invest. 1998;5:88–192.

25. Hamidi Asl L, Fournier V, Billerey C, Justrabo E, Chevet D, Droz D, et al. Fibrinogen Aα chain mutation (Arg554Leu) associated with hereditary renal amyloidosis in a French family. Amyloid Int J Exp Clin Invest. 1998;5:279–84.

26. Uemichi T, Liepnieks JJ, Benson MD. Hereditary renal amyloidosis with a novel variant fibrinogen. J Clin Invest. 1994;93:731–36.

27. Alexander F, Atkins EL. Familial renal amyloidosis, case reports, literature review and classification. Am J Med. 1975;59:121–28.

28. Mornaghi R, Rubinstein P, Franklin EC. Familial renal amyloidosis: case reports and genetic studies. Am J Med. 1982;73:609–14.

29. Uemichi T, Liepnieks JJ, Alexander F, Benson MD. The molecular basis of renal amyloidosis in Irish-American and Polish-Canadian kindreds. Q J Med. 1996;89:745–50.

30. Uemichi T, Liepnieks JJ, Yamada T, Gertz MA, Bang N, Benson MD. A frame shift mutation in the fibrinogen Aα-chain gene in a kindred with renal amyloidosis. Blood. 1996;87:4197–203.

31. Hamidi Asl L, Liepnieks JJ, Uemichi T, Rebibou J-M, Justrabo E, Droz D, et al. Renal amyloidosis with a frame shift mutation in fibrinogen Aα-chain producing a novel amyloid protein. Blood. 1997;90:4799–805.

32. Bybee A, Hollenbeck M, Debusman E, Gopaul D, Gilbertson J, Lachmann H, et al. Hereditary renal amyloidosis in a German family associated with fibrinogen Aα-chain Glu540Val. In: Grateau G, Kyle RA, Skinner M, editors. Amyloid and amyloidosis. Boca Raton, FL: CRC Press; 2005. p. 367.

33. Bybee A, Kang HG, Ha IS, Park MS, Cheong HI, Choi Y, et al. A novel complex indel mutation in the fibrinogen Aα-chain gene in an Asian child with systemic amyloidosis. In: Grateau G, Kyle RA, Skinner M, editors. Amyloid and amyloidosis. Boca Raton, FL: CRC Press; 2005. p. 315.

34. Gillmore JD, Lachmann HJ, Rowczenio D, Gilbertson JA, Zeng CH, Liu ZH, Li LS, Wechalekar A, Hawkins PN. Diagnosis, pathogenesis, treatment, and prognosis of hereditary fibrinogen A alpha-chain amyloidosis. J Am Soc Nephrol. 2009;20:444–51.

35. Gillmore JD, Booth DR, Rela M, Heaton ND, Rahman V, Stangou AJ, et al. Curative hepatorenal transplantation in systemic amyloidosis caused by the Glu526Val fibrinogen α-chain variant in an English family. Q J Med. 2000;93:269–75.

36. Zeldenrust S, Gertz M, Uemichi T, Bjo"rnsson J, Wiesner R, Schwab T, et al. Orthotopic liver transplantation for hereditary fibrinogen amyloidosis. Transplantation. 2003;75: 560–561.

37. Pepys MB, Hawkins PN, Booth DR, Vigushin DM, Tennent GA, Soutar AK, et al. Human lysozyme gene mutations cause hereditary systemic amyloidosis. Nature. 1993;362: 553–57.

38. Zalin AM, Jones S, Fitch NJS, Ramsden DB. Familial nephropathic non-neuropathic amyloidosis: clinical features, immunohistochemistry and chemistry. Q J Med. 1991;295: 945–56.

39. Lanham JG, Meltzer ML, DeBeer FC, Hughes GRV, Pepys MB. Familial amyloidosis of Ostertag. Q J Med. 1982;201:25–32.

40. Booth DR, Sunde M, Bellotti V, Robinson CV, Hutchinson WL, Fraser PE, et al. Instability, unfolding and aggregation of human lysozyme variants underlying amyloid fibrillogenesis. Nature. 1997;385:787–93.

41. Valleix S, Drunat S, Philit J-B, Adoue D, Piette J-C, Droz D, et al. Hereditary renal amyloidosis caused by a new variant lysozyme W64R in a French family. Kidney Int. 2002;61:907–12.

42. Yazaki M, Farrell SA, Benson MD. A novel lysozyme mutation Phe57Ile associated with hereditary renal amyloidosis. Kidney Int. 2003;63:1652–57.

43. Röcken C, Becker K, Stix B, Rath T, Kähne T, Fändrich M, et al. Systemic ALys amyloidosis presenting with gastrointestinal bleeding. In: Grateau G, Kyle RA, Skinner M, editors. Amyloid and amyloidosis. Boca Raton, FL: CRC Press; 2005. p. 368.

44. Weiss SW, Page DL. Amyloid nephropathy of Ostertag with special reference to renal glomerular giant cells. Am J Pathol. 1973;72:447–60.

45. Ostertag B. Familiere amyloid-erkrankung. Z Menschl Vererbungs Konstit Lehre. 1950;30:105–15.

46. Benson MD, Liepnieks JJ, Yazaki M, Yamashita T, Hamidi Asl K, Guenther B, et al. A new human hereditary amyloidosis: the result of a stop-codon mutation in the apolipoprotein AII gene. Genomics. 2001;72:272–77.

47. Yazaki M, Liepnieks JJ, Yamashita T, Guenther B, Skinner M, Benson MD. Renal amyloidosis caused by a novel stop codon mutation in the apolipoprotein A-II gene. Kidney Int. 2001;60:1658–65.

48. Yazaki M, Liepnieks JJ, Barats MS, Cohen AH, Benson MD. Hereditary systemic amyloidosis associated with a new apolipoprotein AII stop codon mutation Stop78Arg. Kidney Int. 2003;64:11–16.

49. Rowczenio D, Gilbertson JA, Bybee A, Hernández D, Hawkins PN. Hereditary amyloidosis in a Spanish family associated with a novel non-stop mutation in the gene for apolipoprotein AII. In: Grateau G, Kyle RA, Skinner M, editors. Amyloid and amyloidosis. Boca Raton, FL: CRC Press; 2005. p. 366.

50. Connors LH, Prokaeva T, Akar H, Metayer M, Smith P, Lim A, et al. Familial amyloidosis: recent novel and rare mutations in a clinic population. In: Grateau G, Kyle RA, Skinner M, editors. Amyloid and amyloidosis. CRC Press; 2005. p. 360.

51. Magy N, Liepnieks JJ, Yazaki M, Kluve-Beckerman B, Benson MD. Renal transplantation for apolipoprotein AII amyloidosis. Amyloid J Protein Folding Disord. 2003;10: 224–28.

52. Meretoja J. Familial systemic paramyloidosis with lattice dystrophy of the cornea, progressive cranial neuropathy, skin changes and various internal symptoms. Annals of Clinical Research. 1969,4.173–85.

53. Maury CPJ, Kere J, Tolvanen R, de la Chapelle A. Finnish hereditary amyloidosis is caused by a single nucleotide substitution in the gelsolin gene. Federation of European Biochemical Societies Letters. 1990;276:75–77.

54. Levy E, Haltia M, Fernandez-Madrid I, Koivunen O, Ghiso J, Prelli F, Frangione B. Mutation in gelsolin gene in Finnish hereditary amyloidosis. J Exp Med. 1990;172:1865–67.

55. Sunada Y, Shimizu T, Nakase H, Ohta S, Asaoka T, Amano S, Sawa M, Kagawa Y, Kanazawa I, Mannen T. Inherited amyloid polyneuropathy type IV (gelsolin variant) in a Japanese family. Ann Neurol. 1993;33:57–62.

56. Steiner RD, Paunio T, Uemichi T, Evans JP, Benson MD. Asp187Asn mutation of gelsolin in an American kindred with familial amyloidosis, Finnish type (FAP IV). Hum Genet. 1995;95:327–30.

57. de la Chapelle A, Tolvanen R, Boysen G, Santavy J, Bleeker-Wagemakers L, Maury CP, Kere J. Gelsolin-derived familial amyloidosis caused by asparagine or tyrosine substitution for aspartic acid at residue 187. Nat Genet. 1992;2:157–60.

58. Yin HL, Kwiatkowski DJ, Mole JE, Cole FS. Structure and biosynthesis of cytoplasmic and secreted variants of gelsolin. J Biol Chem. 1984;259:5271–76.

59. Kwiatkowski DJ, Mehl R, Yin HL. Genomic organization and biosynthesis of secreted and cytoplasmic forms of gelsolin. J Cell Biol. 1988;106:375–84.

60. Kwiatkowski DJ, Westbrook CA, Bruns GAP, Morton CC. Localization of gelsolin proximal to ABL on chromosome 9. Am J Hum Genet. 1988;42:565–72.

61. Gudmundsson G, Hallgrimsson J, Jonasson TA, Bjarnason O. Hereditary cerebral hemorrhage with amyloidosis. Brain. 1972;95:387–404.

62. Ghiso J, Pons Estel B, Frangione B. Hereditary cerebral amyloid angiopathy: the amyloid fibrils contain a protein which is a variant of cystatin C, an inhibitor of lysosomal cysteine proteases. Biochemical and Biophysical Research Communication. 1986;136:548–54.

63. Abrahamson M, Grugg A. Increased body temperature accelerates aggregation of the Leu686Gln mutant cystatin C, the amyloid-forming protein in hereditary cystatin C amyloid angiopathy. Proc Natl Acad Sci USA. 1994;91:1416–20.

64. Benson MD, James S, Scott K, Liepnieks JJ, Kluve-Beckerman B. Leukocyte chemotactic factor 2: a novel renal protein. Kidney Int. 2008;74:218–22.

65. Yamagoe S, Yamakawa Y, Matsuo Y, et al. Purification and primary amino acid sequence of a novel neutrophil chemotactic factor LECT2. Immunol Lett. 1996;52:9–13.

66. Yamagoe S, Kameoka Y, Hashimoto K, et al. Molecular cloning, structural characterization, and chromosomal mapping of the human LECT2 gene. Genomics. 1998;48:324–29.

67. Hiraki Y, Inoue H, Kondo J, et al. A novel growth-promoting factor derived from fetal bovine cartilage, chondromodulin II. Purification and amino acid sequence. J Biol Chem. 1996;271:22657–62.

68. Nagai H, Hamada T, Uchida T, et al. Systemic expression of a newly recognized protein, LECT2, in the human body. Pathol Int. 1998;48:882–86.

69. Lachmann HJ, Booth DR, Booth SE, Bybee A, Gilbertson JA, Gillmore JD, Pepys MB, Hawkins PN. Misdiagnosis of hereditary amyloidosis as AL (primary) amyloidosis. N Engl J Med. 2002;346:1786–91.

70. Benson MD, Breall J, Cummings OW, Liepnieks JJ. Biochemical characterization of amyloid by endomyocardial biopsy. Amyloid. 2009;16:9–14.

Index

Note: The letters 'f' and 't' following locators refer to figures and tables respectively.

From: *Amyloidosis*, Contemporary Hematology,
Edited by: M.A. Gertz and S.V. Rajkumar, DOI 10.1007/978-1-60761-631-3,
© Springer Science+Business Media, LLC 2010